BASIC IMMUNOLOGY

BASIC IMMUNOLOGY

BY

E. R. GOLD, M.D.

Research Fellow, Department of Child Health, University of Bristol

AND

D. B. PEACOCK, M.B., CH.B.

Lecturer in Virology and Immunology, University of Bristol

WITH CHAPTERS BY

J. VERRIER JONES, M.B., B.CH., M.R.C.P.

Lecturer in Medicine, University of Bristol

T. E. BLECHER, M.B., B.CH., M.R.C.P. (ED.), M.R.C.PATH.

Consultant Haematologist, Nottingham General Hospital

M. O. SYMES, M.D., CH.B.

Lecturer in Experimental Surgery, University of Bristol

W. J. HARRISON, M.A., D.M., M.R.C.PATH.

Lecturer in Pathology, University of Bristol

BRISTOL: JOHN WRIGHT & SONS LTD.
1970

Distribution by Sole Agents:

United States of America: The Williams & Wilkins Company, Baltimore

Canada: The Macmillan Company of Canada Ltd., Toronto

ISBN 0 7236 0252 2

PRINTED IN GREAT BRITAIN BY JOHN WRIGHT AND SONS LTD.
AT THE STONEBRIDGE PRESS, BRISTOL BS4 5NU

PREFACE

THIS book is intended for students of medicine and allied scientific disciplines who wish to acquire a grasp of the basic concepts of immunology. Since the book's inception the topic of immunity has sprung into prominence because of the way in which transplantation surgery has fired the imagination of the world. As a result there is widespread recognition that the immune mechanisms play a vital role not only by combating infection but also in the maintenance of health. It is becoming widely accepted, therefore, that some familiarity with immunology is necessary for students in the whole field of biology as well as of medicine. We hope that a book of this sort, where the emphasis has been placed on the fundamental aspects that lead to an understanding of the subject as a whole, will be found useful.

The early chapters are devoted to the substances that take part in serological reactions and to the reactions themselves. It is to the study of antigens, antibodies, and, to a lesser extent, of complement, outside the human body, that we owe an understanding of the physicochemical nature of immunological reactions and of their most characteristic feature, specificity.

At this point we turn our attention to the teleologically less satisfactory aspects of immunity, namely the 'immediate hypersensitivities'. Mediated by antibody, these *in vivo* reactions contain an element of damage to the host. The immunological oddity of the Shwartzman reaction concludes this section.

There follows a consideration of 'cell-mediated immunity', a response in which, as its title suggests, humoral antibodies as we know them do not take part. Chapter 9, 'Cell-mediated Immunity and Delayed Hypersensitivity', falls within this area and we hope that the separation of 'Immediate Hypersensitivity' from the two chapters on 'Cell-mediated Immunity' will help to dispel the clouds of obscurity that have hovered around these topics for too long. Our knowledge of cell-mediated immunity is fragmentary compared with the humoral mechanisms, and it is not therefore possible to deal with it in quite the same textual form. Nevertheless, many concepts introduced in the early chapters, such as specificity of immunological reactions and immunogenicity of antigens, are equally relevant to cell-mediated immunity, though the details of their application differ.

The chapters on 'Transplantation Immunology' and 'Tumour Immunology' introduce the wider implications of immunology in which defence against infection is not the primary consideration, but in which *resistance to change* might be regarded as the keynote.

In the final chapter the wheel has turned full circle and we consider the three responses to an immunogenic stimulus; antibody production, cell-mediated immunity, and tolerance, and the way in which such responses can develop so that the immunological system is turned against the host's own tissues.

It cannot have escaped the attention of anyone engaged in the biological sciences that the past decade has witnessed what is popularly called an 'information explosion'. Nowhere is this more evident than in the field of immunology. We are well aware, therefore, that during the course of the final revisions to chapters many interesting and significant facts have emerged in the literature which have not been incorporated in the text. Like other authors before us, we have tried to find ways to remedy this defect so that the latest information, hot from the presses, could be included. Like other authors, too, we have had to accept the limitations of our medium, among which are the impossibility, even in a multiple-author work, of covering the literature in a short space of time and, as a corollary, the unevenness of selected material that would result. For the guidance of the discerning we would say that the text was substantially finished at the end of January, 1969, and the references at the end of each chapter will indicate the period up to which the literature was covered.

We recognize, too, that it is hazardous to predict the future. Nevertheless, certain trends can clearly be distinguished. Progress in the chemical study of immunoglobulins is so rapid that it can be anticipated that the full sequence of amino-acid structure of a number of antibody molecules will soon be known. From this point it would be a relatively short step to defining the antibody-combining site in chemical terms—the culmination of the immunochemist's dream. With the availability of chemically defined antigenic sites (determinants) this would lead to an important advance in our understanding of the interaction between antigen and antibody and the contribution made by the various forces involved. It is not unreasonable to assume that the 'recognition factors' of cell-mediated immunity will soon be biochemically characterized, and possible differences between them and immunoglobulins carrying antibody activity delineated. In a number of other areas, such as immune lysis with complement, the biochemical approach will again lead to greater understanding, and understanding brings in its wake the capacity to manipulate for the benefit of health and the prevention of disease.

Advances of such basic significance as those described above also have their impact on various fields of applied medical science: blood-group serology, for instance, which can itself be used as a research tool in other fields such as cytogenetics. It is just this approach that has allowed a start to be made in the mapping of human autosomes.

Eventually it may become possible to express all immunological reactions in terms of physicochemical parameters, and large parts of the subject will become a specialized branch of biochemistry if, as many biologists assume, the mystery of life can be expressed entirely in chemical and physical terms. Before such concepts are realized we still have an immense distance to travel, as can be seen from the fact that we are still quite ignorant of the processes which control the synthesis of antibody molecules of various specificities.

Finally, as editors, we wish to express our sincere thanks to our collaborating authors for bringing fresh outlooks and new inspiration to chapters that they have contributed. Without them the task of writing a book, even confined to basic immunology, would have become an intolerable burden. On their behalf as well as ours we also extend our grateful thanks to all those friends and colleagues who, in discussion, have contributed so freely in knowledge and ideas, and so helped in bringing this task to fruition.

Bristol, 1970

E. R. G.
D. B. P.

CONTENTS

BASIC IMMUNOLOGY

CHAPTER 1

BASIC NOTIONS OF IMMUNITY

BY E. R. GOLD AND D. B. PEACOCK

I. INTRODUCTION

HISTORICAL records show quite clearly that for many centuries Man has recognized that previous experience of certain infectious diseases confers protection on the individual in the face of subsequent contact with the same disease. It was even the practice in ancient China and in Persia to inoculate vesicle fluid or crusts from cases of smallpox into people who did not show the marks of a previous infection. 'Variolation', as this method of immunization against smallpox is called, has probably been carried on without intermission right up to modern times and is currently employed by some nomadic Arab tribes. However this may be, it is apparent that the concept of immunity to epidemic disease is by no means a new one and that the restricted nature of acquired immunity is inherent in such practices and observations; that is to say that an attack of smallpox protects only against a subsequent attack of smallpox and not against any other infection.

The notion of specificity is the cardinal point in our understanding of the nature of acquired immunity. However, it was not until the germ theory of infectious disease had been established that the full implication of such ideas could be realized. First, therefore, had to come the recognition that certain bacteria caused certain diseases; that *Salmonella typhi* caused typhoid fever and not whooping-cough. Second came the recognition that it was a specific resistance to that bacterium or its toxins that prevented recurrences of the same disease. Third came the discovery that after recovery from an infectious disease protective substances called 'antibodies' could be found in the blood of animals and man that would react with bacteria and their products *in vivo* and *in vitro*. A whole host of serological reactions was devised to detect the presence of specific antibodies in serum, and according to the type of reaction antibodies were given various names: 'agglutinins' for those that clumped cells, bacterial or otherwise, 'antitoxins' for those that neutralized toxins, 'precipitins' for those that aggregated soluble substances, and so on. Substances that give rise to the production of antibodies such as bacteria, their products, and indeed all kinds of chemical and biological molecules, are known as 'antigens'.

Explanation of the reaction between antigen and antibody constituted something of a difficulty at first because it was first visualized as a chemical reaction based on the formation of covalent bonds. It soon became apparent that the number of antibody molecules combining with an antigen depended to some extent on the relative concentrations of the reactants in a mixture. Another way of putting this is to say that antigens and antibodies combine in multiple proportions and this in turn leads on to the hypothesis, now confirmed, that there is more than one reactive site on each antigen and antibody molecule. The nature of the reaction between these sites is also unusual and specificity is achieved by a unique arrangement of weak physicochemical bonds (*see* Chapter 6).

II. RESISTANCE

So far we have been considering only acquired immunity, but immunology as a whole takes account of many other factors that operate at the host–parasite level. It would be quite proper for us to go into the question of virulence of pathogenic bacteria, for instance, but we will confine our approach to the point of view of the host. If we then further confine our attention to immunity from disease for the time being, we find that the subject falls roughly into two compartments, specific immunity and non-specific resistance. Specific immunity arises as the result of an antigenic stimulus and is directed against that antigen.

Non-specific resistance is compounded of an array of mechanisms that come into operation in the face of any, or at least a range of, invasive and pathogenic parasites. In the above definitions the distinction between immunity and resistance is one of specificity, but, as we shall see later, it is not always possible to maintain this distinction absolutely. The classic inflammatory response to infection is, for instance, initially non-specific and ultimately assisted by specific factors; thus phagocytosis can proceed without the intervention of antibody but is both more rapid and more effective in its presence.

The relationship between host and parasite is a complex one ranging from the mutual assistance of symbionts, through the toleration of commensals and indifference towards saprophytes, to defence against pathogens.

Parasites that are saprophytes in one species may be pathogens in another. In such cases the difference lies in the species of animals, of course, and not in the parasite, nor are we concerned in these cases with the development of acquired immunity by the host owing to past infection by the parasite. There is in fact a wide range of factors influencing the susceptibility of animals to disease—factors that are non-specific in character and that can be considered under such general headings as 'genetic constitution' and 'stress', or under more particular ones such as 'physical and chemical factors', 'phagocytosis', and 'competition between parasites'.

A. Genetic Constitution

Native resistance to potentially harmful agents in the environment may be due to (1) the provision of barriers through which the agent cannot penetrate, (2) the failure to provide an environment in which the agent can multiply or elaborate toxins, and (3) the functional absence of receptors susceptible to the action of potentially harmful metabolites elaborated by the agent.

All these aspects can be considered under the heading of 'genetic constitution', but it will be convenient to deal with the first category separately as 'physical and chemical factors'; the second two are more conveniently dealt with under the present heading.

Species differences in resistance are easy to recognize; horses do not catch measles, nor dogs typhoid. But when it comes to differences within a species we find they are much harder to define and normally, of course, they are differences of degree rather than quality. In just a few instances defined abnormalities have been discovered in inbred strains of laboratory animals that have been associated with a heightened susceptibility to bacterial infection. Two or three strains of animals have now been bred that were deficient in a component of blood serum known as 'complement'. Complement is itself a complex of substances (see Chapter 5) that has antibacterial activity in the presence of antibody. Animals deficient in this complex or even in one of its components are unduly susceptible to bacterial infections, and inbred strains carrying this trait tend to die out. In man there is the well-known example of the gene governing the production of the abnormal haemoglobin S. Homozygotic individuals develop sickle-cell anaemia and often die before puberty. Heterozygotes, however, are more resistant to malaria than 'normal' individuals so that where falciparum malaria abounds there is a selective pressure for this abnormal and normally disadvantageous gene.

It is fairly obvious that genetic differences may also be reflected in differences in specific immunological responses. Evidence of this can be seen in inbred strains of animal that form antibodies directed against different parts of an antigenic molecule such as insulin. In man differences in the ease with which antibodies are formed to blood-group antigens have been discovered as a result of repeated transfusions.

In man too there is no doubt that certain congenital disorders of the immunological apparatus are associated with increased and more severe bacterial infections. Among patients with some forms of congenital hypogammaglobulinaemia bacterial infections have regularly and relentlessly claimed their victims, chiefly before but also since the advent of antibiotics. However relevant to genetic control such disorders are, they rather miss the point at issue in two important particulars, since what we are really concerned to do here is to demonstrate, in the first instance, that there are differences in susceptibility between apparently normal individuals, and, secondly, that the differences are in native resistance rather than in acquired immunity. Certainly of more immediate relevance is the case of Algerian sheep which exhibit greater resistance to anthrax than European breeds. In man even more subtle distinctions have been drawn. For instance, a familial susceptibility to tuberculosis is fairly well attested. Admittedly it is not easy to exclude a number of extrinsic factors such as food and environment in such studies, but Kallmann and Reisner [1] record that three out of four homozygotic twins went down with tuberculosis after the corresponding twin had contracted the infection, whereas the figure for heterozygotic twins was only one out of three.

Even more striking, though not necessarily more compelling in evidence, is the incidence of infectious disease in virgin populations. We know from history that armies in the field have more often been defeated by disease than by force of arms, but often enough these fearful epidemics are the result of lack of hygiene inherent in the movement of armies rather than in any innate susceptibility to disease in the stricken men. Nevertheless, enshrined in the history of the movement of European races over the globe there are some remarkable stories of the capture of large countries by small bands of armed men. None of these is more extraordinary than the conquest of Mexico by Cortez. At the time the Mexicans were numerous, war-like, brave, and ably led. How then did Cortez, with a band of soldier-adventurers never numbering more than two thousand and sometimes only a few hundred strong, conquer this rich country? Certainly he made allies of the indigenous population by exploiting existing factions and jealousies. Certainly his methods included diplomacy and even treachery. But at the most critical stage in Cortez's campaign, Montezuma's followers suffered from an appalling epidemic of smallpox, presumably introduced by the Spaniards. The epidemic killed great numbers of fighting men and their leaders and is said to have been exacerbated because of the Mexicans' habit of bathing frequently.

Settlers from the Old World used roughly the same prescription one hundred years later in North America, the Red Indian population proving to be highly susceptible to imported infections, in this case tuberculosis as well as smallpox. Whole tribes were decimated or worse in the early part of the eighteenth century, with populations of tens of thousands being reduced to a few hundreds [2]. Another century later and the Plains' tribes were suffering in the same way, and again Dubos records that in the year 1837 the Crows lost one-third of their number to smallpox.

The suggestion here is quite clear that races that have experienced certain infectious diseases over periods of hundreds, perhaps even thousands, of years acquire a degree of constitutional immunity to them by a process of natural selection. Unequivocal evidence supporting such an ecological concept is not easy to come by, but we come closer to it in the Qu'Appelle valley reservation in Canada where Indian families were collected together and kept under a degree of medical supervision. Here, Dubos [2] reports, 'the annual death rate from tuberculosis reached the fantastic figure of 9000 per 100,000. More than half the Indian families were eliminated in the first three generations of the epidemic. However, some 20 per cent of deaths in the surviving families were caused by tuberculosis.' Continuing observation led to the suggestion that succeeding generations gradually acquired an innate resistance to the disease as judged by the more limited spread and severity of lesions in individual cases among the school population.

Numerous other examples of the disastrous progress of infectious disease through virgin populations are to be found in medical and historical writings. By all accounts the Pacific Islanders were a healthy and happy people when first encountered by Europeans. Their subsequent history has a strong note of tragedy in it with epidemics of venereal diseases, tuberculosis, smallpox, measles, whooping-cough, and influenza sweeping through communities, reducing their numbers drastically and sapping the vitality of the survivors. As an indication of the severity of such diseases in the Pacific Islands, it is said that no baby born in Hawaii in 1848 lived through the whooping-cough, measles, and influenza epidemics that raged in the islands that year [2].

It is sometimes held that genetic factors contributed to the severity of the more recent measles epidemic of 1951 in Greenland. Morbidity and mortality-rates of 999 and 18 per 1000 of population were recorded [3]. Such figures, and the morbidity rate is fantastically high, are not all that surprising given the extremely infective nature of the virus, the sociability of the Greenlanders which made nonsense of any attempt at isolation, and the reported absence of an epidemic in southern Greenland for over a hundred years. Nor does the mortality-rate seem to indicate any great degree of heightened susceptibility when the crowded conditions under which the inhabitants lived and their general state of health and nutrition are taken into account. Certainly far higher mortality-rates have been described in various other parts of the world [4].

In April, 1949, Canadian Eskimoes experienced an outbreak of poliomyelitis with a paralytic rate of 18·5 per cent and a case fatality rate of 24·7 per cent [5], but here we begin more certainly to encounter other influences. The epidemiology of poliomyelitis is rather complex, with the clinical manifestations being more closely associated with communities where infection is relatively uncommon. In other words, the disease is more severe in those who have reached or passed adolescence. Because of their isolation a high proportion of Eskimo adults in this epidemic were presumably quite without previous experience of this virus. A high paralytic rate is to be expected in any community in these circumstances. In any event age brings in its train many changes, both physiological and pathological, that alter a host's susceptibility to and capacity to deal with an infection. Nevertheless, we may be witnessing truly heightened levels of susceptibility in this epidemic.

As far as hereditary factors are concerned, we can say with confidence that there are differences in susceptibility between species that have nothing to do with specific immunological responses, but are simply questions of suitability of host tissues for sustaining a particular parasite or susceptibility of host tissues to elaborated toxins. When we come to consider differences between races of man and breeds of animal, we are on much more difficult ground, and though we have good reasons for supposing that there are differences in innate resistance the burden of proof is somewhat onerous.

B. Stress

At first sight the data from the Qu'Appelle valley reservation would seem to provide fairly convincing evidence of the operation of innate factors of resistance. However, it would be unwise to forget that there are a number of other factors that affect the course of an infection in any individual. Some of these factors are fairly concrete, such as nature of diet, state of nutrition, protection from the elements, and overcrowding; others are more nebulous but can be interrelated, such things as sense of purpose or of despair or simply of confusion. Psychological, social, and dietary factors could all have been operating among the Qu'Appelle valley Indians, but the impact of these conditions could be expected to be less and less severe on each successive generation both by reason of adaptation by the Indians themselves and by experience gained by the supervising authorities.

Both concrete and nebulous causes can be lumped together under the heading of 'stress', and their effect can be seen on the course of tuberculosis in the inmates of concentration camps in the Second World War. Tuberculosis was widespread in these camps, no doubt due in part to the opportunities for spread engendered by overcrowding and lack of isolation of open cases. What is of particular interest from the present point of view though is that the majority of cases of tuberculosis resolved simply with rescue, rest, and food. In other words, the progress of the disease in the individual was arrested and reversed by removing a number of stress factors, although one must recognize that dietary deficiencies, for example, can go well beyond the induction of stress.

Similar conclusions about stress can be drawn from the bizarre story of swine influenza in the Middle West. The causative agent, swine influenza virus, is excreted by infected pigs in the ova of swine lungworms. The ova in turn are ingested by earthworms in which they undergo three developmental cycles. The third stage may be reached within two months and persist for years, during the whole of which time the earthworm remains infective for the pig. After ingestion, the lungworm larvae are released and migrate back to the lungs where they undergo further development to become adult worms. At this stage the 'masked' virus they are carrying can apparently be stimulated into activity. Under natural conditions the appropriate stimulus seems to be the first cold snap of autumn [6], so that what appears to be an epizootic spreading with lightning speed is probably just the unmasking of a widespread latent infection by a geographically widespread stimulus.

C. Physical and Chemical Factors

That skin and mucous membranes afford protection against the penetration of potentially pathogenic micro-organisms is clear to all of us from our experience of the frequency with which infection follows breaks in the skin, however insignificant. Though these surfaces do provide mechanical barriers, they are by no means inert in other respects and with their associated properties and ingredients, such as fats, waxes, pH, mucus, and cilia, are well able to hamper, remove, or destroy a wide variety of potential invaders. Taken together, all these factors therefore assume considerable importance, but it is often very difficult to assess the contribution effected by any one of them.

D. Temperature

The possible role of outside temperature on the general degree of resistance has already been mentioned in connexion with swine influenza, but internal temperature can also assume a critical importance at times. Pyrexial therapy was once widely used in the treatment of late manifestations of syphilis because temperatures well above 37° C. are inimical to the survival of the spirochaete. In similar vein we may note that avian and piscine forms of tuberculosis are harmless to man, it is presumed because 37° C. is not a sufficiently favourable temperature for the organisms to establish and maintain a foothold; also that tetanus toxin is not toxic to a number of cold-blooded vertebrates at ambient temperatures substantially below 37° C. Pathogenic strains of smallpox and poliomyelitis are capable of replicating in tissues at higher temperatures than strains that are less virulent, again illustrating the possibly profound influence of temperature on the course of infections. This provides us with the teleological explanation that pathogenicity in such cases is due to a capacity of the organisms to multiply under the conditions of fever. It is also of interest that at least some of the causative agents of the common cold, rhinoviruses, induce degenerative changes in tissue-culture cells only when the temperature of incubation is lowered from body heat to that obtaining in the mucous membrane of the nose (33° C.).

Consideration in any detail of the vast number of chemical substances possibly linked with non-specific resistance to infection is quite beyond the scope of this book and a brief mention will be accorded chiefly to those that will again be the subject of comment in some other context.

Of all the cell constituents and secretions that have been examined for direct action against bacteria, only substances falling within the class of basic proteins have unequivocally been demonstrated to have activity. Chief among these is lysozyme which is to be found in all body fluids except C.S.F., aqueous humour, sweat, and urine, and which reaches particularly high concentrations in polymorphonuclear leucocytes. Lysozyme is bactericidal and sometimes bacteriolytic as well.

E. Complement

Another well-known factor, this time found in blood-plasma, is the complex of substances known as 'complement'. Here we meet a recurring and unavoidable difficulty owing to the classification of immunity into specific and non-specific compartments. Complement, though quite properly regarded as non-specific in this sense, is usually quite inactive unless preceded by a specific antigen–antibody reaction. It attaches to preformed antigen–antibody complexes and its activity is characteristically seen in the lysis of Gram-negative bacteria and mammalian red cells. Its role in defence is probably considerably wider than this since it has been suggested that not only does it render particles it coats more appetizing to phagocytes (opsonization), but may also be responsible for the specific movement of phagocytes towards antigen–antibody complexes (chemotaxis).

F. Conglutinin

The substance conglutinin [7] enhances the specific agglutination of bacterial and other cells effected by antibody. Originally described as a property of bovine sera, it seems to be found only in the sera of the Bovidae. Biologically it behaves like an antibody to complement, but does not belong, as do antibodies, to the group of proteins known as 'immunoglobulins'.

Its action is in many ways paralleled by *immunoconglutinin*, which is antibody directed against the complement moiety of antigen–antibody-complement complexes. Immunoconglutinin can be prepared by injecting appropriate immune complexes containing heterologous complement into animals, but it may also be formed by a host against its own fixed complement. In the reactions involving conglutinin and immunoconglutinin we again have a strange mixture of specific and non-specific mechanisms operating: the reaction between antigen and antibody we can regard as the truly specific element; between this complex and complement as physico-chemically but not immunologically specific; between the fixed complement and immunoconglutinin as immunologically specific as regards these two reactants, but non-specific with respect to the original antigen, since complement adsorbed to any antigen–antibody complex will suffice as the substrate in the final reaction.

Though there is evidence that conglutinin and immunoconglutinin afford some protection against infection, the extent to which they contribute to a host's defences remains uncertain.

G. 'Natural Antibodies' and Properdin

A few years ago another substance known as 'properdin' enjoyed a considerable reputation as a universal non-specific 'antibody'. This view has since been considerably modified even among properdin protagonists (*see* Chapter 5). In rather similar vein we have the vexed question of 'natural' antibodies, of which perhaps the best known examples are the anti-A and anti-B isohaemagglutinins of man. It is only in the sense that they arise without known antigenic stimulus that they can be regarded as non-immunological since their reaction with antigen is to all intents and purposes a normal immunological phenomenon. The existence of natural antibody is crucial to some theories of antibody production in which the first step is considered to be the capture of antigen by preformed natural antibody. Many so-called 'natural' antibodies display a low degree of specificity for antigens, particularly of intestinal bacteria, and because of this and a degree of heat-lability have been equated by some with properdin.

Apart from specificity they bear all the hall-marks of innate resistance rather than acquired immunity, and this is the reason for discussing them at all here. The question of stimulus is also at the root of the dispute about how such antibodies arise. The absence of stimulus is almost impossible to prove or disprove, but we would suggest that the bulk of the evidence from studies of the mechanism of antibody formation and the development of the specific immune response, particularly in germ-free animals, indicates the necessity for such stimuli.

H. Interferon

Viruses are subject to inimical influences in the host that do not differ in principle from those active against other parasites except in so far as the obligate intracellular relationship imposes new conditions. Anything which prevents or impedes the entry of virus particle into host cell could contribute to resistance in this way. Such a role has been suggested for the inhibitors of influenza viruses. These inhibitors are present in the mucus of the respiratory tract and carry receptors for the attachment of virus. The virus can liberate itself by the action of its own enzyme, neuraminidase, on a sialic acid substrate. Identical receptors are present on red cells and it is presumed on cells capable of supporting replication of the virus, where they might perform some necessary preliminary to the penetration of host cell by virus particle.

Once inside the cell, viruses stimulate the cell to manufacture and secrete interferon, a protein that is capable of inhibiting virus replication in neighbouring cells [8]. Interferon is quite strongly host specific but not specific in its action towards viruses, though some are more readily affected than others. Viruses also vary in their capacity to stimulate interferon production.

The discovery of a totally new system of defence against attack by viruses warrants sufficient attention in itself, but in addition there is some evidence that foreign nucleic acid stimulates interferon production. This opens up the exciting possibility that in interferon we have found the basis of a protective mechanism directed against potentially the most hazardous of all invasions as far as the host is concerned, namely that of a direct attack on the hereditary mechanism of host cells by the introduction of new genetic material.

Interferon is quite distinct from antibody in that it is neither specifically directed against the stimulating virus nor is it produced by cells necessarily associated with antibody production.

I. Phagocytosis

One of the most primitive functions exercised by animal cells is phagocytosis. It is the means by which protozoa ingest their food and serves as one of the principal distinctions between animal and vegetable kingdoms. Its very basic function is reflected in ontogenesis by the ability of cells of all three germinal layers to ingest particles at some stage in development. In multicellular animals the property of phagocytosis is retained only by some cells, and in the vertebrates would appear to be reserved particularly for the elimination of waste host material. Along with this specialization, however, the system also seems to have become adapted for the protection of the host against certain, especially particulate, noxious agents.

It is in this area of defensive mechanisms that the most critical distinctions between non-specific resistance and specific immunity have to be made. Phagocytosis in fact partakes of both elements so that complete separation of these two mechanisms is quite impossible. Phagocytic cells are widely distributed throughout the animal body, as one would expect from a system that has such vital and all-pervading functions to perform. We are taught that bacterial infection and many another insult to body tissues call forth an inflammatory response, but as far as the phagocytic element is concerned it is as well to recognize from the outset that a number of different cell types is involved, and that it is unlikely that the mechanisms and functions of all the types are identical.

Phagocytes of higher animals can be divided into two broad classes, the polymorphonuclear microphages of blood and the mononuclear macrophages of blood and tissues. The phagocytic mononuclear cells of the blood together with certain other phagocytic cells found lining sinusoids and in the reticulum of organs such as the spleen, liver, lung, etc., constitute the reticulo-endothelial system, which is sometimes taken to include lymphocytes and plasma cells as well. The justification for including the latter lies not so much in the possibility that all these cell types derive from a common precursor or that there is some interchange of cell types following initial differentiation, as in the belief that together they form a single functional system devoted, in this context, to the development of specific immunity directed towards specific immunogens (antigens). Though this may well be true, at any rate for the development of humoral immunity, little would seem to be gained by lumping together cells that seem to perform very different functions in detail. Indeed by analogy and on some evidence microphages could be included in the same system, since it has been suggested that polymorphonuclear leucocytes may first process antigen before it is taken up by monocytes in the chain of events leading to antibody production.

However this may be, it is plain that we are already in something of a dilemma since the same cell types are being involved in both non-specific resistance and specific immunity. This does not in any way invalidate the classification of immunity into these sections, but it does perhaps remind us how often Nature will adapt existing systems to perform new functions. We are also faced with the question of what determines the ultimate fate of phagocytosed material. Is it to be breakdown and excretion? Or is it to be breakdown and immunological response? We are unable to answer these questions at present, but they imply first of all a mechanism of recognition operating at this level in order that immunogenic material may be distinguished from host material. We also know that the immunological response may take any of three pathways: immune tolerance, humoral immunity (antibody production), or cell-mediated immunity (delayed hypersensitivity-type response). It is quite possible that different kinds of antigen, soluble or particulate, carbohydrate or protein, may follow different routes of phagocytosis and processing terminating in different immunological responses. The same could be true of antigens given in different doses or by different routes.

We are, however, considering specific responses rather than phago-cytosis alone. What is clear at this stage is that in general the different cell types play different phagocytic roles. In the inflammatory response the granular leucocytes are first on the scene, at any rate in large numbers. They may be sufficient to deal with a minor bacterial invasion, for instance. If, however, the bacteria are unduly toxic and there is sufficient tissue damage the granulocytes may themselves succumb in enormous numbers under adverse conditions of pH and so on. Macrophages are so wide-spread that in many situations they will already be present, but nevertheless they accumulate more slowly in an area of inflammation than do granulo-cytes. They are, however, more hardy in the face of adverse conditions and at sites of chronic inflammation come to be the predominant cell type. They are responsible for clearing up the debris left by the heat of previous battle. Macrophages have the advantage over microphages in that they can multiply at the site as well as form multinucleate giant cells to deal with really large particles.

Both sets of phagocytes are capable of ingestion and digestion, and it must be accepted, therefore, that they are both part of the non-specific defensive system. It must be admitted that there are innumerable experi-ments that show unequivocally that specific antiserum enhances phago-cytosis considerably. As far as microphages are concerned, this may be their only connexion with specific immunity. In the case of macrophages this is almost certainly not so and phagocytosis of foreign material is a preliminary to the passing of information to immunologically competent cells, i.e., cells that are capable of a specific immune response. The role of the reticulo-endothelial system in defence is extremely complex and our understanding of it is by no means complete.

1. BLOCKADE OF THE RETICULO-ENDOTHELIAL SYSTEM

The function of the phagocytes of the reticulo-endothelial system can be studied by injecting particulate matter into the vein of an animal and determining the parameters connected with its disappearance from the blood-stream. It is an old observation that such particles may sub-sequently be found in the sessile phagocytes of organs such as the liver, spleen, lung, etc. That the blood-clearing mechanism can be inhibited has also frequently been shown by injecting massive doses of either antigenic or 'inert' particles. Whatever the type of particle, an initial period of a few hours, during which clearance of new particles from the blood-stream is inhibited, is followed by a period of enhancement, sometimes lasting as long as two weeks. It seems fairly certain that the period of enhancement supervenes too quickly for there to be any question of the development of specific immunity; and experimentally a vaccine of *Bordetella pertussis* induces an immunity in mice several days before specific antibodies can be detected in serum [9]. The immunity might conceivably be associated with a non-specific increase in phagocytosis. It is of interest that an increased rate of phagocytosis is not necessarily confined to the material injected, and this is again evidence of the non-specificity of the response. One must not be in too great a hurry either to equate an increase in phagocytosis with a higher level of immunity; the fate of the ingested particle must also be taken into account. It is remarkable all the same to find that the period of enhanced phagocytosis is associated with increased levels of immunity to bacterial infections when antigenic particles have been used to blockade the system, but not when so-called 'inert' particles such as carbon, dyes, kaolin, etc., have been used.

We are still left with a puzzling element of non-specificity when the reticulo-endothelial system is stimulated by antigenic substances, a mechanism that is just hinted at in the old observations that the macrophages of animals infected with tubercle bacilli show enhanced uptake of carbon particles. The period of heightened immunity may be similarly non-specific, i.e., directed against a different bacterium from that used to stimulate the system.

It is clear that both resistance and immunity are the end-products of mechanisms that begin with phagocytosis. However, phagocytosis itself is a complex process beginning with ingestion which may or may not be followed by digestion. We will now consider these two processes separately.

2. INGESTION

In 1903 Wright and Douglas [10] demonstrated the presence of factors in normal serum that enhanced the uptake of bacteria by phagocytes, and which they called 'opsonins'. Subsequently it was shown that both heat-stable and heat-labile components might be involved in this reaction, and even at this distance in time the nature of opsonins is still being debated.

Some authors have reserved the term for the heat-labile component of serum, and others have assumed that because of its heat-lability it must be 'complement'. Still others take the view that opsonins are antibodies, either 'natural' or 'immune', or that opsonins are any substance or complex of substances that enhance phagocytosis. What is not in doubt is that a specific antiserum exerts a very great opsonizing effect on its homologous antigen and, consistent with the view that this effect is due to antibody, is little affected by the application of heat. The nature of heat-stable opsonins in 'normal' sera remains somewhat obscure. To say that they are 'natural' antibodies simply begs the question since there is no general agreement on what natural antibodies are, nor on how they originate, though specificity is implied. Evidence for heat-labile elements of serum apart from complement has also been adduced [11].

From an immunological standpoint we might perhaps think that the unique role of phagocytes is to make the initial recognition of 'foreign' material, and this poses the question, Is this recognition due to a chance meeting or is it in some sense directed? It is true that a wide range of substances, not all of them of biological origin, appear to attract phagocytes [12], i.e., are chemotactic, and it is probable that in some cases chemotaxis is not dependent on serum factors. Conversely it would be unwise to regard any particles as 'inert' in this respect since as long ago as 1921 Fenn showed that phagocytosis of carbon particles was enhanced by serum [13], and the adsorptive capacity for proteins of a number of substances that are readily ingested is well known. In recent years a heat-stable principle has been described which is released from fresh serum by the addition of antigen or antigen–antibody complexes and which is chemotactic for rabbit polymorphonuclear leucocytes [14, 15]. Sub-sequently chemotactic activity has been ascribed to certain components of complement [16]. It might be noted in passing that the *lytic* activity of complement is destroyed by heating at 56° C. for 30 minutes and in serology this is what is generally meant by 'heat-labile', but lytic activity requires all the components of complement whereas chemotactic activity apparently does not. Since the ease with which different components of complement are inactivated by heat varies, the fruitlessness of trying to equate heat-stability with the activity of complement in chemotaxis, without specifying which components are involved, becomes apparent.

Whatever the additional factors that influence phagocytosis, there is no doubt that the most effective opsonins are antibodies. This is reflected in the extremely small amounts of antibody that can be detected *in vivo*—as little as 0·001 μg. of antibody nitrogen, a sensitivity that is paralleled only by the most sensitive serological tests available, such as passive cutaneous anaphylaxis. Opsonization may nevertheless affect two distinct processes: attraction and engulfment. For instance, before ingestion can take place in the absence of antiserum encapsulated pneumococci have to be trapped against a surface; coated with antibody they can be snatched, as it were, out of mid-stream by any passing leucocyte. It has been suggested that opsonization of this sort is due to an alteration in the net electrical charge at the surface of bacteria. An alternative explanation for enhanced phagocytosis could be that the phagocytes themselves become more active. It is perhaps rather difficult to rule out this possibility purely on the basis of microscopical evidence, and at first sight it would appear that the non-specific stimulation of the reticulo-endothelial system by bacterial endotoxins, etc., that we have already noted, would support such a possibility. However, on more detailed examination it appears that the main effect of injecting such substances is to increase the production of new phagocytes. In addition, a concurrent rise in serum opsonins has often been observed.

The picture of events initiating ingestion thus remains very confused with antibody, complement, or some components of complement, and possibly other serum factors, either heat-stable or heat-labile, all exerting some influence on the outcome.

3. Digestion

We have taken note that ingestion is not sufficient either for the disposal of effete host materials or for defence against micro-organisms. Digestion in many cases succeeds ingestion and in order that it should do so a train of metabolic events has to be set in motion. The process of digestion is immediately preceded by an event described as 'degranulation' which has been equated with the rupture of lysosomes into vacuoles containing ingested material. Lysozyme and phagocytin are two enzymes that probably play a leading part in the dissolution of bacteria and other particles; a process that may be completed by other hydrolytic enzymes of which lysosomes are known to contain a number. Degranulation is very much less marked, or absent altogether, when 'virulent' bacteria are ingested, and this observation can be correlated with an absence of specific antibody in serum. For example, avirulent pneumococci, which lack the strain-specific polysaccharide capsules of virulent members and which are therefore coated by the much more widely distributed group-specific antibodies, are also much more readily ingested and digested. Antibody is thus seen to take part in both processes, and the same can probably be said of complement. Red blood-cells 'sensitized' with the so-called IgG class of antibodies fail to 'fix' complement and though ingested are not lysed. The same cells 'sensitized' with IgM antibodies do 'fix' complement and are lysed [17]. Lysis is accompanied by degranulation.

Possibly nowhere else in the field of immunology is a phenomenon so readily observable and the elucidation of its mechanism so baffling. Studies can be undertaken *in vitro* and *in vivo*, but the devising of valid experimental procedures is fraught with pitfalls, as has been pointed out in a number of recent reviews on the subject [12, 15, 18]. For instance, well-washed phagocytes have been used to study ingestion in the absence of serum, but whether such cells are still in anything approaching a physiological condition is open to grave doubt. The type of phagocytic cell, the class of antibody, the role of complement, and other as-yet-undefined plasma constituents all have to be considered. Even the phylo-genetic relationship between phagocyte and ingested particle may influence the outcome since distantly related erythrocytes have been shown to be more readily phagocytosed in the absence of antibody than those more closely related [19]. Some 'inert' particles, e.g., polystyrene, can be ingested in the absence of serum; others, e.g., starch, cannot. It is presumed that the surface of the particle has a decisive bearing. These are but some of the conditions that have to be observed if meaningful experi-ments are to be devised, and it comes as no surprise to find that the literature on the subject abounds in conflicting statements. Nevertheless, the fact that so many of these problems are now recognized offers hope that future investigations will prove more rewarding.

III. Specific Immunity

With phagocytosis we reached a half-way house between resistance and immunity where both factors operate. The development and operation of acquired immunity may certainly involve phagocytosis, but what distinguishes acquired immunity from resistance is the specificity of the response towards the stimulating antigen. Specific immunity may be acquired in a number of ways and the simplest subdivision is as follows:—
　1. Natural: (*a*) Passive; (*b*) Active.
　2. Artificial: (*a*) Passive; (*b*) Active.
By 'passive immunity' is meant that a normal or susceptible animal receives material from an immune animal that confers a specific immunity on the recipient. By 'active immunity' is meant the development of an

immune response by the host's own immunological system to an antigenic stimulus.

The transfer of maternal antibodies to the offspring via the placenta is an example of natural passive immunity; the injection of serum or gamma-globulin from an immune animal into another animal constitutes artificial passive immunity. Active immunities result from accidental infection (natural) and purposeful administration of antigenic substances (artificial).

Once an individual has received an antigenic stimulus and responded, its subsequent reaction to that antigen is altered. This state of 'altered reactivity' was the meaning von Pirquet originally gave to *allergy*, a term that is now generally used to indicate a state of hypersensitivity. Basically this altered reactivity is expressed in either humoral or cellular forms. Classically the administration of a soluble antigen stimulates an animal to produce circulating (humoral) antibody. The antibody reacts specifically with antigen, and *in vivo* either neutralizes it or increases the rate at which is catabolized and excreted. Antibody production may also result in a state of heightened susceptibility in the host animal, known as 'immediate hypersensitivity', in which the subsequent administration or continued presence of the stimulating antigen engenders a state of shock (*see* Chapter 7).

It is still easy to visualize how antibodies can exert a protective effect on the organism as a whole. This is not so in the case of cell-mediated immunity. Here we are characteristically dealing with a phenomenon known as 'delayed hypersensitivity', of which the very name suggests that we are dealing with anything but an immune phenomenon. It is indeed a matter of considerable difficulty to demonstrate that delayed hypersensitivity or the mechanism from which it derives is in any way protective. What is certain is that delayed hypersensitive responses cannot be correlated with circulating antibody levels. These are in truth two quite separate states of altered reactivity that are consequent on antigenic stimulation.

How can we resolve the paradox that a hypersensitive reaction is the result of an immune response? First, we must make it clear that no proof exists as yet that the acquisition of a state of delayed hypersensitivity confers protection on an animal—we are in this sense no farther forward than the bacteriologists of the last century who originally described the phenomenon. Second, that the two phenomena, humoral immunity and delayed hypersensitivity, are mediated by quite distinct mechanisms. Proof of this lies in the fact that humoral immunity can be transmitted from one animal to another by means of blood-serum, whereas delayed hypersensitivity can be transmitted only by cells (of the lymphoid series). Nevertheless, although these two types of response are quite distinct they can sometimes, and perhaps would usually if we had the means to detect them, be seen to occur together. Indeed, they are sometimes so interrelated that it appears that they must share some common pathway in their development. This is most clearly seen when a small dose of native protein is used to induce a state of delayed hypersensitivity in an animal. After a suitable interval of time a second dose of antigen can be used to elicit the delayed hypersensitivity reaction. But the secondary stimulation afforded by the antigen is also sufficient to push the immunological apparatus over into antibody production. The first dose thus induced a state of cell-mediated immunity, the second dose a state of humoral immunity on top of it. The relationship between these mechanisms can be seen if the second dose consists of slightly denatured antigen instead of native antigen. The hypersensitivity reaction is then obtained but not the antibody response.

We must deduce from this that the first dose is sufficient (1) to induce a state of cell-mediated immunity so that a second dose elicits a hypersensitivity reaction, and (2) to prime the antibody-forming mechanism so that on secondary stimulation it can go into production. If the second dose consists of altered antigen it is still sufficiently similar to the native antigen to elicit the immunological reaction of delayed hypersensitivity, but at the same time it is too different to provide the stimulus needed for antibody production.

Taken in conjunction these facts quite clearly distinguish between the two types of response. They also indicate that the responses are in some way interconnected since the same dose of antigen primes both mechanisms.

In addition, we can draw a number of other conclusions from the same evidence. First is the point already partly made that an immunological *reaction* is less demanding with respect to specificity than an immunological *response*. In this case the reaction is one of delayed hypersensitivity, although the same would probably apply equally well to an antigen–antibody reaction. The immune response, of course, was one of antibody production, and since this mechanism requires the native rather than the denatured antigen for its operation it must be presumed that it functions at a different level.

This brings us to the second point: that there must also operate a system of memory in order that the antibody-forming mechanism should distinguish between native and denatured antigen. Since memory is not deceived by the slightly altered antigen, a third point would be that memory is more highly specific than the immune reactions that ultimately result from its operation.

Memory is thus seen to form an important link in the chain of events leading to a specific immunological response. It should not be confused with *recognition*, which serves only to distinguish between antigenic and non-antigenic substances. Cells which are capable of reacting to an immunogenic stimulus are said to be *immunologically competent*; they might be said to be associated with *recognition*. Those that have already been in contact with an immunogen, directly or indirectly, and are ready to respond specifically to another stimulus from the same immunogen are said to be *immunologically committed*. They might be said to be associated with *memory*.

Returning to the foregoing experiment once more, we might have found that if a larger first dose of antigen had been given the second dose would not have elicited the reaction of delayed hypersensitivity, and indeed circulating antibodies might already have made their appearance. Are we to conclude from this that it is only the size of antigenic dose that determines whether the response is cell-mediated or humoral immunity? Size of dose is certainly important but is equally certainly not the only criterion that determines the nature of a response to an immunogenic stimulus. That antibody production classically follows the intravenous administration of soluble antigens has already been remarked on. Conversely the administration of antigen into the dermal or subcutaneous tissues, accompanied by the slow release of antigen, appears to favour the development of cell-mediated immunity. These conditions are probably mimicked to some extent by skin and whole-organ homografts, the rejection of which can be regarded as a consequence of the development of cell-mediated immunity (see Chapter 10). If Gowans [20] is right, the small lymphocyte plays a very prominent role in the rejection of homografts. This cell type is certainly an immunologically competent cell whereas phagocytic cells are not, so it may be that the way in which an immunogen is presented to the small lymphocyte, and through it to other cells of the lymphoid series, determines whether the immune response is one of cell-mediated or humoral immunity.

A. Local Immunity

Throughout the foregoing discussion we have used the term 'cell-mediated immunity' and eschewed that of 'cellular immunity' because the latter has been given so many meanings by so many writers—ranging from 'phagocytosis', through 'delayed hypersensitivity' and 'homograft rejection', to 'local (or tissue) immunity'. The last-named are again phrases of somewhat imprecise meaning which we would prefer to restrict to the sense of specific immunity to reinfection acquired by certain tissues. Examples can be found in the spreading lesions of ringworm and erysipelas; rather more uncertain is the oft-recorded failure of smallpox vaccination to 'take', only for a subsequent inoculation at a new site to succeed. Convincing explanations based on immunological grounds have been difficult to sustain in the past. It is all the more interesting, therefore, to find that in recent years a new class of antibody molecule, called IgA, has been discovered that is often locally produced and is particularly associated with mucous membranes. The way in which such antibodies might act is well illustrated by comparing the results of vaccination with the two types of poliomyelitis antigen. The killed (Salk-type) vaccine is injected and stimulates the production of circulating antibodies which protect the individual against the clinical disease, but do not prevent him from becoming infected and excreting the virus in large numbers. The live (Sabin-type) vaccine is swallowed and like the wild virus produces a gut immunity as well as humoral antibodies. It is possible that the freedom of the intestinal wall from further infection by the virus could be due to the local production of antibody. Whatever the mechanism, the effect is that those people who have taken oral vaccine do not subsequently become infected by and excrete wild strains and are therefore less of a danger to their fellow-men.

B. Herd Immunity

The concept that the immune status of an individual reflects the susceptibility of the population as a whole to certain infections is inherent in the idea of herd immunity. Any parasite has a greater chance of establishing itself in a community containing a relatively large number of susceptible hosts. Given that defence against a particular infection is the result of specifically acquired immunity, susceptibles may arise in a number of ways: by introduction from without either by birth or immigration; by loss of acquired immunity through the absence of repeated or continuing infection; and by alteration in the antigenic structure of the infectious agent as with the influenza virus. Herd immunity is thus seen as an epidemiological concept with a foundation in the development of specific immunological defences.

C. Development of Specific Immunity

So far we have dealt with the subject-matter of immunology almost wholly in the context of infectious disease. We have only strayed from this path to mention certain examples, for instance of homograft rejection, in order to shed light on particular problems. While there can be no doubt that the specific immune response to foreign invasion is of vital importance to many animal species, it is nevertheless worth exploring the possibility that this is not its primary purpose. Or if that is put in too teleological a manner, then that possibly the exploration of the development of the immune apparatus might show us how it came to be adapted to resist invasion from without.

The study of this aspect of immunology may be approached from the point of view of ontogeny or phylogeny, since we see an accelerated version of evolution in embryological development in a manner of speaking. According to Gesner [21], 'the development of immunological competence coincides phylogenetically and embryologically with the appearance of lymphocytes'. Part of the evidence on which this statement is based is that in the opossum embryo the accelerated elimination of an injected bacterial virus is correlated with both the appearance of small lymphocytes and with antibody production [22]. This bears the implication that before the development of this cell type injected antigen is slowly excreted, perhaps no quicker than host protein. But here we have introduced a new topic. Why should host material be any different from 'foreign' material, since it would in fact be 'foreign' to another host? The concept that an animal does not react immunologically against its own antigens was recognized by the earlier immunologists and is enshrined in the term 'horror autotoxicus'. We shall see later (Chapter 12) that this aversion is not always maintained and that the pathological lesions of so-called 'atuo-immune diseases' can result. It has also been suggested that the physiological production of auto-antibodies assists, or is necessary for, the normal scavenging process associated with the excretion of worn-out body materials.

Under normal circumstances it would seem at the moment that the distinction between antigen and host material is made principally on the basis of dose and continuing presence. It can be verified experimentally that very heavy doses of antigen induce a state of acquired immunological *tolerance* which continues so long as there is a sufficient concentration of antigen present to enforce it. Tolerance towards the host's own immunogens can then be looked upon as resulting from the saturation of its immunological apparatus by those immunogens. Saturation with 'foreign' antigens is much easier to achieve during the perinatal period than in adult life, and this explains in part why tolerance was first induced regularly and with certainty under such conditions. Nevertheless, tolerance can be induced in adult animals providing adequate doses are administered and maintained.

In this manner the vexed question of how the immunological apparatus can distinguish between 'self' and 'not-self' has been rather neatly side-stepped with the explanation that it is inherent in the nature of the immune response.

We have still to deal with the fundamental questions posed above, namely, what has called the immunological system into existence and why has it been retained? The mere fact that we can trace it down the phylogenetic scale, at least as far as the teleost fishes, only tells us that these functions developed or were adapted a fairly long time ago and have presumably proved to be of survival value in vertebrates. In fact we have independent evidence of survival value in the early demise of congenital hypogamma-globulinaemics in the face of bacterial infection, at least until the advent of antibiotics.

It is, of course, quite easy to recognize the benefit that accrues to an animal from the presence of humoral antibody, especially if we consider only reactions such as agglutination, precipitation, bacteriolysis, and opsonization. With reactions of immediate hypersensitivity, also mediated by antibody, and of cell-mediated hypersensitivity the benefit to the host is by no means obvious. Indeed immediate hypersensitivities can kill the host and delayed hypersensitivity has not been proved to have a protective function. However, the part played by antibodies in recovery from viral infections is not nearly so marked as it is in bacterial infections; and this at least opens the door to explanations of the type that the tissue destruction that accompanies delayed hypersensitivity might militate against viral replication.

Possibly of greater significance is the rejection of grafted tissues by cell-mediated immunity. It is very tempting to extend such observations to the speculation that this type of immunity is particularly associated with maintaining the integrity of the host. The concept that multicellular organisms are constantly replacing worn-out cells, and in the process mutations of suicidal or perhaps only harmful consequence are occurring, is one that Sir MacFarlane Burnet has made peculiarly his own [23]. The connexion between 'forbidden' mutants of any cell type and uncontrolled tumour growth is easy to draw; and there is abundant evidence that tumour cells differ from parent cells morphologically, genetically, and antigenically. It is a reasonable assumption that early mutants with new antigens on the cell surface stimulate an immune response and are destroyed. The suggestion that the immunological apparatus is, though competent, less flexible at the extremes of life is perhaps sufficient to account for the higher incidence of malignant neoplasms at these ages.

The considerable threat to the host's integrity posed by viruses has already been mentioned, and it is of interest that tumour viruses characteristically alter the surface antigens of the cells they infect. From this point of view the postulated immunological attack against these 'mutant' cells is more in the nature of maintaining integrity than an attack directed against virus replication.

Though largely speculative, the view that the whole breadth of resistance and immunology is concerned with the maintenance of a host's integrity does form a unifying concept in a field where there are many complicated mechanisms and confusing factors operating. It is, however, with the consideration of mechanisms as well as principles that immunology is concerned and it is to the more detailed study of those aspects and their application that we shall now turn.

REFERENCES

1. KALLMANN, F. J., and REISNER, D. (1943), 'Twin Studies on the Significance of Genetic Factors in Tuberculosis', *Am. Rev. Tuberc. pulm. Dis.*, **47**, 549.
2. DUBOS, R. J., ed. (1958), *Bacterial and Mycotic Infections of Man*. Philadelphia: Lippincott.
3. CHRISTENSEN, P. E., SCHMIDT, H., BANG, H. O., ANDERSEN, V., JORDAL, B., and JENSEN, O. (1953), 'An Epidemic of Measles in Southern Greenland, 1951. Measles in Virgin Soil, II', *Acta med. scand.*, **144**, 430.
4. CHRISTENSEN, P. E., SCHMIDT, H., JENSEN, O., BANG, H. O., ANDERSEN, V., and JORDAL, B. (1953), 'An Epidemic of Measles in Southern Greenland, 1951. Measles in Virgin Soil, I', *Acta med. scand.*, **144**, 313.
5. PEART, A. F. W. (1949), 'An Outbreak of Poliomyelitis in Canadian Eskimoes in Wintertime. Epidemiological Features', *Can. J. Publ. Hlth*, **40**, 405.
6. SHOPE, R. E. (1955), 'Swine Lungworm as a Reservoir and Intermediate Host for Swine Influenza Virus. V, Provocation of Swine Influenza by Exposure of Prepared Swine to Adverse Weather', *J. exp. Med.*, **102**, 567.
7. LACHMAN, P. J. (1967), 'Conglutinin and Immunoconglutinins', *Adv. Immun.*, **6**, 480.
8. FINTER, N. B., ed. (1966), *Interferons*. Amsterdam: North-Holland.
9. EVANS, D. G., and PERKINS, F. T. (1954), 'The Ability of Pertussis Vaccine to produce in Mice Specific Immunity of a Type not associated with Antibody Production', *Br. J. exp. Path.*, **35**, 322.
10. WRIGHT, A. E., and DOUGLAS, S. R. (1903), 'An Experimental Investigation of the Role of Blood Fluids in Connection with Phagocytosis', *Proc. R. Soc. Med.*, **72**, 357.
11. HIRSCH, J. G., and STRAUSS, B. (1964), 'Studies on Heat-labile Opsonin in Rabbit Serum', *J. Immun.*, **92**, 145.
12. SUTER, E., and RAMSEIER, H. (1964), 'Cellular Reactions to Infection', *Adv. Immun.*, **4**, 117.
13. FENN, W. C. (1921), 'The Phagocytosis of Solid Particles. III, Carbon and Quartz', *J. gen. Physiol.*, **3**, 575.
14. BOYDEN, S. V. (1962), 'The Chemotactic Effect of Mixtures of Antibody and Antigen on Polymorphonuclear Leucocytes', *J. exp. Med.*, **115**, 453.
15. BOYDEN, S. V., NORTH, R. J., and FAULKNER, S. M. (1965), 'Complement and the Activity of Phagocytes', in *Complement* (ed. WOLSTENHOLME, G. E. W., and KNIGHT, J.), p. 190. Ciba Foundation Symposium. London: Churchill.
16. WARD, P. A., COCHRANE, C. G., and MÜLLER-EBERHARD, H. J. (1966), 'Further Studies on the Chemotactic Factor of Complement and its Formation *in vivo*', *Immunology*, **11**, 141.
17. GERLINGS-PETERSEN, B. T., and PONDMAN, K. W., (1964), 'Function of Antibody and Complement in Phagocytosis', *Nouv. Rev. Fr. d'Hematol.*, **4**, 593.
18. ROWLEY, D. (1962), 'Phagocytosis', *Adv. Immun.*, **2**, 241.
19. PERKINS, E. H., and LEONARD, M. R. (1963), 'Specificity of Phagocytosis as it may relate to Antibody Formation', *J. Immun.*, **90**, 228.
20. GOWANS, J. L. (1965), 'The Role of Lymphocytes in the Destruction of Homografts', *Br. med. Bull.*, **21**, 106.
21. GESNER, B. M. (1965), 'The Life-history and Functions of Lymphocytes', in *The Inflammatory Process* (ed. ZWEIFACH, B. W., GRANT, L., and McCLUSKEY, R. T.), p. 286. New York: Academic.
22. KALMUTZ, S. E. (1962), 'Antibody Production in the Opossum Embryo', *Nature, Lond.*, **193**, 851.
23. BURNET, Sir F. MACFARLANE (1966), *The Integrity of the Body: A Discussion of Modern Immunological Ideas*. New York: Atheneum.

CHAPTER 2

ANTIGENS

By E. R. Gold and D. B. Peacock

I. Introduction

    A. Haptens
    B. Partial antigens
    C. Pro-antigens

II. Antigenicity

    A. Molecular size
    B. Chemical structure
    C. Chemical composition

III. Specificity

    A. Protein antigens
        1. Specificity of natural proteins
        2. Species specificity
        3. Organ specificity
        4. Chemically altered proteins
           Nitration and iodination
        5. Conjugated proteins
           a. Influence of acid radicals
           b. Influence of neutral radicals
           c. Influence of spatial configuration
           d. Influence of aliphatic side-chains
           e. Influence of peptide side-chains
        6. Configuration
        7. Chemical structure
        8. Size of determinants

    B. Polysaccharide antigens
        1. Size of determinants
        2. Structure of determinants
           a. Blood-group antigens
               i. Biochemistry of soluble ABH and Lewis substances
               ii. Antigens of the MNSs system
               iii. Other blood-group antigens
           b. Bacterial polysaccharides
               i. Pneumococcal capsular antigens
               ii. Somatic antigens of enterobacteria

I. Introduction

IF 'antigen' is defined in terms of 'antibody', as it used to be, then it is true to say that an antigen is any substance that stimulates the production of antibody that is complementary to and reacts with the antigen. Such a definition is incomplete as will become immediately apparent, but from it follows that immunogenicity of antigen, i.e., its ability to stimulate the production of antibody, and specificity, i.e., its ability to react with the antibody produced, are the two most important attributes of an antigen.

In the light of more recent knowledge it is clear that antigens provoke responses other than the production of humoral antibody, such as delayed hypersensitivity and tolerance. Therefore we would now say that the main property of an antigen is its ability to change the reactivity of certain cells; first in ways that are general to all antigens and second in ways that are specific to the particular antigen. The same criteria of immunogenicity and specificity are inherent in both definitions, but immunogenicity now takes on a rather wider meaning.

As far as is known at present, the commonest response to an antigenic stimulus culminates in the production of specific antibody. Specificity is determined by a small patch on the antibody molecule that is complementary in configuration to a site on the antigen molecule. The fact that these reactive sites are comparatively small has important consequences. A large antigen such as a cell or even a molecule of protein has a number of such sites, not all of which are necessarily the same, indeed the contrary is the rule rather than the exception. Failure to recognize the diversity of stimuli represented even by chemically pure antigens has been responsible for much confusion in the past and probably still is. Immunogenicity is thus seen as a property of a whole molecule or cell, or at any rate of a substantial part of it, whereas specificity is determined by relatively small areas.

In most instances all the essential properties of antigen are found together, though sometimes they become separated. This has led to the evolution of the concept of *complete* and *incomplete* antigens. The latter lack one or more of the properties of complete antigens and though the term has been used as a synonym for partial antigens and complex haptens (q.v.), we feel that the broader definition given here should be retained, including as it does all haptens and pro-antigens.

A. Haptens

Haptens are substances that react serologically with antibodies but are unable to stimulate their production; they may be simple or complex. Simple haptens are not precipitable by antibody but they will inhibit precipitation of a corresponding whole antigen or complex hapten. That portion of an antigen which actually combines with an antibody is known as a 'determinant' or 'determinant group', 'group' in this sense being intended to convey the idea of an arrangement of physicochemical forces which together form a determinant. It should be noted that a determinant group is not the same thing as a group of determinants. It will become clear in succeeding pages that a simple hapten consists of a single determinant group, or even part of a determinant, but also perhaps with enough of the antigen molecule attached to hold the structure of the determinant in its correct steric configuration. Complex haptens consist of portions of

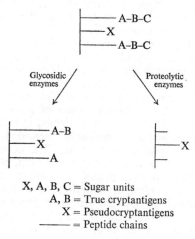

X, A, B, C = Sugar units
A, B = True cryptantigens
X = Pseudocryptantigens
——— = Peptide chains

Fig. 1.—Cryptantigens and pseudocryptantigens. *After Uhlenbruck* [2].

antigen molecules that retain two or more determinant groups; they are precipitable by antibody. The difference between simple and complex haptens is also expressed by the terms 'univalent' (unifunctional) and 'polyvalent' (polyfunctional). According to one well-known theory precipitation should follow the formation of a lattice-like structure resulting from the interaction of polyvalent hapten and divalent antibody. Under these conditions univalent haptens would form complexes with only one antibody molecule and divalent haptens would form chains but not lattices. It is interesting to note, therefore, that it has recently been found that the two monosaccharides 3-O-methyl-D-fucose and 3-O-methyl-D-galactose behave like simple haptens at low concentrations, but are precipitable by antiserum at higher concentrations [1]. The precipitate is apparently immunologically specific since it obeys serological 'rules' in that the amount of precipitate is proportional to the hapten concentration, and decreases in the zone of 'antigen' excess.

Cryptantigens are chemical structures present but 'unavailable' in a native antigen because they are not terminal.

Pseudocryptantigens are also 'unavailable' in the native molecule, not because they are subterminal, but because they cannot react due to steric hindrance by other groups (*Fig.* 1) [2]. These last two concepts are also covered by the terms 'hidden' or 'buried' antigenic determinants.

B. Partial Antigens

Wilson and Miles [3] equate partial antigens with haptens, but in blood-group serology the term 'partial antigen' simply means part of a larger antigen from which it can be distinguished serologically, but not yet chemically.

C. Pro-antigens

The expression 'pro-antigen' is principally used in connexion with the hypersensitivity reactions of skin. It denotes all the low molecular weight substances that induce hypersensitivity and that acquire immunogenicity probably by combining with autologous protein *in vivo*. A great variety of such substances has been found, ranging from simple ions like iodine, mercury, and nickel, through still fairly simple compounds such as formaldehyde, iodoform, mercaptan, picryl chloride, and dinitro chlorobenzene, up to more complex substances like resins and sterols. The simplest of them lack the inhibitory power of haptens but all of them possess one fundamental property of antigens, specificity, although the whole antigenic determinant is probably formed by the pro-antigen plus adjacent parts of autologous protein. The development of hypersensitive reactions to iodine in guinea-pig and man, presumably through coupling to autologous protein *in vivo*, is perhaps comparable to the iodination of protein *in vitro*, a situation in which the specificity of protein is also changed (p. 35). For some of these simplest substances there may be alternative explanations, i.e., idiosyncrasies due to defective enzyme mechanisms in the host, or some other non-immunological cause.

Finally, as pointed out by Wilson and Miles [3], it must not be forgotten that all the above definitions are artificial in the sense that there is in reality a gradual transition from complete antigens, with all the properties of antigen intact to the simplest pro-antigens, with only one property, specificity, left.

Somewhere in between is the *minimal antigenic determinant*—the simplest chemical structure with a configuration complementary to the combining site of antibody and which may comprise only a small part of an antigen molecule.

II. Antigenicity

In spite of continued investigation over the years we are still not able to state unequivocally the indispensable properties that confer antigenicity on a substance. We can only list those properties that an antigen usually possesses, mention exceptions, and point out some of the unsolved problems.

A. Molecular Size

Complete antigens are large organic molecules. Very large molecules, e.g., haemocyanin with a molecular weight of nearly $6\frac{3}{4}$ million, are highly antigenic. So too are viruses and organized structures such as intact bacteria and human and animal cells; but because of their complex structure they possess a great variety of different antigens that are situated in many different parts of the cell. Even macromolecules like the globular proteins have antigenic determinants both at the surface and within the depths of the molecular structure; but even if we consider only the surface it should not be supposed that the whole of it is concerned with determining specificity.

The influence of size is suggested by the fact that non-antigenic or weakly antigenic substances can be made actively antigenic by adsorbing them to particulate substrates, e.g., bentonite, collodion, kaolin. Such particles sometimes enhance the antigenicity of even strong antigens, but their effect may be due only in part to an increase in size, or to other factors altogether (see ADJUVANTS, p. 149). Some proteins of low molecular weight are reputedly antigenic, e.g., ribonuclease (M.W. 13,683), insulin (M.W. c. 6000), and dinitrophenylated bacitracin A (M.W. 1928). This is all the more surprising in the case of the first two because they are substances widely distributed in nature and certainly in the case of a number of insulins derived from a variety of animal species it is known that they differ little in composition. However, such substances are almost invariably injected with adjuvants or in a form likely to enhance immunogenicity, and since we do not altogether understand the mechanism of enhancement some doubt must remain about their antigenicity. It is also usually impossible to rule out the possibility that they form complexes with autologous protein *in vivo*.

Early attempts to shed light on the nature of antigenicity were naturally directed towards proteins that could be obtained in relatively pure form and that were reasonably well characterized chemically. Protamines and gelatin fall into this category and display a number of features of interest.

Clupein is a protamine obtained from herring sperm and is the protein part of its nucleoprotein. Little more than a large polypeptide, though still twice the size of bacitracin A, it is strongly basic, consisting mainly of the basic diamino-acids arginine and lysine. It is not antigenic by itself but can be made so very simply by coupling it to phenylisocyanide. Antisera to conjugated clupein react with the unconjugated protamine or with phenylisocyanide conjugated to another protein carrier. Phenylisocyanide thus confers antigenicity on clupein and does not necessarily form part of the determinant. The acquisition of antigenicity is not due to an increase in molecular weight since this is raised by only five hundred up to four thousand five hundred; but it may be due to the introduction of an aromatic ring structure into the molecule. The complete structure of clupein has now been determined and it should be possible in any future studies to correlate immunological findings with structure.

Since an increase in molecular size did not seem to be a likely explanation of the antigenicity of conjugated clupein, it was reasonable to assume that the deficiency supplied by phenylisocyanide was its ring structure. But against this it was found that it was not possible to make gelatin, a protein that also contains very little in the way of aromatic amino-acids, antigenic by conjugation with phenylisocyanide. Then again, albumin, normally antigenic, is rendered non-antigenic by alkali denaturation, although it still retains its quota of aromatic amino-acids such as tyrosine. Other protamines (M.W. 5000–8000) which like clupein are devoid of tyrosine and tryptophane are also not antigenic. This has usually been put down to their low molecular weight, but it might equally be due to their essentially basic reaction, and the importance of acid radicals will be discussed under the heading of SPECIFICITY (p. 29).

The problem of the lack of antigenicity of gelatin is still not solved. A denatured protein and derived from collagen, gelatin contains only small amounts of the aromatic amino-acids phenylalanine and histidine, and little or no tyrosine. Again, it was thought originally that this paucity of aromatic residues was responsible for the lack of antigenicity, strengthened by the fact that the introduction of additional tyrosine conferred antigenicity on gelatin. However, as we have seen, phenylisocyanide is not effective in this respect so that the lack of aromatic amino-acids as such is not likely to be the cause. Among other suggestions that have been put forward are that gelatin is too rapidly excreted and that it does not possess a sufficiently rigid structure. Many good antigens, however, are quickly excreted and yet enough must remain to provide an antigenic stimulus. On the other hand, it has long been thought that rigidity of structure plays an important part in determining antigenicity, and recently support for this outlook has come from the finding that polycyclohexanylalanyl coupled to gelatin renders it antigenic [4]. Collagen is antigenic even if gelatin is not, and antibodies to it which appear in certain auto-immune diseases also react with gelatin. In fact it is now considered that gelatin itself is weakly antigenic, but this does not alter the basic proposition that collagen and gelatin differ markedly in antigenicity. It is this difference which remains something of a puzzle.

B. Chemical Structure

Nevertheless, there does not seem to be any generally valid correlation between the rigidity of particular areas on the surface of antigen molecules or of the presence of aromatic amino-acids in them, on the one hand, and antigenicity, on the other, although both are important in certain cases. However, the concept of immunological tolerance has made possible a new approach to the problem of antigenicity [5]. If it is assumed that every healthy animal possesses an acquired immunological tolerance to autologous macromolecules, antigenicity can be related to the chemical differences between these molecules and antigens. A 'bad' antigen is then a substance which differs only slightly from the autologous molecules, whereas a 'good' antigen differs very greatly. These assumptions and a knowledge of the species specificity of serum proteins (q.v.) can be used to explain the results of experiments in which animals of one species are immunized with sera from closely or distantly related species. If, for instance, a rabbit is immunized with the serum of another rodent, a mouse, antibodies that are specific for mouse serum will be produced; but if a rabbit is immunized with chicken serum, it will produce antibodies that fail to distinguish chicken serum from the serum of any other bird. In the first case a rabbit would produce antibodies directed against those few amino-acid sequences which are different in the two rodents, whereas in the second case it would produce antibodies directed against the many determinants or amino-acid sequences that are shared by all birds but are absent in mammals. The validity of such an interpretation was elegantly confirmed by showing that a rabbit made tolerant to hen antigen would subsequently produce antibody specific for turkey antigen [6]. The implication is that the rabbit is rendered tolerant to all those antigens present in chicken serum which distinguish avian species from mammalian species, so that only those antigens which distinguish turkey from chicken give rise to the production of antibody.

The experimental evidence quoted above illustrates differences in 'perspective' that are related to the taxonomical position of the immunized animal vis-à-vis the donor of antigen. In general a close relationship is necessary in order that small differences in structure should be detectable; but this is not always so and the occasional rabbit antiserum will detect as fine a distinction of antigenic structure in human globulin as the more general run of monkey antisera.

The recent availability of synthetic amino-acid polymers has made yet another approach to the problems of antigenicity possible. In contrast to older ideas on the subject Maurer points out that too high a negative charge on the molecule may even prevent an antigen from exercising antigenicity, and that the role of molecular weight is also minor [7, 8]. In accordance with current ideas on these matters, Maurer stresses the importance of a number of other factors. Foremost among these is the capacity of the immunological mechanism itself, which in turn depends principally on the genetic constitution of the host, and to a lesser degree on the host's previous immunological experience.

The genetic constitution of the individual assumes even greater significance than might be predicted by considerations of immunological tolerance (see Chapter 4) when it is appreciated, as Maurer has shown, that synthetic polymers are antigenic in some strains of animal and not in others. One of the mechanisms through which an antigen might act could well be the capacity of the host to metabolize the antigen, with antibody production being directed mainly against those areas of the antigen molecule that are accessible to the action of hydrolytic enzymes. This would also explain the 'unmasking' of 'hidden' determinants; a modern concept dealing more particularly with specificity, though antigenicity could well operate at this level too. Even if the postulate is inverted and antibody production held to precede catabolism the relevance of genetic constitution is not thereby lessened.

Another factor more certainly applicable to antigenicity is diversity of structure. Artificially produced homopolymers of amino-acids are not antigenic in themselves, though they can be made so by coupling them to proteins, and rather more unexpectedly to small haptens, like 2,4-dinitro-aniline, indicating that it is not simply high molecular weight that confers antigenicity on proteins. The importance of diversity of structure is also suggested by the observation that co-polymers, e.g., of glutamic acid (G) and alanine (A), are antigenic even when the polymer is composed of as few as 20 units, i.e., smaller than clupein and about the size of bacitracin A [9]. Co-polymers in the proportions $G_{60}A_{40}$ and $G_{40}A_{60}$ are better antigens than $G_{90}A_{10}$ or $G_{75}A_{25}$, which suggests that, rather than relative proportions of G and A, it is again diversity of structure that is important.

Interesting and suggestive though these results are, it is possible that the immunogenicity of low molecular weight synthetic polyamino-acids may be due in some cases to their contamination with high molecular weight polymers of the same substance. Such a criticism probably does not apply in cases where diversity of structure has deliberately been introduced as in the following: to a non-antigenic poly-L-lysine chain short co-polymers of tyrosine and glutamic acid are added. The resulting branched polymers are now antigenic. If monomers of say 20 D,L-alanine residues are then added to the short side-chains the polymer again becomes non-antigenic, probably because the tyrosine-glutamic acid peptides are now masked. If the experiment is repeated in a different order so that alanine monomers are first added to a polylysine backbone to yield a branched structure, the molecule is again non-antigenic, even though molecular weights of 20,000–200,000 can be achieved. The addition of tyrosine and glutamic acid to this structure will again result in an antigenic molecule, even when the chemical content of the final molecules in the first and second experiments is identical. The presumption is that the difference is due to the presence of the tyrosine-glutamic acid peptides in the interior or on the exterior of the molecule, and illustrates the importance of structure as well as of composition. The importance of the latter is indicated by the fact that the addition of glutamic acid alone will not confer antigenicity, whereas it will enhance the antigenicity conferred by tyrosine.

It is of considerable interest too that if tyrosine-glutamic acid co-polymers are again masked by monomeric D,L-alanine, as in the first experiment, but this time the co-polymers are attached to a backbone consisting of a lysine-alanine co-polymer, we once more get an antigenic substance. A likely explanation would seem to be that because the side-chains are attached to alternate amino-acid residues they are spaced sufficiently widely apart for the tyrosine-glutamic acid structures to be sterically accessible—another illustration of the importance of structure.

C. Chemical Composition

Both animal and vegetable proteins stimulate the production of anti-bodies and it was once thought that only proteins were antigenic. Mostly they make very good antigens. It is now appreciated that carbohydrates certainly and lipids possibly are antigenic, but they are both more concerned in specificity and will be discussed under that heading.

The amino-acid spectrum of many proteins has been investigated and it has been shown that several non-aromatic amino-acids are inessential for antigenicity.

As we have seen, treatment of albumin with alkalis destroys its antigenicity, but can be restored by nitration of the denatured protein. There are indeed several instances of the acquisition of antigenicity following small changes or additions to chemical substances, or the combination of two non-immunogenic substances. Clupein and phenylisocyanide are a case in point, and a more recent example is penicillin combined with polylysine.

A prerequisite for immunogenicity that is often quoted is that a substance should be 'foreign' to the animal producing antibody, but this rule has many exceptions. For instance, insulin of foreign species is a poor antigen and this also applies to other substances that perform the same function in different species and which therefore might be expected to have similar structures. The chemical structures of insulins from a number of species are now known and show only very slight differences in amino-acid composition. The concept of 'foreign', as indicated under CHEMICAL STRUCTURE, must be used to convey the sense of difference in structure of substances in donor and recipient, invader and host, but also in the sense of 'foreign' to the immunological apparatus, a view that is further developed in Chapters 4 and 12.

We may perhaps conclude that the role of size in antigenicity has not been proved; that diversity, rigidity of structure, and possibly capacity to be metabolized are important. Some of these attributes are certainly more likely to be found in large molecules than in small ones. After these criteria have been fulfilled a protein antigen must still differ from host protein in amino-acid composition or sequence, or in spatial configuration in order to stimulate an immunological response, i.e., be foreign.

III. SPECIFICITY

Specificity depends on antigens and antibodies having structures that are complementary to each other. The majority of natural antigens are macromolecules and as such their specificity in serological reactions is due to one or more determinants on the surface of a molecule. These determinants are structures which display a high degree of chemical and spatial correspondence with structures forming part of the antibody molecule. How this correspondence comes about and what forces are active in bringing about the interaction of antigen and antibody will be discussed in Chapter 6.

A. Protein Antigens

The concept of specificity has always excited the curiosity of immunologists. Why are serological reactions so specific, and why sometimes are they not as specific as we would expect? Can specificity be altered and what happens if it is? Such understanding as we now have of the remarkable degree of specificity displayed by protein antigens has been achieved by approaching the problem from two quite different directions.

Historically the first approach was to introduce substances of defined chemical composition into protein molecules and observe their capacity to influence or determine specificity. These were the methods used by Landsteiner and it was he who placed immunology on a sound chemical basis. The second approach was of much more recent origin and had to await the development of refined techniques of chemical analysis. This work is still in its infancy and our knowledge of the detailed composition of proteins is still fragmentary, though that of a number of proteins is now fully known. It is to be expected, therefore, that knowledge of the chemical structure of antigenic determinants will soon follow.

1. Specificity of Natural Proteins

The earliest studies on specificity were conducted mostly with mixtures of naturally occurring proteins. Bacterial and animal cells, body fluids, plant cells, and juices all contain a heterogeneous collection of antigenic material. The bacterial cell, for instance, may contain flagellar, somatic, and capsular antigens, and there will be more than one antigen at all or some of these loci. An antiserum prepared against the whole bacterial cell will therefore contain antibodies directed at several antigens, and when mixed with antiserum the bacterial cell will react with several kinds of antibody. Some of the determinant groups present on these antigens may be the same as, or very similar to, determinant groups on related bacteria. The related bacteria will then also react with the antiserum. Such a reaction is termed a *cross-reaction*. If a bacterium 1, containing antigens A and B, is used for immunization, the corresponding antibodies anti-A and anti-B will be produced. If a bacterium 2, containing antigens B and C, is mixed with the antiserum to bacterium 1 it will react with anti-B. The bacterial cells can be separated from the antiserum by centrifugation, anti-B will remain attached to them and the supernatant fluid will contain only anti-A. This process is known as absorbing out an antibody.* The resulting absorbed antiserum will now react specifically with bacterium 1, but not with bacterium 2. Wide use is made of this principle in the preparation of mono-specific antisera. If instead of identical B antigen components we postulate that bacteria 1 and 2 contain similar components B_1 and B_2 respectively, then an antiserum to B_1 will react with its homologous antigen at a higher dilution than with heterologous antigen B_2.

The principle of cross-reactions is an important one in immunology. Antibodies to protein antigens can nearly always be shown to cross-react with some heterologous proteins. Sometimes at least this is because part of the amino-acid sequences of different macromolecules is identical. Antibodies to simple haptens can display a much sharper specificity; for instance, antiserum to 3-aminobenzoic acid fails to react with a number of similar determinants (*Table V*, p. 40).

Sometimes cross-reactions are quantitatively reciprocal, and equal amounts of antibody are found in precipitates with homologous and heterologous protein [10]. That this is not always so is shown in *Table VII*, p. 41, where it can be seen that an antiserum to 2-aminobenzoic acid reacts strongly with 2-aminobenzenesulphonic acid, while the reciprocal cross-reaction is non-existent. The whole subject of cross-reactions is dealt with under a separate heading in Chapter 6; here we are concerned only to show how specificity can be expressed as a non-reciprocal cross-reaction. This kind of situation is illustrated diagrammatically in *Fig. 2* where antibody A can be seen to 'fit' antigen B, though less well than homologous antigen A, but antibody B is unable to form any sort of 'fit' with antigen A. It is important to recognize that the issue of cross-reactions is only clear-cut when single determinants or simple haptens are

---

* The physicochemical process by which antibody is joined *to* antigen is probably correctly described by *ad*sorption. In serology where this mechanism is made use of in order to remove an antibody *from* a mixture of antibodies we shall use the term *ab*sorption.

under consideration. In the bacterial cell we have seen that the several determinants may be found on different organisms; the same is true of mammalian cells and the concept has been expressed in the terms 'antigenic mosaic' and 'mosaic structure' (*see* PARTIAL ANTIGENS, p. 24).

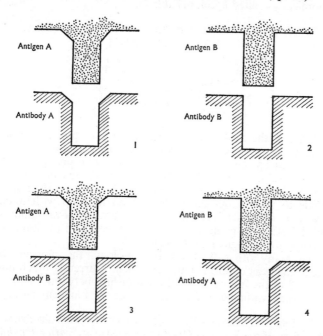

Fig. 2.—Reactions of homologous and heterologous antigen–antibody systems. 1, Homologous system A. 2, Homologous system B. 3, Heterologous system. Antigen A will not 'fit' antibody B. 4, Heterologous system. Antigen B will form partial 'fit' with antibody A.

2. SPECIES SPECIFICITY

From the taxonomical point of view three kinds of antigen and antibody are distinguishable.

A *hetero-antigen* is an antigen derived from a species other than that of the immunized animal. It stimulates the production of homologous hetero-antibody that may also react with antigens from animals of the same species (*iso-antigens*), or even with antigens from the immunized animal itself (*auto-antigens*).

An *iso-antigen* is an antigen that elicits the production of iso-antibodies in an individual of the same species that differs genetically from the donor. Rarely, an iso-antibody may also react as an *auto-antibody* with the animal's own tissues, or even as a hetero-antibody with antigens from a foreign species, e.g., thyroid antigen.

An *auto-antigen* is an antigen derived from the unaltered or slightly altered tissues of an animal that stimulates the production of antibodies against its own tissues. Exceptionally such an auto-antibody will also react with iso- and hetero-antigens. In transplantation immunology and more generally the prefix iso- is used in a different sense (*see* Chapter 10).

It has long been observed that natural proteins, such as serum proteins, exhibit species specificity. This specificity is not absolute, but encroaches on taxonomically related species (*Table I*).

Table I.—CROSS-PRECIPITATIONS WITH PRIMATE SERA.
After Landsteiner [11]

	Per cent
Man	100
Orang-utan	47
Cynocephalus mormon	30
Cercopithecus petaurista	30
Ateles vellarosus	22

Percentages in the table relate to the volume of precipitate obtained. All the reactions were performed with antiserum against human serum and 100 per cent has been assigned to the volume of precipitate obtained with human serum. The strength of the precipitin reaction decreases in the order Anthropoid apes, Old World apes, New World apes, which corresponds to their supposed zoological relationship with man. In a similar way Landsteiner [11] showed that anti-hen-ovalbumin gave a larger precipitate with galliform than with anseriform ovalbumin, again corresponding to zoological relationships.

As in so many other fields of immunology, the pioneer work of Landsteiner has been confirmed and extended. Currently much interest is being devoted to the immunological relationships between man and other primates. Much valuable information about the biochemical aspects of

Table II.—PRECIPITATION OF VARIOUS NATIVE AND HEATED SERA BY AN IMMUNE SERUM TO HEATED (100° C.) OX SERUM. *After Furth* [13].
Antigens diluted 1:1000

	WHOLE SERUM ANTIGEN					
	Ox	Sheep	Horse	Man	Rabbit	Guinea-pig
Heated	+++	+++	++	++	+	±
Unheated	+++	++	−	−	−	−

− : No precipitation.   ± to +++ : Degrees of precipitation.

evolution, complementing previous taxonomical knowledge, has been obtained by comparing immunological reactions of both soluble and cellular antigens derived from such sources [12]. It has been pointed out, however, that similarities in each kind of parameter (physical characters, serum proteins, red-cell antigens, etc.) between other primates and man vary according to the yardstick of comparison chosen, and this is probably true of all taxonomical comparisons. Also it should not be forgotten that similarities in structure occur throughout the vegetable and animal kingdoms, of which the Forssman antigen is among the best known and earliest examples.

Much broader specificities than those described above have been obtained when denatured serum proteins are used as antigens. In the case of heated (100° C.) mammalian serum proteins an antiserum reacts with heated serum from a wide range of mammalian species [13], the so-called 'mammalian reaction', including even heated serum from the species in which the antiserum was raised. Cross-reactions between such an antiserum and native (unheated) whole-serum antigen range far less widely (*Table II*).

3. ORGAN SPECIFICITY

Differences in function are generally linked with differences in structure, so it is not altogether surprising to find that serum albumins and globulins of the same species are serologically more distinct than serum albumins of related species. In fact albumin from species as distinct as ox and man are not all that different serologically, though they can, of course, be distinguished. Similarly different organs from the same animal have different structures and are serologically distinct. This is one expression of organ specificity but it goes farther than this. As indicated above, the same organs in animals of one species or of different species may carry the same specificities. This is likely to be particularly true in the case of organs that have undergone relatively little change in the course of evolution. Such an organ might be the lens of the eye, but the question then arises how can we raise antibodies to 'antigens' that are virtually the same in all animals? In this particular instance the peculiar isolation of the organ from the blood-stream comes to our aid, for tissues so isolated often behave as though they were 'foreign', even in the host animal.

In fact antisera prepared against lens proteins often fail to distinguish between species, although a very broad division into classes or groups of classes is possible. For instance, antisera to ocular lenses of sheep, pig, and chicken cross-react with all three antigens in spite of the great phylogenetic differences between birds and mammals (*Table III*). The strengths of the

Table III.—CROSS-PRECIPITATIONS BETWEEN VARIOUS EYE-LENS ANTIGENS.
After Landsteiner [11]

ANTISERA MADE AGAINST	ANTIGENS DILUTED 1 : 40,000			
	Sheep Lens	Pig Lens	Hen Lens	Fish Lens
Sheep lens	+++	+++	+	−
Pig lens	+++	++++	+	−
Hen lens	+±	++	++++	−
Fish lens	−	−	++	++++

reactions, particularly of the more distantly related species, do, however, vary and antisera to mammalian and avian lens proteins fail to react at all with fish lens, though the reverse situation does not quite hold, since there is some reaction between anti-fish and hen lens.

In the case of lens antigens then we have the situation where organ specificity dominates species specificity. Even so, modern serological

2

techniques can demonstrate quite definite differences between mammalian species: of the eight antigens found in bovine lens, three are present in sheep, two in pig, and only one in horse and human lenses [14, 15]. In addition, five antigens of rabbit lens have been compared with lens antigens from a number of other vertebrates: four or five being common to man, monkey, guinea-pig, and rat; two shared with fowls; and only one with the single salt-water fish tested [16].

We have already noted that unicellular organisms like bacteria possess a number of antigens. Even more must this be so of multicellular organs. It is to be expected that not all the antigens display organ specificity, but of those that do the species specificity is also likely to vary. Antisera to thyroid antigens detect two kinds of antigen in this respect. One of these antigens displays organ specificity but is also found in thyroid extracts of other individuals of the same species, i.e., it is organ specific *and* species specific; the second antigen is much more widely distributed among different species, i.e., is organ specific but *not* species specific.

Similar studies have been conducted with partly purified extracts of adrenal medulla that contain at least three such antigens [17]. One is again organ and species specific; another is organ but not species specific; but the third, though showing a high degree of species specificity, is not organ specific, being found in spleen, liver, kidney, etc., as well as adrenals. There would appear to be minor antigenic differences, however, in the category of antigens that are not species restricted; differences that can be detected by employing antisera to adrenal tissue from horse, pig, ox, and man, and a number of different serological reactions.

It is axiomatic that only those antigens normally well separated from the blood-stream stimulate the formation of antibodies in the autologous host. Such antigens are the lens of the eye and spermatozoa, and less obviously brain tissue and thyroglobulin. They are particularly suitable for studies of organ specificity so long as account is taken of the multiplicity of antigens in each organ. Nevertheless, somewhat unexpected results, quite different from those obtained with thyroid and adrenal antigens, have been observed with extracts of rabbit pancreas [18].

Immunization of a rabbit with the pancreatic extract from another rabbit resulted in the production of antibody that did not react with the recipient's own pancreas, but did with some, though not all, pancreatic extracts of other rabbits. Antisera prepared against extracts of single organs also reacted with pooled extracts. In other words, these antigens behaved more like histocompatibility antigens or the antigens of red blood-cells and immune globulins that express individual characteristics rather than organ or species differences.

Such results also provide confirmation of the opening statements in this section in the sense that very small differences in the structure of substances that perform the same physiological function are reflected in differences in immunological specificity. This concept is of fairly recent origin when applied at the molecular and subcellular levels but is now widely accepted, has opened up a vast field of exploration in the realms of molecular biology, and is also relevant to transplantation of organs.

4. CHEMICALLY ALTERED PROTEINS

Chemical treatment of proteins may produce a partial or total loss of specificity, or it may create new and sharply defined specificities. It may result in disruption of disulphide and other bonds leading eventually to a total loss of secondary and tertiary structure in the protein molecule. Alternatively, the protein may be denatured in the manner effected by physical agents such as heat, with the formation of new bonds leading to a loss of the molecule's hydrophilic qualities so that it precipitates out of solution and even coagulates. Both processes are reversible in the early stages, but beyond this point a protein begins to lose its species specificity, and an antiserum prepared against such a protein, e.g., heat denatured, also reacts with other heated proteins (*see* MAMMALIAN REACTION, p. 33). With lesser degrees of alteration new specificities arise which may nevertheless be species specific, though there is a concomitant loss of specificities of the native protein. The effect of chemical denaturation is probably much the same, but it is the effect of chemical treatment and alteration falling far short of denaturation that is of so much interest to immunologists, since it has led to an understanding of the nature and scope of specificity in immunological reactions.

Nitration and Iodination

Nitration and iodination were among the first methods to be used for introducing defined chemical groupings into proteins and observing the effect on specificity. The process is not one of denaturation but simply the substitution of hydrogen by new chemical groupings, leading to a partial or total loss of species specificity in the treated protein, depending on how far the reaction is allowed to proceed. Landsteiner was of the opinion that although characteristic groupings in the proteins had been altered by nitration and iodination, the new chemospecificity was also due to a masking of native chemical structures. It is indeed a remarkable fact that an antiserum to one such protein also reacts with proteins similarly treated but derived from other species of animals, even though the basic structural differences between the various proteins have not been altered. Rabbits can even be immunized against their own nitrated serum proteins, and an antiserum to animal xanthoprotein (nitrated proteins are so called because of their yellow colour) cross-reacts with plant xanthoprotein. This is not to say that antibodies formed against such proteins are directed solely towards the introduced groups. In the case of nitration, nitrotyrosine and nitrotryptophane are formed, and in iodoproteins the formation of 3,5-di-iodo-4-hydroxytyrosine appears to be of chief importance. It is these altered residues that determine the new specificities, and it is evidence such as this that has led to an appreciation of the considerable part played by aromatic amino-acids in determining specificity.

Nevertheless, antibodies of several different specificities can result from immunization with iodinated proteins. Protein containing small amounts of iodine, perhaps up to 18 atoms per globulin molecule, behaves as unchanged protein, i.e., it stimulates the formation of anti-native protein antibody only. As soon as all the tyrosine residues are saturated antibodies are formed against iodinated protein only. In between these two extremes antibodies against both native protein and iodinated protein are produced. It is from evidence of this sort that the diversity of antigenic stimulus provided by a single kind of protein molecule came to be recognized. Nor should it be forgotten that animals are subject to individual variation in the way they respond to identical stimuli. Thus antibodies to iodinated protein may be species specific, may react with all iodoproteins, or with those of a limited number of species.

5. CONJUGATED PROTEINS

Landsteiner made many notable contributions to immunology, but none was greater than his demonstration, over the years, of the chemical basis of serological specificity. We have already considered the effect of iodination and nitration on specificity; treatment of proteins with alkalis and acids also leads to loss of original specificity and ultimately to loss of antigenicity as well, even before the size of the molecule is greatly diminished. These were merely beginnings, however, and Landsteiner went on to study the effect of altering the fine structure of proteins on specificity. For this purpose he used the method of diazotization for coupling aromatic amines to proteins. The system provided him with an immensely flexible approach for making relatively minor alterations in the composition of proteins, and since the highly reactive ring structure can accommodate an almost limitless range of chemical substituents attached to various carbon atoms, he was able to study the effect on specificity not only of precise changes in chemical composition but also of chemical configuration.

The steps involved in coupling atoxyl to a protein (through a tyrosine residue) are set out diagrammatically in *Fig.* 3. Substances so formed are known as conjugated proteins or azoproteins.

Landsteiner conjugated those substances he wished to investigate to proteins simply because proteins make excellent antigens; and on the advice of Doerr he used the precipitation reaction to test the effect of conjugation on serological specificity. Similar results could no doubt have been obtained using complement fixation or any other serological test, but precipitin tests are simple to perform and give results that are just as clear-cut. Diazotization is not the only way in which defined chemical groupings can be conjugated to proteins; essentially similar results have been obtained with other methods. Conjugation through sulphydryl groups is particularly appropriate for proteins like keratin which contain many disulphide bridges that can be reduced to sulphydryl groups. It is also possible to conjugate to protein by peptide bridges and this method has been considered more 'natural' and causes little or no denaturation.

When azoproteins are used for immunization the resulting antiserum may contain antibodies directed at three types of determinants: (1) those associated with the protein carrier only; (2) those associated with the introduced group only; and (3) those formed from both carrier and conjugate. All three possibilities are not equally likely because the specificity of an antibody is not usually directed against the introduced group only but also against adjacent parts of the protein, though this may well be due in part at least to the fact that usually small haptens are used for conjugation experiments and that they do not occupy the whole of the available space in an antibody-combining site. The existence of all three types of determinant and of antibodies directed specifically towards them is clearly shown following immunization with polypeptidyl proteins (peptides linked through peptide bonds to protein). Absorption of such an antiserum successively with the peptide and the protein leaves the antiserum still capable of precipitating the conjugated protein. Nor is this

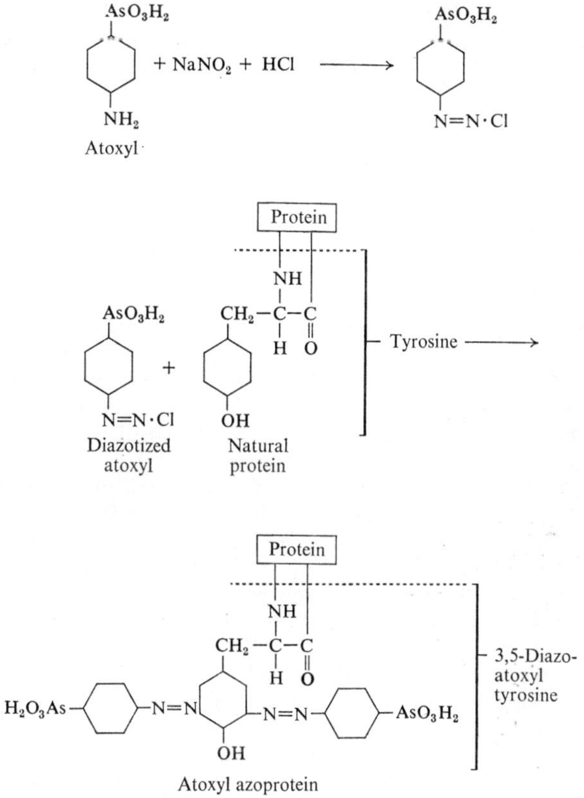

Fig. 3.—Diazotization. *After Carpenter* [19].

type of response confined to antibody production; studies undertaken with delayed hypersensitivity also suggest that the whole determinant may consist of one or more amino-acid residues in addition to an introduced haptenic group [20].

There are, of course, many reasons for heterogeneity of specificity displayed by antibodies even when they are directed against small haptens. One of these is that a hapten can have different points of attachment either on the same or different molecules of protein. Diazotization normally results in the coupling of diazonium compounds to tyrosine and histidine, each residue accommodating one or two compounds (*see Fig. 3*). These are not the only residues involved, however, because more molecules of hapten can be introduced into a molecule of protein than can be accounted for by all the tyrosine and histidine residues together. The possibility therefore exists that there is a real heterogeneity of antigenic determinants in azoproteins since, although the haptens are identical, their environment, i.e., point of attachment, is not. The introduction of about ten azo-groups per molecule of protein is usually considered optimal for the production of a highly specific antiserum. Even under these conditions we are still faced with the possibility that antibody specificity will be directed at more than one of the three types of determinant mentioned above. Landsteiner was therefore careful to point out that it must not be assumed that every laboratory animal will produce antibodies of the required specificity [11].

The question remains, To what extent do introduced haptens alter the specificity of proteins and how far are they distinguishable from each other? Obviously if antibody specificity is directed towards the protein carrier as well as the diazonium compound this will obscure the interpretation of any precipitin tests carried out with the antiserum and immunizing azoprotein. Landsteiner solved this problem very elegantly by using horse-serum protein as the carrier for immunization, and chicken-serum protein as the carrier for precipitation. In this way he virtually eliminated the possibility of reactions due to the protein moiety because of the great distance, taxonomically speaking, between mammalian and avian species. Any precipitation observed in the *in vitro* tests could therefore be attributed to the introduced hapten and its homologous antibody. The principle formulated by Landsteiner therefore was to use two distantly related proteins for the separate procedures of immunization and precipitation. The single exception to this rule would be if the protein carrier was derived from the same species as the immunized animal since such proteins would form a poor immunological stimulus.

Experiments of this sort suggested to Landsteiner that his introduced groups were acting as determinants. In order to confirm these findings he applied an old technique in a new way. In the presence of a large excess of antigen a mixture of antigen and antibody does not precipitate. Instead of antigen Landsteiner used a large excess of hapten and, as expected, no precipitate was formed with the immune serum. To this mixture was then added an amount of hapten-protein conjugate that would have given a precipitate without the previous addition of hapten. Once again no precipitate was formed. In this way Landsteiner showed that even though a simple hapten was not precipitated it nevertheless combined with antibody and prevented precipitation of the complete antigen. Although there is probably no strict analogy between the inhibition of precipitation seen in the zone of antigen excess and precipitin-inhibition by hapten, an excess of hapten may nevertheless be necessary in the latter case if its binding affinity for antibody is less than that of whole antigen.

Since its introduction by Landsteiner the precipitin-inhibition test has been widely used in different fields and with different techniques. In recent years particular use has been made of it for elucidating the structure of proteins and carbohydrate determinants. Examples will be found in later sections dealing with bacterial antigens, blood-group substances, and immunoglobulins.

a. Influence of Acid Radicals

Landsteiner immunized rabbits with azoproteins coupled to aniline or to one of a number of acid derivatives of aniline. In *Table IV* can be seen the results of cross-precipitation tests with these haptens. The acid radicals, although they are all in the para position, confer an absolute

Table IV.—ACTION OF STRONG ACID RADICALS ON THE SPECIFICITY OF AZOPROTEINS. *After Landsteiner* [11]

ANTISERUM AGAINST AZOPROTEIN COUPLED WITH THE HAPTEN	AZOPROTEINS COUPLED WITH			
	Aniline NH_2 (benzene ring)	4-Aminobenzoic acid NH_2 / $COOH$	4-Aminobenzene sulphonic acid NH_2 / SO_3H	4-Aminobenzene arsonic acid NH_2 / AsO_3H_2
Aniline	+ + +	−	−	−
4-Aminobenzoic acid	−	+ + + ±	−	−
4-Aminobenzene sulphonic acid	−	−	+ + + ±	−
4-Aminobenzene arsonic acid	−	−	−	+ + + +

degree of specificity on the antisera, i.e., there are no cross-reactions, either between them or with aniline. It follows that the *chemical composition of acid radicals is of decisive influence on the specificity*. The absence of any reaction between the derived haptens and aniline illustrates a general rule that antisera to azoproteins which contain acidic groups give negative, or occasionally very weak, reactions with 'neutral' antigens.

b. Influence of Neutral Radicals

The influence of methyl, halogen, and other non-acid substituents is often only slight. In *Table V* is shown the effect of substituting methyl, chlorine, and bromine radicals in the para position in 3-aminobenzoic acid.

i. The antiserum to the chlorine-substituted hapten cross-reacts strongly with the other three haptens, though there is a faint suggestion of halogen specificity.

ii. The antisera to the methyl and bromine substituted haptens, in addition to homologous specificity, cross-react with the other two substituted haptens. They do not cross-react with aminobenzoic acid, however, which shows that the introduction of neutral radicals does alter the specificity of a hapten, but that the chemical composition of the radical itself confers relatively little specificity. In the case of antiserum to 3-amino-4-bromobenzoic acid the cross-reaction with 3-amino-4-chloro-benzoic acid is stronger than the reaction with the homologous hapten.

Cross-reactions that are stronger than reactions with the homologous substance are not restricted to conjugated chemically defined antigens but have also been found in natural antigens.

Table V.—INFLUENCE OF HALOGEN AND METHYL RADICALS ON THE SPECIFICITY OF AZOPROTEINS SUBSTITUTED IN THE BENZOL RING. *After Landsteiner* [11]

ANTISERUM AGAINST AZOPROTEIN COUPLED WITH THE HAPTEN	AZOPROTEINS COUPLED WITH			
	3-Amino-benzoic acid $COOH$ NH_2	3-Amino-4-methylbenzoic acid $COOH$ NH_2 CH_3	3-Amino-4-chlorobenzoic acid $COOH$ NH_2 Cl	3-Amino-4-bromobenzoic acid $COOH$ NH_2 Br
3-Aminobenzoic acid	+ + + +	−	−	−
3-Amino-4-methyl-benzoic acid	−	+ +	+ ±	±
3-Amino-4-chloro-benzoic acid	+ + +	+ + +	+ + + +	+ + + +
3-Amino-4-bromo-benzoic acid	−	±	+ + ±	+ +

Table VI.—ACTION OF CHLORO-, METHYL-, AND NITRO-GROUPS ON THE SPECIFICITY OF ANILINE AZOPROTEINS. *After Landsteiner* [11]

ANTISERUM AGAINST AZOPROTEIN COUPLED WITH THE HAPTEN	AZOPROTEINS COUPLED WITH				
	Aniline NH_2	2-Chloro-aniline NH_2 Cl	4-Chloro-aniline NH_2 Cl	4-Methyl-aniline NH_2 CH_3	4-Nitro-aniline NH_2 NO_2
Aniline	+ + ±	+ ±	+ + ±	+ ±	+
2-Chloroaniline	+ +	+ + ±	+	+	Trace
4-Chloroaniline	+	Trace	+ +	+ +	+ +
4-Methylaniline	+ ±	+	+ +	+ +	+ ±
4-Nitroaniline	+	±	+ ±	+	+ +

iii. The antiserum to aminobenzoic acid reacts only with the homologous antigen and confirms that the addition of a neutral radical to haptens which already carry neutral and *acid* radicals alters specificity markedly.

Though the antiserum to aminobenzoic acid does not cross-react with 3-amino-4-chlorobenzoic acid, antiserum to the latter does cross-react with aminobenzoic acid. This is a clear-cut example of a non-reciprocal cross-reaction.

In *Table VI* the effect of substituting neutral radicals in aniline is seen. In this case there is no acid radical present, and neither the substitution of a second neutral radical *per se* nor its chemical composition has such a profound effect on the specificity. Antiserum to aniline reacts to some extent with all the haptens and vice versa.

In addition, comparison of the results in *Tables IV* and *VI* shows that whereas the introduction of acid radicals alters the specificity of aniline completely the introduction of neutral radicals alters the specificity slightly or not at all.

c. Influence of Spatial Configuration

In *Table VII* are shown the reactions between aniline, its carboxylic and sulphonic acid derivatives, and their antibodies. As we would expect, aniline displays no cross-reactions with these derivatives. The introduction of a carboxylic acid group in the ortho, meta, or para positions of aniline

Table VII.—EFFECT OF SPATIAL CONFIGURATION OF ACID RADICALS ON THE SPECIFICITY OF AZOPROTEINS. *After Landsteiner* [11]

ANTISERUM AGAINST AZOPROTEIN COUPLED WITH THE HAPTEN	AZOPROTEINS COUPLED WITH						
	Aniline	2-Amino-benzoic acid	3-Amino-benzoic acid	4-Amino-benzoic acid	2-Amino-benzene sulphonic acid	3-Amino-benzene sulphonic acid	4-Amino-benzene sulphonic acid
Aniline	+++	−	−	−	−	−	−
-Aminobenzoic acid	−	+++	−	−	+++	−	−
-Aminobenzoic acid	−	−	++++	−	−	−	−
-Aminobenzoic acid	−	−	−	+++±	−	−	−
-Aminobenzene sulphonic acid	−	−	−	−	++++	+++	−
-Aminobenzene sulphonic acid	−	−	−	−	+++	++++	−
-Aminobenzene sulphonic acid	−	−	−	−	−	+	+++±

results in haptens of three completely distinct specificities. However, the antiserum to 2-aminobenzoic acid reacts strongly with 2-aminosulphonic acid, though the reverse cross-reaction does not occur. This is an instance of spatial configuration taking precedence, in one direction only, of chemical composition. Of interest too are the cross-reactions shown between the sulphonic-acid-substituted compounds. In this case cross-reactions are seen between haptens where the acidic group is substituted at positions 2 or 3, and 3 or 4, but not between the sterically more dissimilar 2- and 4-aminobenzene sulphonic acid haptens.

The influence of spatial configuration is even more striking with optical isomers. *Table VIII* shows the results of cross-precipitation tests with laevo-, dextro-, and meso-tartaric acids. The laevo and dextro forms

Table VIII.—EFFECT OF STEREO-ISOMERISM OF DETERMINANTS ON THE SPECIFICITY OF AZOPROTEINS. *After Landsteiner* [11]

ANTISERUM AGAINST AZOPROTEIN COUPLED WITH THE HAPTEN	AZOPROTEINS COUPLED WITH		
	Laevo-tartaric acid COOH | HOCH | HCOH | COOH	Dextro-tartaric acid COOH | HCOH | HOCH | COOH	Meso-tartaric acid COOH | HCOH | HCOH | COOH
Laevo-tartaric acid	+ + +	Trace	+
Dextro-tartaric acid	−	+ + +	+
Meso-tartaric acid	Trace	−	+ + +

hardly cross-react at all. The meso form cross-reacts slightly with anti-bodies against both the other forms. This is probably due to the fact that meso-tartaric acid differs from the other two forms only at one asymmetric carbon atom, whereas the dextro and laevo forms differ from each other at two asymmetric atoms. Other optical isomers can also be distinguished immunologically, but this is not always the case, e.g., D- and L-fucose derivatives [21, 22].

d. Influence of Aliphatic Side-chains

The length of the chain in the lower dicarboxylic acids has a very marked influence on specificity. Diazotized proteins conjugated with

Table IX.—EFFECT OF TERMINAL AMINO-ACIDS AND LINKAGE OF AMINO-ACIDS ON SPECIFICITY OF AZO-PEPTIDE PROTEINS. *After Landsteiner* [11]

ANTISERUM AGAINST AZOPROTEIN COUPLED WITH	AZOPROTEINS COUPLED WITH			
	Glycyl-glycine	Glycyl-leucine	Leucyl-glycine	Leucyl-leucine
Glycyl-glycine	+ + ±	−	−	−
Glycyl-leucine	−	+ + ±	−	Trace
Leucyl-glycine	+	−	+ + +	−
Leucyl-leucine	−	+	−	+ +

4-amino-aniline in which the free amino group was substituted with oxalic, malonic, and succinic acids display no cross-reactions. However, the higher dicarboxylic acids with more than 4 carbon atoms cross-react strongly with each other and the addition of two or even three carbons to the length of the chain makes little difference to the specificity [11].

e. Influence of Peptide Side-chains

In *Table IX* can be seen the results of cross-precipitation tests with some simple dipeptides coupled to protein by diazotization. The influence of the terminal amino-acid is immediately apparent. Weak cross-reactions occur where the subterminal amino-acid is different but the terminal acid is the same. No cross-reaction occurs where the subterminal amino-acids are the same but the terminal amino-acids are different. More elaborate experiments with tri- and penta-peptides show unequivocally that other links in the chain of amino-acids influence specificity.

6. CONFIGURATION

Changes in the tertiary structure of a protein molecule, though not necessarily involving a determinant site, may nevertheless result in the alteration of the structure of such a site. For instance, structural differences between intracellular and extracellular penicillinases are reflected in differences in serological specificity [23]. Equally disruption of the disulphide bonds of ribonuclease leads to complete loss of tertiary structure and the oxidized ribonuclease fails to react with antiserum to the native molecule [24]. If the broken bonds are re-formed serological specificity is restored, but if incorrect disulphide bridges are remade the newly formed structures differ from native ribonuclease in configuration only and do not then react with antiserum to the native protein.

Insulins also provide us with very striking examples of the influence of configuration on specificity. Antiserum to native beef insulin reacts, in part at least, with amino-acid residues 8–10 of chain A; the separated A chain, however, is serologically inactive. Separation of the chains involves rupturing a disulphide bond between residues 6 and 11 of the A chain, so here again configurational changes can be seen to alter serological specificity. We can deduce from evidence such as this that in a native protein molecule with its bent and coiled polypeptide chains the amino-acid residues that go to make up a determinant need be neither sequentially adjacent in a chain length nor indeed present in the same chain.

Though it has been held that tertiary structure of a protein is determined by its primary sequence of amino-acids this may not always be so. We have in fact seen that it is not under experimental conditions where incorrect disulphide bonds are formed in the disrupted ribonuclease molecule. Possibly the same conclusions can be drawn from the evidence that although sperm whale and pig insulins are identical in amino-acid sequence they inhibit the reaction between beef insulin and homologous antiserum to different degrees [25].

In a so-called three-component system, antibody–enzyme–substrate, the possibility is considered that the inhibitory action of antibody on enzyme activity is sometimes effected even when the site of union is at a distance from the catalytic site. A postulated mechanism would be that union between antibody and enzyme results in a rearrangement of hydrogen bonds in the latter with a concomitant distortion of the catalytic site [26].

That tertiary structure is not always paramount in determining specificity is suggested by the fact that degraded thyroglobulin lacking secondary and tertiary structure is still able to inhibit the reaction between the native globulin and homologous antibody. This leads us to the recognition that determinants on the surface of proteins may be formed either from a straight sequence of amino-acids constituting part of the primary structure or from an area in which different parts of the same or different polypeptide chains come together as a result of tertiary configuration.

7. CHEMICAL STRUCTURE

Probably the smallest difference found so far in the chemical structure of a protein that alters its specificity concerns the amido group. The two iso-enzymes ribonuclease A and B probably differ only in the amidation of a single carboxyl group, and show slight but definite differences in serological reactivity [27]. Deamination of the terminal lysine residue of bovine ribonuclease also results in a greatly diminished precipitate with antibody to unaltered ribonuclease, but in this case a local alteration in the tertiary structure cannot be excluded. That the limit of serological resolution has been reached here is likely, not only because of the very small chemical differences involved but also because such findings are not consistently obtained when other systems are investigated. For instance, it has not proved possible to distinguish between normal and desamido-insulin immunologically. Even when considerably greater differences are present, involving perhaps a whole amino-acid, distinctions often prove difficult. For instance, haemoglobins A, S, C, and E differ from each other by a single amino-acid only. Nevertheless S, C, and E could not be distinguished serologically [28], though with the use of chicken antisera and conditions ensuring maximum precipitation A and S could be distinguished [29]. Similarly it has proved difficult or impossible to distinguish between the various insulins that differ by only one amino-acid residue, such as beef and sheep or horse and pork; though some human sera do distinguish between the first and second pairs where there is a difference of at least two amino-acids. Such differences in insulins from various animal sources may be of more than academic interest. In the past indiscriminate use has been made of beef and pork insulins in the treatment of diabetics. Apart from the fact that pig insulin seems to be less antigenic in man than beef insulin and would therefore seem to be the most suitable choice, a change from beef to pig insulin could produce hypoglycaemic shock in a patient already somewhat immune to beef insulin.

Although we may be approaching the limit of serological discrimination with differences of one amino-acid, when the protein molecule as a whole is considered it still seems remarkable at first that splitting off the valine residue at the C-terminal end of ribonuclease does not alter its specificity at all. This example is of particular interest since it suggests that the terminal residue of a polypeptide chain is not necessarily the terminal residue of a determinant. Landsteiner's demonstration of the decisive role of terminal and subterminal amino-acids on the specificity of conjugated oligopeptides, which was intended to throw light on their role in serological specificity, is not necessarily of universal application. Indeed, Kaminski even states [30]: 'As to the role played by the ends of peptide chains, they seem scarcely involved in globular proteins.'

In this connexion an interesting comparison can be drawn between the immunological and pharmacological activity of terminal amino-acids. In the case of bradykinin, angiotensin, and other peptides it has been convincingly shown that pharmacological action depends on the C-terminal, though not the N-terminal residue [31]. On the other hand, the terminal carboxyl and amino groups of angiotensin II can be blocked by polylysine without affecting its capacity to stimulate the production of specific antibody to the unaltered molecule [32]. This would suggest that internal units of the chain can be responsible for specificity, as indeed has been shown to be the case with carbohydrate structures [33]. (*See also* SOMATIC ANTIGENS OF ENTEROBACTERIA, p. 65.)

The study of ribonuclease is also interesting in that it has already proved possible to correlate antigenic sites with amino-acid sequence. Two major antigenic regions have been found; one is in the four-peptide sequence 120–123, and the other consists of at least 14 residues in the segment 38–61.

The crux of the matter would seem to be that it is not so much a terminal or subterminal position in a polypeptide chain that decides whether a sequence of amino-acids acts as a determinant, but rather the position of a sequence with respect to the molecule as a whole. In other words, in *serological reactions* with native protein it is the accessibility of a determinant on the surface of the molecule that is of primary importance.

8. SIZE OF DETERMINANTS

Progress in the field of protein chemistry is now extremely rapid. Synthetic polypeptides and cleavage products of proteins are both being used to probe into the structure of the antigenic site.

Investigations with antibodies directed against polypeptides of lysine and glutamic acid have shown that these antibodies precipitate some natural proteins. It is likely that their reactive sites are directed against paired lysine or glutamic acid residues, combinations known to occur in proteins. If single lysine or glutamic acid residues formed determinant sites one would expect to find cross-reactions between virtually all proteins. It is now possible to synthesize complex polypeptides with molecular weights of up to 200,000, and variations in the structure of these molecules will make it possible to study more closely the relationship between chemical structure and antigenicity and specificity.

Polypeptide fragments with molecular weights ranging from 7000 to 23,000 have been obtained by enzymatic cleavage of serum albumin at an inhibitor/antigen molar ratio of 1·5 : 1·0 [34], but are not themselves precipitable. Much smaller fragments of protein than these are, however, still capable of inhibiting precipitation—for instance, octa- and dodeca-peptides of silk fibroin [35]—but in such cases the molar ratio of inhibitor to antigen is often 1000 or more. This is not to say that an antigenic determinant consists of sixty rather than a dozen amino-acids. Indeed we have independent evidence that the antideterminant site is of the order of 10–20 amino-acids [36]. The wide discrepancy observed between the inhibitory capacities of large and small simple haptens is more probably a function of differences in their configuration. In the larger fragments we would expect the original three-dimensional structure to be mostly retained, whereas in the smaller fragments it might be partly lost. Ultimately these differences could be expressed in terms of dissociation constants for the respective antibody-hapten reactions, and because this value would be much greater for the smaller molecules they would need to be in much higher concentration than the large fragments in order to achieve the same level of inhibition.

Alterations in specificity and combining power due to such changes in configuration are supported by a number of other serological observations. First, we must not forget that the reaction of the active site of an enzyme with its substrate can change the configuration of antigenic sites at a distance from the catalytic site. Secondly, in ABH blood-group substances specificity depends on terminal and subterminal sugars and not on the polypeptide backbone. Nevertheless, digestion of the polypeptide part destroys serological activity probably because the configuration of the oligosaccharide is altered. Thirdly, the Gm(4) antigenic determinant of immunoglobulins, though situated in the heavy chain of the molecule, still requires the light chain for a full expression of its serological activity, probably for the same reason.

In recent years then the serological specificity of cleavage products of proteins, and particularly of globulins, has been widely studied. Multiple determinants have been found in and on antigens such as serum and egg albumins, diphtheria toxin, fibrinogen, gamma-globulins, thyro-globulin, and tobacco mosaic virus (TMV) protein. 'A' protein, derived from TMV by treatment with alkali, has been shown to possess at least six different specificities, all apparently present in the intact molecule [37]; but cleavage of antigenic molecules may also lead to the appearance of a number of hitherto unsuspected specificities, either by virtue of unmasking determinants buried in the interior of the intact molecule, or by the acquisition of new specificities due to changes in configuration caused by the denaturing processes [30]. For these reasons, and because even chemically purified proteins often consist of physical, structural, and serological populations of molecules, it has proved difficult to obtain definite evidence regarding the size of antigenic determinants with methods that involve cleavage. We shall return to the subject of size in the next section dealing with polysaccharide antigens and in Chapter 3, IMMUNOGLOBULINS.

B. Polysaccharide Antigens

In general it might be said that polysaccharides provide a poorer antigenic stimulus than do proteins, but it is now conceded that some purified polysaccharides uncontaminated with protein are antigenic in a number of mammalian species such as man, horse, and mouse. Some polysaccharides such as dextran are essentially simple and highly repetitive structures, consisting largely of glucose units linked 1,6 with some cross-links: of high molecular weight, they can stimulate the production of antibodies. Other species of animal, e.g., rabbit and guinea-pig, fail to respond immunologically to such stimuli so that here we have a good example of a different biological response in an immunological field as between different species, just as with protein antigens we noted differences in qualitative and quantitative responses between individuals within species. Here we have the situation where complete antigens in some species behave as haptens or complex haptens in others.

Large polysaccharide molecules are slowly catabolized compared with proteins of similar size and can be detected in animal tissues for months and even years after being introduced into the tissues. They could therefore

ANTIGENS 47

be expected to provide a prolonged antigenic stimulus and thereby
presumably enhance their prospects of provoking a detectable antibody
response in the injected host (*see* Chapter 4). Small doses of pneumococcal
polysaccharide of the order $0 \cdot 1–1 \cdot 0$ μg. give rise to good antibody responses
in mice. An interesting anomaly has been demonstrated when much larger
doses, 50–100 μg., are injected [38]. In these circumstances adult mice fail
to produce any demonstrable antibody at all over their whole life-span.
This refractory state, originally called 'immunological paralysis', is now
considered to be one of the manifestations of 'tolerance', a subject dealt
with in more detail in Chapters 4 and 10. It is sufficient here to say that
when a state of tolerance has been induced in an animal by the administration of antigen, the animal does not respond with the production of
antibody to further doses of the same antigen. Originally thought to be a
property peculiar to polysaccharide antigens, it is now known that the
same effect can be achieved with massive doses of protein antigens.
Possibly the slow rate of catabolism associated with polysaccharides
renders it easier to achieve an overwhelming concentration with them.

Following the discovery that pneumococcal capsular material was
polysaccharide in nature, it became apparent that these carbohydrates
determined the serological specificity of the various pneumococcal type
strains. That specificity as opposed to antigenicity is determined by
carbohydrates is not very surprising since if we take into account all the
configurational possibilities of a disaccharide formed from the various
stereo-isomers of glucose we are already dealing with very large numbers.
Nevertheless, it was soon noted that serological cross-reactions occurred
both between pneumococcal types and between these and polysaccharides
from a wide variety of living organisms in the animal and vegetable
kingdoms. No doubt this is due largely to the repetitive nature of their
structure so that there is less variety than in the case of proteins. It is
perhaps worth noting at this point that cross-reactions are often loosely
ascribed to the sharing of antigens whether from closely or distantly related
or even unrelated species. This is, of course, usually quite wrong and in
most cases the sharing is limited to small bits of molecules that include a
common determinant or part of a determinant. It is not necessary then to
implicate a whole antigen, whether protein or polysaccharide, when a
cross-reaction has been detected even in those cases where homologous
and heterologous reactions are of equal strength.

Under natural conditions polysaccharides often occur complexed with
protein, and with or without an attached lipid fraction. In these circumstances the whole molecule is antigenic even though the isolated polysaccharide is not. Nevertheless, the carbohydrate moiety frequently
determines specificity. Indeed, it is becoming increasingly apparent that
the specificity of lipids, proteins, and lipoproteins is often determined by
quite small carbohydrate components.

1. SIZE OF DETERMINANTS

The size of reacting sites in antigen–antibody complexes is fundamental
to our understanding of the scope and nature of specificity in serological
reactions. At the moment there appear to be striking similarities between
the specificities displayed by antibodies for antigens, by viruses for their

cellular receptors, and by enzymes for their substrates. The virtual absence of covalent bonds in such reactions has led to the conclusion that a number of individually weaker forces must be responsible for the primary union of the reactants, and that this allows for a variety of patterns of intermolecular forces, and that specificity is the expression of unique patterns built up in this way.

We have already seen how Landsteiner coupled known chemical groupings to proteins, but the use of these artificial antigens has not contributed a great deal to our knowledge about the size of the reacting sites because much of the reactivity of such determinants can be attributed to those amino-acid residues of the carrier adjacent to the substituted group. Landsteiner and van der Scheer [39] did, however, substitute succinanilic acid and arsanilic acid in positions 3 and 5 of the aniline ring. After coupling this relatively bulky compound (*Fig.* 4) to protein by diazotization, antisera were prepared against the introduced group. The

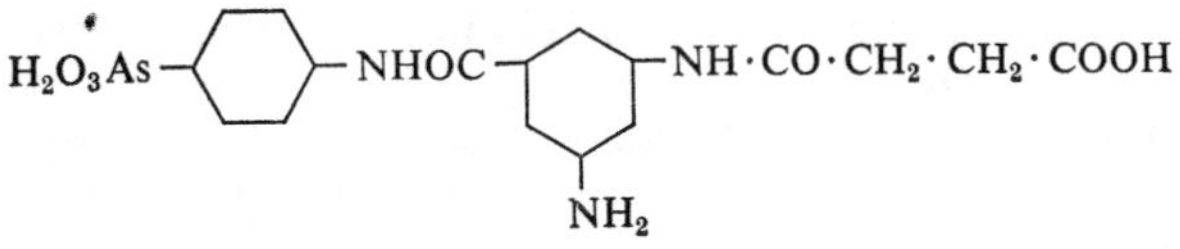

$$H_2O_3As - \langle \bigcirc \rangle - NHOC - \langle \bigcirc \rangle - NH \cdot CO \cdot CH_2 \cdot CH_2 \cdot COOH$$
$$NH_2$$

Fig. 4.

antisera contained antibody capable of reacting with either the succinanilic part or the arsanilic part, suggesting that antibody sites were not large enough to accommodate both.

Calculations made subsequently on the basis of this experiment indicated that the upper limit of the combining area was in the region of 700 Å². An alternative explanation would be that there is some restriction on the shape which an antibody site can assume.

The fact that the structure of carbohydrates is relatively easily analysed compared with proteins led Kabat and his colleagues to use them for studying the size of antigen determinants [40]. They investigated the capacity of glucose units linked 1→6 to inhibit the precipitation of dextran by antisera obtained from human beings who had been injected with various natural and synthetic dextrans. Calculations based on equimolar concentrations of a number of glucose oligosaccharides showed that the inhibitory capacity of the small chains rose to a maximum when 6 or 7 hexose units were linked together. The experimental methods available are not precise enough to show whether the heptaose was more inhibitory than the hexaose.

When equimolar concentrations of members of the glucose series were compared, it could be seen that the capacity of the disaccharide to inhibit precipitation was less than double the capacity of the monosaccharide. Similarly the triaose, tetraose, pentaose, and hexaose each caused more inhibition than the preceding member of the series but the percentage increase became less and less. A study of the binding energies (*see* Chapter 6) involved when the antibodies and oligosaccharides combined tended to confirm these findings. Thus if the effect of 6 units was taken to be 100 per cent the contribution of the first unit was 40 per cent and of the sixth unit a mere 2 per cent. The conclusion may be drawn that the terminal residue of a sugar determinant plays proportionately the greatest part in determining specificity and is the component having the greatest capacity to inhibit precipitation of homologous antigen by antibody. By determining the capacity of each sugar residue in a determinant to inhibit precipitation, either alone or combined with others, it is possible, in theory at least, to identify the position of each residue along the chain. Possible pitfalls in this line of reasoning have already been pointed out in the section on protein antigens. Nevertheless, this principle has been successfully applied to the elucidation of the structure of a number of carbohydrate determinants.

As we have seen, Landsteiner's work led to an estimate of 700 $Å^2$ as the maximum size of a reactive site. The dimensions of the hexaose used in the above experiments are $34 \times 12 \times 7$ Å, a volume of 2856 $Å^3$ and a maximum area in one plane of 408 $Å^2$. An area of this size corresponds to a comparatively small portion of the surface of an IgG antibody molecule, and there is ample space for two combining sites, so that there is no inherent difficulty in accepting this estimate of size for antigenic determinants provided by studies on the dextran–antidextran system. A substantially similar estimate, $36 \times 10 \times 6$ Å, has emerged from studies on synthetic polymers of amino-acids [7].

2. STRUCTURE OF DETERMINANTS

Precipitation techniques have also been widely used to examine the chemical structure of carbohydrate determinants with a more complicated composition than dextran. Although it might appear at first sight that qualitative chemical analysis would yield decisive information, it is frequently found that determinants of related classes of antigens are composed of exactly the same monosaccharide units. Chemical analysis can, of course, be taken further and sometimes the complete structure, i.e., composition, order of residues, and the way they are linked, can be determined. But more often in the past it has been necessary to use immunological methods to suggest or confirm particular structures.

a. Blood-group Antigens

In 1900 to 1901 Landsteiner and his colleagues [41–43] showed that human beings could be divided into four groups on the basis of two antigenic characters in their red blood-cells (*Fig.* 5). Since that time a third

Blood group	Antigen	Isoagglutinin
O	—	Anti-A and Anti-B
A	A	Anti-B
B	B	Anti-A
AB	A and B	—

Fig. 5.—The ABO system.

antigen, 'H', falling within the same genetic system, has been characterized; it is present in all four groups but in relatively larger amounts in group-O cells and it distinguishes quantitatively such cells from those of the other three groups. Together the three antigens form the ABH system.

H antigen is not the same as O antigen and though it is felt that group-O cells may possess a specific O antigen of their own its existence has not been proved.

Antibodies present in human sera that agglutinate human red blood-cells are by definition *iso-agglutinins* (p. 31).

Originally blood transfusion practice took account of ABO groups only. Later it was found that in cases where there should have been no in-compatibility on the basis of this system transfusion reactions still occurred. The presence of other antigens had therefore to be assumed. Some of these proved to be of great importance clinically and are grouped together in the Rh system. Approximately 100 antigens, arranged in at least 14 independent systems, have now been discovered, and the number of possible antigenic patterns is so great that the erythrocyte is probably just as distinctive of an individual as his finger-prints.

The blood-group antigens that have been most widely investigated chemically are A, B, H, and the antigens of the Lewis system. Their study has necessitated the use of large amounts of purified blood-group antigens, though the amount available from red blood-cells is strictly limited. Progress was therefore hampered until it was discovered that approxi-mately 80 per cent of Europeans are 'secretors' of A, B, and H blood-group substances. Present in saliva, meconium, gastric juice, urine, and fluid from pseudomucinous cysts, large cysts are by far the most prolific source of these materials, and the large amounts that have become available in this way have greatly facilitated the investigation of blood-group antigens, Lewis^a (Le^a) blood-group substance is found in the corresponding fluids of 'non-secretors'. Materials with the same or similar serological specificity have been obtained from the mucin-secreting glands of other animals, e.g., gastric mucosa of horse and pig, and from plants.

Such antigens, or at any rate antigenic determinants, are widely dis-tributed in nature. Equally widely distributed are a variety of haem-agglutinins specific for human blood-group antigens. It is sufficient to state here that extracts of seeds of many plants have the capacity to agglutinate red blood-cells, sometimes with a specificity rivalling that of specific antibody. Such extracts are known as 'phytohaemagglutinins' or 'lectins'. Substances with a similar action are found to occur naturally elsewhere as well, e.g., eel serum, with anti-H specificity. Both classes of reagents have been and are extensively used in routine blood-group serology and in the study of the structure of blood-group antigens. It is of particular interest that some lectins, for instance, though specific for certain blood-group antigens, do not necessarily react with structures identical with those against which specific antibody is directed. Even this apparent anomaly has been turned to good account in elucidating the composition and structure of red-cell antigens. Many examples of the use of these reagents will be found in the succeeding pages.

i. Biochemistry of Soluble ABH and Lewis Substances

It is only in very recent years that any progress has been made in defining the composition of blood-group antigens on erythrocytes as such. Nearly all that is known on the subject derives from investigations of soluble blood-group substances, i.e., of materials with the same serological specificity as red-cell antigens but found free in solution in various body fluids. The biochemistry of ABH blood-group substances has been reviewed recently by Watkins [44]. In this section we shall first consider the evidence derived from studies of the ABH and Lewis soluble blood-group substances and then deal with the materials obtained directly from erythrocytes; but in the case of ABH and Lewis substances in red cells under the separate heading of GLYCOLIPIDS (p. 83).

Chemically ABH and Lewis soluble substances are carbohydrate-protein compounds. After purification they have molecular weights ranging from 200,000 to 1,000,000, about 85 per cent of which is accounted for by the carbohydrate fraction. The teams of workers led by Morgan and Kabat who are mainly responsible for our present-day knowledge of the biochemistry of these substances have called them 'mucopolysaccharides'. Unfortunately, the classification and nomenclature of macromolecules of this sort are by no means uniform. The term 'mucopolysaccharide' is usually taken to refer to a class of substances composed of sugars, amino-sugars, uronic acids, and sugar-like compounds. They are widely distri-buted in nature, generally performing some supportive function. Large polymeric structures are sometimes built up using the same 'brick' over and over again. Examples are the polyhexosamines of chitin and shells of crustaceans, and the polyuronides of plants and bacteria. Sometimes more than one brick is used as, for instance, sugars and uronic acids in pneumococci, and repeating units of N-acetyl-glucosamine and glucuronic acid in hyaluronic acid. ABH and Lewis blood-group substances are compounds consisting of mucopolysaccharides as defined above combined with polypeptides.

Uhlenbruck, who works with similar compounds but within the human MNSs blood-group system, describes them as 'mucoids' and eschews the term 'mucopolysaccharides' altogether [45]. He divides carbohydrate-protein compounds into four types:—

α. The *mucins* consisting of a protein chain with many short, unbranched side-chains with terminal N-acetyl-neuraminic acid and subterminal N-acetyl-hexosamine. The same structural units are used as in the blood-group-active mucoids of type $β$ below, but the structure as a whole is more monotonous (*Fig. 6*).

β. The *mucoids* also have a protein chain but the carbohydrate side-chains are longer than in mucins and also branched (*Fig. 6*).

γ. The *glycoproteins*$_{ss}$ (*sensu strictiori*) consist of a protein chain that bears side-chains of both the above types, but just a few scattered over the length of the chain. Usually the side-chains are rather simpler structures than in $β$. In principle every carbohydrate-protein complex could be designated a glycoprotein but the meaning here is restricted in the above sense (*Fig. 6*).

δ. *Gamma-globulins* are also glycoproteins in the general sense but differ in that they have still fewer carbohydrate prosthetic groups (*Fig. 6*).

Already there is perhaps sufficient initial evidence to justify us in thinking that an infinite gradation leads from mucopolysaccharides with little or nothing in the way of amino-acids in their composition to proteins with little or no carbohydrate. As far as the blood-group substances of the ABH and Lewis systems are concerned, we are interested in molecules falling into Uhlenbruck's second category of mucoids. We know that the carbohydrate fraction confers specificity on the whole molecule in serological tests, so it is somewhat surprising to find that degradation of the polypeptide part also results in a lowering of activity. It must be assumed that the latter somehow orders the configuration or orientation of carbohydrate residues. The polypeptide fractions of all ABH and Lewis blood-group active substances are composed of the same eleven

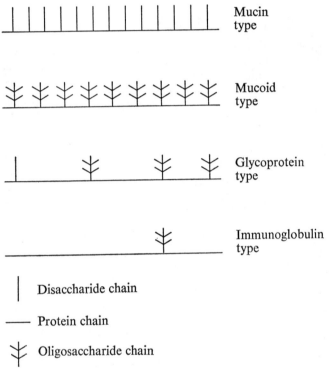

Fig. 6.—A proposed scheme for carbohydrate-protein compounds by Uhlenbruck [45].

amino-acids, but the similarity between them goes beyond the qualitative aspect. It is possible to induce a different kind of immunological response from antibody production in animals by injections of soluble substances, namely delayed hypersensitivity. In these cases it is the polypeptide fraction that determines the specificity of the response. Animals sensitized with A substance respond to subsequent injections of B substance which points to an immunological similarity, i.e., of detailed structure as well of overall composition. Thus the polypeptide not only influences the serological specificity of the carbohydrate moiety but also has an immunological function and specificity of its own. This quite simply illustrates the complexity of immunological responses in the host and serves as a warning to the unwary that nothing can be taken for granted.

Turning now to the chemical analysis of the carbohydrate fraction we again find that all the soluble substances are qualitatively the same; containing the sugars L-fucose and D-galactose, and the amino-sugars N-acetyl-D-glucosamine and N-acetyl-D-galactosamine. In addition, various amounts of N-acetylneuraminic acid are found, but it is not implicated in ABH and Lewis blood-group specificities.

Though characteristically soluble in water, the solubility of blood-group substances varies considerably. The more soluble preparations consist of mucopolysaccharides with molecular weights of 200,000–500,000, whereas the gel-like substances obtained from ovarian cyst fluids are giant macromolecules built up from the more soluble molecules with intermolecular disulphide bonds.

At present the detailed structure of neither the polypeptide nor the carbohydrate part is known, but a reasonable estimate is that each molecule contains some 350 oligosaccharides of which each chain contains a minimum of 7 sugar units [46, 47]. Although we may be ignorant of the overall structure of the molecule, considerable progress has been achieved in the past few years in elucidating the arrangement of the terminal 5 or 6 hexoses that make up each determinant. Such progress has been due to a concentric attack by a battery of methods and to recent technical advances. The methods employed involve chemical, enzymatic, and serological approaches.

Partial acid hydrolysis yields a variety of mono- and oligosaccharides from blood-group substances. With the use of a new hydrolytic agent, a macromolecular water-soluble form of polystyrene sulphonic acid, neutral oligosaccharide fragments are split off. With the reaction carried out in dialysis tubing the fragments quickly diffuse through the membrane and are preserved from further hydrolysis. A good yield of tri-, tetra-, and pentasaccharides can be obtained largely in their original N-acetylated form. Alkaline hydrolysis is also used to yield oligosaccharides and to separate carbohydrate and protein fractions. The O-glycosidic link joining them is probably between an internal N-acetylgalactosamine and the hydroxyl group of an oxyamino-acid (threonine or serine) [48]. There may be many such bonds since large amounts of these two amino-acids are found in blood-group active mucoids. The same bonds are also present in the active mucoids of the MNSs system.

A wide variety of enzymes has been used to attack specific bonds, though the precise substrate of a particular preparation is not always known at the outset. Glycosidases can be used to split off terminal mono-, di-, or oligosaccharides, proteinases to degrade the polypeptide part. If neuraminidase is used to treat bovine red cells, pneumococcus type XIV specificity is exposed; and strong agglutination of such cells takes place with anti-XIV serum. New specificities arise either because an oligosaccharide from which the terminal sugar or sugars has been removed presents a different configuration and therefore specificity (cryptantigen), or because the same process exposes side-chains of different specificity that were previously sterically masked (pseudocryptantigen) (*Fig.* 1, p. 23).

The serological activity of blood-group substances can be tested before and after treatment with glycosidases; subsequently the specific action of the enzyme can be confirmed by inhibiting its activity with known sugars.

Serological tests are, of course, used in conjunction with both chemical and enzymatic methods. Precipitation in agar gels because of its power to resolve antigens in mixtures of antigens and inhibition of precipitation, agglutination, and haemolysis because of their sensitivity and precision are methods particularly suited to the characterization of antigenic determinants. Inhibition tests can be performed not only with enzymatic cleavage products of blood-group substances but also with natural and synthetic sugars; for instance, the rare sugars isolated and identified by Kuhn and his colleagues [49] have been helpful in defining the structure of some determinants.

It is worth re-emphasizing at this point that our knowledge of the detailed structure of blood-group substances is confined to the terminal 5 or 6 units of an oligosaccharide side-chain that go to form a determinant, and not at all to their ordering in the molecule as a whole except in so far as they are presumed to be superficially placed. Reference to *Fig.* 7 will show that the same determinant structure could be repeated over and over again in a single molecule, and, though no doubt this is so, it is thought that there must also be other determinants present to account for the exposure of pseudocryptantigens.

We can summarize our present knowledge of the detailed structure of ABH and Lewis substances by saying that they all have a common precursor carbohydrate chain to which is attached one or more sugars that determine the various specificities. It is unnecessary to make any assumptions about how many such structures appear on a single molecule or whether other serologically specific structures are present in the depths of the molecule. The common precursor is a tetrasaccharide that exists in two forms which differ only in that N-acetylglucosamine (GNAc) is linked (1→3) in type I and (1→4) in type II chains to the terminal galactose (*Fig.* 7) [44]. Normally both precursors are present in each individual. Type-II chains cross-react with antiserum to pneumococcus XIV by virtue of a common terminal disaccharide, N-acetyl-lactosamine, that they share with that polysaccharide. This serologically active grouping is therefore present in all ABH and Lewis blood-group substances as a cryptantigen; pseudocryptantigens of the same or other specificities are probably also present.

Cross-reactivity with pneumococcus XIV is not, of course, an exclusive property of human blood-group substances. The oligosaccharide, lacto-N-neotetra-ose, isolated from bovine red cells has the formula

$$\beta\text{-Gal-}(1\rightarrow4)\text{-}\beta\text{-GNAc-}(1\rightarrow3)\text{-}\beta\text{-Gal-}(1\rightarrow4)\text{-Glu}$$

from which it will be seen that it shares a terminal trisaccharide with the type II chain (*Fig.* 7) and therefore the terminal disaccharide with pneumococcus XIV. As we would expect, weaker cross-reactions occur when the steric configuration is changed by replacing the terminal 1→4 bond between galactose and GNAc with a 1→3 bond, or by replacing the subterminal GNAc with N-acetyl-mannosamine.

Degradation experiments with enzymes have had a considerable influence on the development of the concept of sequential build-up of blood-group substances from a common 'precursor' substance. It is not, indeed, known at present whether sugar units are added singly or as preformed oligosaccharides, but for the sake of clarity in exposition we will presume a sequential addition. As techniques are now being rapidly

Carbohydrate Chains in Precursor Substance

Type I   β-Gal-(1→3)-β-GNac-(1→3)-β-Gal-(1→3)-GalNAc
Type II   β-Gal-(1→4)-β-GNac-(1→3)-β-Gal-(1→3)-GalNAc

Chain Type	Terminal Structure	Specificity
I	β-Gal-(1→3)-GNAc - - -	—
II	β-Gal-(1→4)-GNAc - - -	S XIV
I	β-Gal-(1→3)-GNAc - - - ↑ α1,2 Fuc	H
II	β-Gal-(1→4)-GNAc - - - ↑ α1,2 Fuc	H
I	β-Gal-(1→3)-GNAc - - - ↑ α1,4 Fuc	Le^a
II	β-Gal-(1→4)-GNAc - - -	S XIV
I	β-Gal-(1→3)-GNAc - - - ↑ α1,2 ↑ αl,4 Fuc Fuc	Le^b
II	β-Gal-(1→4)-GNAc - - - ↑ α1,2 Fuc	H

Fig. 7.—Precursor substance and derived structures. GalNAc: *N*-acetyl-D-galactosaminopyranose. Gal: D-galactopyranose. GNAc: *N*-acetyl-D-glucos-aminopyranose. Fuc: L-fucose. *After Watkins* [44].

developed for investigating the biosynthesis of heteropolysaccharides, it is to be hoped that the enzymes that actually produce blood-group substance *in vivo* will very soon be identified, and so the biosynthetic mechanisms of these substances clarified.

The first presumed step leads to the production of Le^a substance and is the enzymatic addition of fucose linked α1,4 to the subterminal GNAc in a type I chain (*Fig. 7*). Such an addition is not possible in type-II chains because the terminal sugar already occupies this position. In Le^a molecules, therefore, type II chains retain their pneumococcus XIV specificity.

If fucose is linked α1,2 to the terminal galactose instead of 1→4 to subterminal GNAc, H substance is formed. This addition can take place in both chain types (*Fig. 7*).

Mention has already been made of the fact that reagents with the same specificity do not always react with the same structures. An excellent example is provided by H antigen and eel serum anti-H. Whereas, as we have seen, human H substance has a terminal L-fucose, 3-O-methyl-D-fucose specifically inhibits eel serum anti-H [1]. It seems that in this case the minimal antigenic determinant is smaller than a monosaccharide and consists of a methyl radical equatorially attached to a pyranose ring with an adjoining ether oxygen and an oxygen-carrying substituent on a contiguous C atom *cis* to the methyl group. Similar conclusions have been drawn with regard to size of reactive sites in the case of reactions between eel serum 'antibodies' and H-active polysaccharides from *Taxus* and *Sassafras*. The active determinant is said to be part of the molecular structure of two very rare natural sugars, 2-*O*-methyl-fucose and 3-*O*-methyl-D-galactose [50].

The addition of both molecules of fucose, characterizing individually H and Le^a determinants, gives rise to Le^b specificity. It is evident that only chain I can be altered in this way so that in individuals with Le^b specificity chain II retains H specificity (*Fig. 7*).

H substance can be further transformed to yield A and B substances (*Fig. 8*). In the case of A substance *N*-acetyl-galactosamine is linked α1,3 to the terminal galactose, whereas in B substance the final addition is galactose, also linked α1,3 (*Fig. 8*). Although these two terminal sugars are characteristic for A and B activity, the antigenic determinant probably includes fucose as well, since oligosaccharides that contain it are the more powerful inhibitors.

Gene	*Structure*	*Specificity*
—	β-Gal-(1→3 or 4)-GNAc - - - ↑ α1,2 Fuc	H
A	α-GalNAc-(1→3)-β-Gal-(1→3 or 4)-GNAc - - - ↑ α1,2 Fuc	A
B	α-Gal-(1→3)-β-Gal-(1→3 or 4)-GNAc - - - ↑ α1,2 Fuc	B

Fig. 8.—Additions to H active chains controlled by A and B genes. Abbreviations as in *Fig. 7*. *After Watkins* [44].

Progressive degradation of both A and B substances therefore leads back through H specificity, then possibly Le^b and Le^a, and ultimately to the precursor substance with pneumococcus XIV specificity in the case of type II chains. When we come to consider the genetic pathways by which the specificity of blood-group substances could be controlled we simply have to reverse this procedure. Once the existence of blood groups in man had become established it soon became evident that they were inherited. Indeed, it is the inheritance of these antigens that defines the different systems, ABH, Lewis, MNSs, Rh, and so on. We are not so much concerned with this aspect, however, as with the genetic pathways through which specificity is expressed biochemically. In this connexion genetics is both servant and master of blood-group serology since each in turn is used as a tool for the study of the other.

In a proposed scheme of genetic pathways [44] a fucosidase under the control of the Lewis gene (Le) adds fucose in the appropriate position in a type I chain. Fucose is also added under the control of the H gene by a, presumably different, fucosidase to type I and II chains to give the H determinant. In order to account for the presence of H, A, and B antigens in secretions a secretor gene (Se) is also postulated. In its absence H gene is not able to initiate the addition of fucose to precursor or Le^a substances in secretions. An individual who possesses Se as well as both H and Le genes can add both fucoses to chain I with the formation of Le^b substance. Similarly, individuals with Se and H genes can, under the influence of A and B genes, add N-acetyl-galactosamine and galactose respectively to form A and B substances (*Fig. 9*).

To sum up: Three gene systems, Lewis, ABH, and secretor, collaborate in the sequential addition of sugars to produce Lewis and ABH substances in secretions. All three systems are necessary for the secretion of Le^b, two or three for A, B, and H, and only one for Le^a. It has been observed that the secretions of individuals possessing Le gene carry in addition to A and/or B determinants, also determinants of Le^a, Le^b, and H specificity. It is presumed, therefore, that, although a full set of genes and enzymes is present, all precursor substance is not completely transformed and intermediate steps are secreted. The same situation obtains in H secretions where Le^a and Le^b specificities may also be present.

It must be stressed at this point that the genetic pathways governing the production of soluble ABH substances are not identical with those governing red-cell antigens (*see* GLYCOLIPIDS, p. 83). The A and B genes each control the manufacture of at least two distinct products: A and B substances of secretions, and A and B antigens of red cells. In secretors both pathways are present, in non-secretors only one. It is the blood-group specificity exhibited by mucopolysaccharides in secretors that has led to the postulation of a secretor gene. In order to account for those rare cases in which H antigen is absent another gene, 'x', is also postulated. In non-secretors (sese) or in people with a double dose of gene x no H and therefore no A or B substance is formed in secretions. If an individual also lacks the Lewis gene (lele) then only precursor substance is found. Non-secretors and individuals with a double dose of gene x differ in that the former lack A, B, and H antigens in secretions only, whereas in the latter these antigens are also lacking in their red blood-cells.

Furthermore, it must not be forgotten that for the moment the O gene is considered to be an amorph, i.e., no true 'O substance' has so far been found in group O human red cells. H substance is *not* the product of the as yet hypothetical O gene, and so-called 'anti-O' sera are defined as sera that are not neutralized by H substance, in contrast to anti-H sera.

From the above 'facts' it follows that the action of the ABH and Le gene systems is a very limited one; far from controlling the building of the huge macromolecules of ABH and Lewis substances, they govern only a few terminal steps. It can now be readily appreciated that a single macromolecule could possess A and B and Lewis specificities at the same time, since each molecule carries numerous small carbohydrate chains; different specificities are then attributed to different chains. Indeed, we have already seen that chains of types I and II in the same macromolecule carry different specificities.

We are left with a picture in which macromolecules of soluble blood-group substances are seen as possessing many oligosaccharide chains of differing length; A and B determinants representing the longest and most complex of them, and A and B substances possessing in addition to

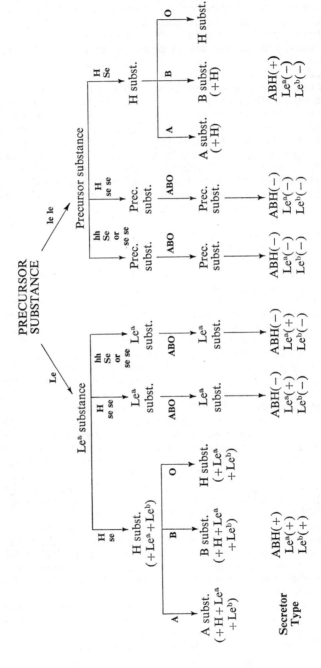

Fig. 9.—Possible genetical pathways for the biosynthesis of A., B, H, and Le^a substances. Gene systems: (1) **Le le**, (2) **Hh**, (3) **Se se**, (4) **ABO**. *After Watkins* [44].

complete chains, incomplete chains with H, Le^a, Le^b, and pneumococcus type XIV specificities.

The view presented thus far is perhaps the simplest that can be proposed for the genetic control and structure of blood-group substances. It does not take into account the recognized subtypes and variations even within the systems discussed, nor the many anomalies and contradictions that are to be found in the literature. For instance, A antigen is not irrevocably the substance depicted above, since oligosaccharide fragments have been obtained by alkaline hydrolysis that are tens of times more inhibitory than trisaccharides obtained previously by acid hydrolysis [51, 52]. None of them has been fully identified but the most active fragment may have the formula

$$\alpha\text{-D-GalNAc-}(1\rightarrow3)\text{-}\beta\text{-D-Gal-}(1\rightarrow3 \text{ or}1 \rightarrow4)\text{-D-GNAc-R,}$$

where R is a reduced sugar or sugar fragment [53]. It is not yet clear why this substance should be more active in haemagglutination inhibition tests than the fucose-containing tetrasaccharide described earlier [54], but it may be due to differences in the test systems, or, more importantly, to the size and/or exact configuration of the respective fragments.

In carbohydrates as in proteins minor changes in composition as well as structure can profoundly alter serological reactivity. In the case of A blood-group substance deacetylation renders it completely inactive in haemagglutination inhibition tests, though it is still able to precipitate with substantial amounts of antibody from the same serum [55]. Perhaps this anomalous finding can best be explained by invoking a very much higher dissociation constant for the altered substance so that it is displaced by the native antigen in inhibition tests, whereas in straight precipitation there would be no competition for antibody sites. We shall see later that a similar difference in structure is found in blood-group active glycolipids though initiated by a different mechanism. In the present case the loss of serological activity might be caused either by a modification in configuration or by the appearance of a positive charge at this previously uncharged site.

So we find that, on the one hand, penta- or hexasaccharides are necessary for maximum reactivity, but, on the other, even a small alteration to the terminal sugar can have a striking effect on specificity.

Even allowing for the possibility that fucose is not part of the A determinant, the various theories of genetic pathways deal only with one A antigen without distinguishing between the subspecificities A_1 and A_2. Wiener postulates a structural difference between these subgroups [56]. He also assumes that in the soluble blood-group antigens the carbohydrate side-chains are relatively mobile, whereas on the red-cell surface they are held rigidly in position. This difference would account for the readily detectable H specificity in the soluble substances of A and B as well as O secretors. In red cells the rigidly held side-chains of A_2 cells are thought to be considerably shorter than those of A_1 cells and therefore to cause much less steric hindrance; consequently reactions with anti-H reagents are stronger with A_2 cells, though still less than with soluble substances where anti-H can be used to distinguish between secretors and non-secretors. Other authors have assumed that the reaction of anti-H with A_2

is stronger because less H is transformed into A substance; in any case the two explanations are not mutually exclusive. It would also seem that AB individuals have fewer A and B specific side-chains than homozygous A or B individuals.

It will be of interest too to see whether the various anti-A reagents are better adapted to A substance formed from chain I or chain II. Work along these lines is in progress using oligosaccharides linked 1→3 and 1→4 in inhibition tests [57]. Meanwhile one might speculate that no difference will be detected by the phytohaemagglutinin of *Dolichos biflorus* since in this case, as with many lectins, the reactive site is small and directed mainly against the terminal sugar, so that the different bonds between the second and third sugars will not influence the reaction.

The concept of stepwise formation of blood-group antigens has been extended to the A subgroups and weak A antigens [58]. It is postulated that there are at least four partial A antigens and that A_1 is synthesized in four consecutive steps. Such speculations may be tempting but, as far as we know, are unsupported by experimental evidence as yet.

We have seen that soluble blood-group substances have carbohydrate and polypeptide fractions, and that specificity is determined by branching oligosaccharide side-chains. Some carbohydrates though present do not seem to form part of the determinant structures. Thus sialic acid is present in varying amounts in soluble substance but does not apparently affect specificity. Similarly, although the polypeptide backbone displays immunogenic properties in delayed hypersensitivity, a number of constituents, cystine, aspartic and glutamic acids, are found in different amounts in blood-group substances of similar or identical immunological activity [59].

Finally, it is remarkable that, as in many other instances in nature, similar patterns are observable in the arrangement of genetic pathways leading to the production of blood-group antigens. Here we have seen how the addition of terminal and subterminal groups to a large macromolecule can result in the appearance of a number of distinct specificities, all under genetic control. Recently Race [60] has shown that this 'terminal sugar icing', although not always done with sugars perhaps, may manifest a general pattern as indicated by the Rh and P systems, where several genes again participate in the 'making of the cake'. A similar pattern can also perhaps be recognized in the cell walls and antigens of bacteria (*see* p. 68).

ii. Antigens of the MNSs System

The antigens of the MNSs system are discussed here in spite of the fact that they are derived from red blood-cells and not secretions because they are mucoids (Uhlenbruck) or mucopolysaccharides (Morgan), just as the soluble antigens of the ABH system are. In the following account we have made extensive use of an excellent review by Uhlenbruck [45].

The immunochemical investigation of these antigens is still in its infancy but interesting results have already been obtained.

The polypeptide part is similar in MNSs and ABH systems in that it does not determine specificity and that serine and threonine are major components. In MNSs antigens, however, 15 amino-acids have been described and there is an abundance of glutamic acid rather than proline. Neur-aminic acid again is present in both, but whereas in ABH substances its amount is very variable and it is not involved in serological specificity, in the MNSs system it is serologically important.

Technically the same methods can be used as for the study of ABH mucopolysaccharides. Once again the advent of polystyrene sulphonic acid has marked a substantial advance in the technique of partial acid hydrolysis. In addition, alkaline hydrolysis, enzymes such as glycosidases and proteinases, and serological methods can all be used. There is no detailed knowledge yet of the structure of the carbohydrate moiety but interesting facts have nevertheless emerged.

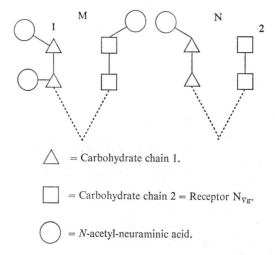

△ = Carbohydrate chain 1.

☐ = Carbohydrate chain 2 = Receptor N_{Vg}.

◯ = N-acetyl-neuraminic acid.

Fig. 10.—Basic structures in MN-antigens. *After Prokop and Uhlenbruck* [61].

The blood-group active substances of human red cells can be divided into 'genuine' and 'acquired' substances. The former are part of the structure of the red-cell surface and are presumably formed through their corresponding genetic pathway; the latter are passively taken up by red cells from the plasma. Lewis substances fall into the second category and biochemically speaking are fucomucoids, i.e., are mucoids with many terminal fucose residues.

The 'genuine' antigens are further subdivided into glycolipids and neuramino-mucoids. The former are represented by the A and B glyco-lipids of human red blood-cells (q.v.), and the latter by MNSs substances and are so called because they possess many terminal neuraminic acid residues. Neuramino-mucoids consist of a protein chain to which are attached many, high molecular weight, branching oligosaccharides of differing structures.

It is evident from serological reactions that M and N substances are very alike. Thus anti-N, whether in the form of immune serum from rabbits or human beings or of phytohaemagglutinin, is absorbed by ordinary M cells. U-negative M cells, i.e., those that contain neither S nor s, are an exception. Cross-reactivity between M and N has been taken by Prokop and Uhlenbruck [61] as supporting their thesis that a basic structure of two carbohydrate chains is common to both M and N substances. In *Fig.* 10 the two carbohydrate chains are depicted diagrammatically; in chain II M substance has an additional *N*-acetyl-neuraminic acid (NANA) compared with N substance, and similarly in chain I there is again an extra NANA in M substance. Removing the terminal NANA from chain II renders M substance inhibitory to the anti-N phytohaemagglutinin obtained from *Vicia graminea*, and chain II without terminal NANA is referred to by Uhlenbruck as *V. graminea* receptor (N_{Vg}). It is assumed that as in ABH and Lewis systems a basic precursor is present in the MNSs system.

It is clear from the foregoing that the chemical structure of 'ordinary' M cells must differ from that of U-negative M cells. How it differs is not known with any certainty. One can speculate, however, in accordance with Uhlenbruck's scheme and drawing an analogy with soluble ABH substances, that 'ordinary' M cells possess some chains of type II without terminal NANA, whereas U-negative cells do not. U-negative cells become reactive with *V. graminea* anti-N after the removal of the terminal NANA by receptor-destroying enzyme (neuraminidase) [62]. In other words, N_{Vg} is present in such cells as a cryptantigen.

The great similarity between M and N substances is again shown by the fact that M substance is only slightly more inhibitory for so-called anti-M phytohaemagglutination from *Iberis amara* than N substance. It is worth noting that the difference between A and B specificities is determined solely by the introduction of an *N*-acetyl group at position 2 in the terminal hexose of the oligosaccharide. The difference between M and N specificities as far as lectins are concerned may be equally subtle. At the same time one must not forget that great though this similarity may be, it is only between M and N. With respect to the other antigens of the red cell differences are just as great as are needed to make serological distinctions. As Romanowska has shown [63] M substance, even devoid of NANA, is a thousand times more inhibitory for *I. amara* anti-M than blood-group substances of the ABH and Lewis systems or their sugars.

A further parallel with ABH substances can be drawn in that the specificity of M and N phytohaemagglutinins is not directed against the same structures as that of antibodies. In this connexion it should be appreciated that 'specificity' is used in two slightly different senses in describing immunological reactions. By the first is meant the degree of complementarity between antigen and antibody or lectin, and the extent to which the 'fit' determines the uniqueness of such a reaction. By the second is meant the recognition of a character; thus a reagent which consistently agglutinates M cells, and others not at all or to a lesser extent, is said to have M specificity. The structure against which it is directed is not defined, and it could be a part of the M determinant or another structure constantly associated with it. In the case of some phytohaemagglutinins it can be said that their specificity is narrower than that of antibody according to the first definition, because they react with only part of the determinant, and yet broader, by the second definition, because there is more likelihood of finding a similar small structure elsewhere than a similar large structure.

The anti-A reactivity of *D. biflorus* has already been mentioned, and its specificity is narrow in the sense that it can be inhibited by a mono-saccharide whereas a disaccharide is necessary in order to inhibit anti-A antibody. A different situation is illustrated by M and N substances in which N-acetyl-neuraminic acid is essential for reactions with rabbit and human sera of anti-M and anti-N specificity. But, in the case of *I. amara* anti-M and *V. graminea* anti N, treatment of M and N substances by neuraminidase increases their inhibitory capacity 50–100 times. To complicate the picture still further even lectins with the same 'specificity' seem to react with different structures. Enzymatic digestion of N substance with a crude extract of *Trichomonas foetus* has no effect on its reactivity with *Bauhinia variegata* anti-N, but destroys its inhibitory capacity for *V. graminea* anti-N.

iii. Other Blood-group Antigens

The study of the structural basis of specificity of blood-group antigens of other systems is at an even more rudimentary stage than that of the MNSs system. We mention a paper by Rule and Boyd [64] not so much because it suggests that N-acetyl-neuraminic acid is a determinant for the D antigen of the Rh system as because it extends the concept, familiar from the biochemical study of ABH and Lewis systems, that numbers of antigenic determinants are found in the same macromolecule. In other words it is suggested that if a red cell possesses, for instance A, B, M, N, D, etc., specificities they are so closely linked that it will be impossible to isolate 'pure' A, M, D, etc. A similar inference can perhaps be drawn from the evidence that I antigen has β- and possibly also α-galactoside receptors [65]. This not only confirms the known serological relationship between Ii and ABH systems, but also renders it conceivable that these receptors also form part of the same macromolecule.

Somewhat more is known about P antigen of the red-cell surface [66, 67] since material of the same specificity is obtainable from the fluid of hydatid cysts in sheep. This mucopolysaccharide is similar in many respects to the soluble human blood-group substance. As in B substance, α-D-galactoside units play an important role in determining specificity. It has been possible to prepare powerful anti-P agglutinins by coupling partially purified P_1 substance to *Shigella shigae* protein, a procedure that has proved successful with ABH substances, but the P_1 substance was still antigenically heterogeneous.

b. Bacterial Polysaccharides

The recent serological investigation of bacterial polysaccharides has followed in broad outline the manner of investigation of blood-group substances. Originally crude extracts of bacteria were made and examined chemically and serologically. Subsequently purified polysaccharides and their degradation products have been characterized, again chemically and serologically.

It is well recognized that many bacterial species have in addition to their protein antigens, group or species specific polysaccharide antigens or haptens. This aspect of their antigenic structure is currently engaging a good deal of attention, but we shall confine ourselves here to discussing representative organisms from among the pneumococci and salmonellae where progress in relating structure to immunological behaviour is already fairly well advanced.

i. Pneumococcal Capsular Antigens

A striking morphological feature of the virulent pneumococcus is its polysaccharide capsule which gives a mucoid appearance to colonies of the organism. It is also responsible for the specificities displayed by some 74 serological types of pneumococci. In the following account the symbols S I, S II, etc., will be used to denote the specific polysaccharides of pneumococcus type I, type II, and so on.

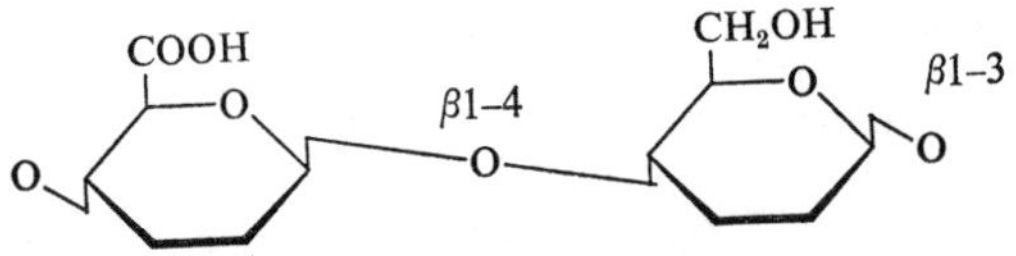

Fig. 11A.—Cellobiuronic acid.

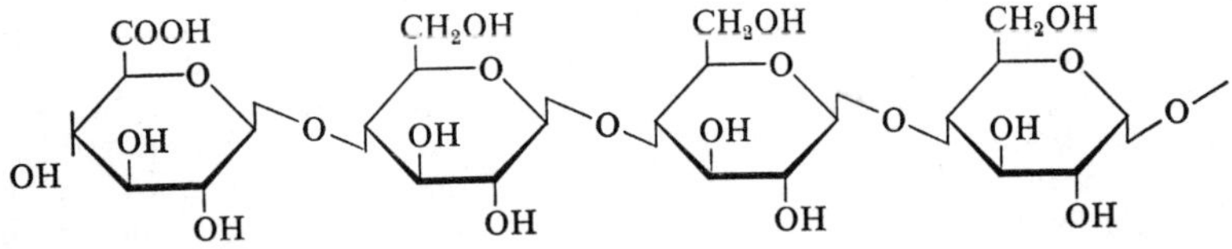

Fig. 11B.—Proposed structure for pneumococcal polysaccharide S VIII [75].

Among the first immunologically significant polysaccharides to have their structure investigated, much of the early evidence about them came from observations of the way in which antisera to them cross-reacted with synthetic and vegetable polysaccharides of which the structure was known in whole or in part. More recent studies have followed closely those used for the analysis of blood-group substance antigens, with hydrolysis products and known sugars being used in serological inhibition tests with native or partly degraded polysaccharides.

The polysaccharides that have been most fully characterized are S II, S III, S VIII, and S XIV. S II is estimated to have a molecular weight of 240,000 and on breakdown yields the components L-rhamnose (48 per cent), D-glucose (35 per cent), and D-glucuronic acid (16 per cent) [68]. Glucuronic acid residues occupy most if not all non-reducing terminal positions and play a dominant role in determining the specificity of anti-S II horse serum. However, glucose and rhamnose are also concerned with determining specificity. In the intact molecule glucosyl residues are involved in 1:4:6 branch-points and antisera to S II cross-react with glycogens and amylopectins known to contain the same structure. In particular, cross-reactions with tamarind seed polysaccharide, in which glucose occupies the same relative position but the other components are D-galactose and D-xylose, indicate that this structural feature forms part of the determinant of S II [69].

The chemical basis of the cross-reactions observed between the specific polysaccharides S III and S VIII lies in the fact that they both contain cellobiuronic acid [70]. The structure of S III is shown in *Fig.* 11A and consists of cellobiuronic acid residues linked 1→3. The repeating unit of S VIII is a tetrao-uronic acid and the probable structure is shown in *Fig.* 11B. The disaccharide 4-*O*-β-D-glucopyranosyl-(1→4)-D-galacto-pyranose, found in partial acid hydrolysates of S VIII, forms the link between cellobiuronic acid residues. The precise nature of the link between successive tetrao-uronic acid residues is not known with certainty [70].

Of considerable interest, intrinsically and for the study of polysaccharide structure, has been the induction of the specific depolymerases, D3 and D8, in bacterial strains grown in the presence of S III and S VIII respectively as the only sources of carbon [70].

β-D-galactose
(1→6) |
β-D-galactose(1→4)β-*N*-acetyl-glucosamine(1→3)β-D-galactose
(1→6) |
→4)β-D-glucose(1→4)β-*N*-acetyl-D-
glucosamine (1→

Fig. 12.—Structure of *Pneumococcus* S XIV [71].

The investigation of S XIV has been of particular interest to medicine because of the cross-reactions of antisera with this polysaccharide and the ABH blood-group substances. Study of these reactions, combined with chemical analysis, has led to the proposed structure of S XIV [71] shown in *Fig.* 12. Comparison with type-II chain of blood-group substance will show that these two oligosaccharides have in common a terminal lactos-amine structure. Subsequent evidence, derived principally from the induction of enzymes in *Klebsiella aerogenes* but also from inhibition studies, suggests that this is not the whole story and the proposed structure of S XIV given above will need modification [70].

In considering antigenic determinants so far we have in general implied that cross-reactions are due to identity or similarity of terminal structures. In the following section on the determinants of *Salmonella* O antigens an alternative explanation is given in which it is suggested that any accessible unit in a chain may present as the dominating structure in determining specificity. This also accords well with evidence from pneumococcal polysaccharides where observed cross-reactions are not always associated with terminal structures, e.g., L-rhamnose in the case of S II and S VI.

ii. Somatic Antigens of Enterobacteria

The family of Enterobacteriaceae comprises a number of different genera among which are *Salmonella*, *Shigella*, *Arizona*, and *Escherichia*. All its members are Gram-negative, rod-shaped bacteria, many of which are motile, and many of which have their natural habitat in the gut of man and animals. The *Salmonella* species have been subdivided into 'serotypes' on the basis of their somatic (O) and flagellar (H) antigens. In the Kauff-mann-White scheme the serotypes are arranged in groups according to their common somatic antigens, one of the antigens in each group being specific for that group, e.g., *9* in group D (*see Table X*) [72]. The other O antigens present in a group are also found in other groups and cannot therefore be said to be group specific, but they indicate the likelihood of cross-reactions occurring between groups. The flagellar antigens are said to be species specific and any one organism may possess an antigen or group of antigens in either phase 1 or phase 2; it is then said to be in that phase. Generally speaking a culture of bacteria, though predominantly in one phase, will always contain some individuals in the other phase. Some species of salmonellae are monophasic, however, and do not have an alternative phase. More than 70 specificities associated with flagellar antigens of salmonellae have been described. In various combinations these provide the genus with a virtually unlimited number of 'serotypes' (species), and already over one thousand are defined. This brief résumé

Table X.—A SELECTION OF MEMBERS FROM THE KAUFFMANN-WHITE SCHEME

GROUP	*Salmonella* SEROTYPE	O FACTORS	PHASE 1	PHASE 2
A	*S. paratyphi A*	1, 2, 12	a	—
B	*S. paratyphi* B	1, 4, 5, 12	b	1, 2
	S. typhimurium	1, 4, 5, 12	i	1, 2
	S. bredeney	1, 4, 12, 27	l, v	1, 7
C_1	*S. paratyphi* C	6, 7, Vi	c	1, 5
	S. montevideo	6, 7	g, m, s	—
	S. mbandaka	6, 7	z_{10}	e, n, z_{15}
	S. mbandaka var. 25	1, 6, 7, 25	z_{10}	e, n, z_{15}
C_2	*S. newport*	6, 8	d	1, 2
	S. bovis-morbificans	6, 8	r	1, 5
D_1	*S. typhi*	9, 12, Vi	d	—
	S. enteritidis	1, 9, 12	g, m	—
	S. panama	1, 9, 12	l, v	1, 5
E_1	*S. anatum*	3, 10	e, h	1, 6
	S. uganda	3, 10	l, z_{13}	1, 5
E_2	*S. newington*	3, 15	e, h	1, 6
E_3	*S. illinois*	(3), (15), 34	z_{10}	1, 5
E_4	*S. senftenberg*	1, 3, 19	g, s, t	—

simply indicates some of the vast complexities of the antigenic structure of this group of organisms and we shall now confine our attention to some of those somatic antigens associated with O specificity.

Gram-negative bacteria are frequently characterized by their possession of a toxic component known as 'endotoxin'. As the name implies, endotoxins are an integral part of the cell; they are released in large amounts only after the death of the organism, in contrast to exotoxins which are released during life. A number of the more generalized manifestations of infection by enterobacteria are due to the action of endotoxins and can be elicited by the injection of killed bacteria. Endotoxins have occasionally found their way into water or saline used in the preparation of materials for injection or transfusion, and the mean pyrogenic dose has been estimated at 0.001–0.004 μg. per kg. body-weight in both man and rabbit.

Endotoxins are part of the bacterial cell wall and can be extracted in the form of Boivin antigens by trichloroacetic acid. Composed of lipid, polysaccharide, and protein fractions, their interest for us stems from the fact that the polysaccharide moiety determines the specificity of the group antigens of salmonellae and related genera. A number of different methods is now available for obtaining serologically active preparations of polysaccharide, either whole or slightly degraded [73]. The most refined preparations of polysaccharide, which by themselves are not immunogenic, have molecular weights of between 10,000 and 20,000, but in the form of the readily extractable lipopolysaccharide of between 1 and 5 million.

Methods of chemical analysis have been supplemented during the past decade by biosynthetic studies, and in particular by the use of mutants in order to determine how changes in specificity are brought about. As a result considerable insight has been gained into the structures of O factors. For a more detailed account than is presented here the reader cannot do better than consult the authoritative review by Lüderitz, Staub, and Westphal [73], who are among the leading workers in this field.

Superimposed on the rigid framework of the cell wall of enterobacteria is a lipopolysaccharide–protein–phospholipid complex, the polysaccharide moiety of which largely, if not totally, determines O specificity. Qualitative chemical analyses of the O antigens of wild-type *Salmonella* strains show that they all contain five to eight sugars of which five are common to them all. This would suggest an inner core of five basal sugars on which are built carbohydrate structures specific for individual O factors.

α. *Basal Core Structure*: The composition and structure of the basal core of O antigens has been studied principally in 'rough' mutants of salmonellae. Rough or R mutants arise spontaneously during laboratory cultivation and besides alterations in colonial morphology, agglutinability in saline, etc., they are found to have lost the O specificity of the parent strain and acquired a new 'R' specificity. Chemical analysis of R mutant polysaccharides at first showed that they were all composed of the same five sugar units: a heptose, probably in the form of a phosphate ester, 2-keto-3-deoxy-octonate (KDO), glucosamine, glucose, and galactose. It is thought that all O antigens of salmonellae probably contain this core of basal sugars arranged in the form of a backbone of heptose and KDO, to which side-chains of glucose, galactose, glucose, and *N*-acetyl-glucosamine, in that order, are attached to one of the heptoses; a short side-chain of galactose is also linked to the first glucose unit (*Fig.* 13) [73]. The almost universal cross-reactivity of R mutants, irrespective of the wild-type parents from which they were derived, lends further support to this concept of a common structure to the inner core. Eventually, however, R mutants were found that lacked one, two, three, or four of the five basal sugars. The general structure of four of these, named Ra to Rd in decreasing order of complexity, is also shown in *Fig.* 13. The fifth, Re, contains KDO only.

β. *Structure of O Factor Determinants*: Specificity of O factors is achieved by the addition, to the side-chains of the basal core, of oligosaccharides composed of sugars already found in the core, or these plus

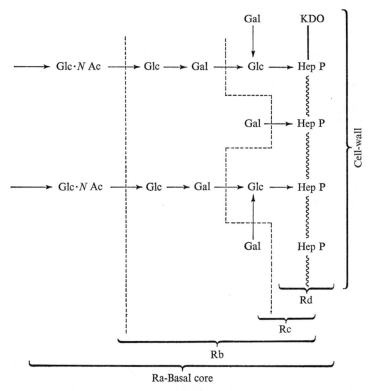

Fig. 13.—Possible structure of *Salmonella* O and R antigens. *After Lüderitz, Staub, and Westphal* [73].

one, two, or three extra sugars. In the complete O antigen the core forms only a small fraction of the polysaccharide moiety and it is assumed that the major portion consists of chains of repeating oligosaccharide units containing the specific determinants (*Fig.* 14) [73]. Heptose and KDO have not been detected in this part of the molecule.

In the Kauffmann-White scheme we have seen that *Salmonella* species are arranged on the basis of serotypes. It now becomes possible to rearrange them according to their content of sugars. Kauffmann et al. [74, 75] have done this and find that all the members so far tested fall into sixteen 'chemotypes' (*Table XI*). The simplest of these, those that belong to chemotype I, yield only the five basal sugars on chemical analysis.

Chemotype I is therefore identical in qualitative composition with chemotype Ra of the R mutants. The small number of cross-reactions between
smooth strains of chemotype I and rough mutants of chemotype Ra is
presumably due to the presence of additional oligosaccharide side-chains
in smooth strains. In general, the higher the chemotype the wider is the
variety of sugars, up to a maximum of eight (*Table XI*).

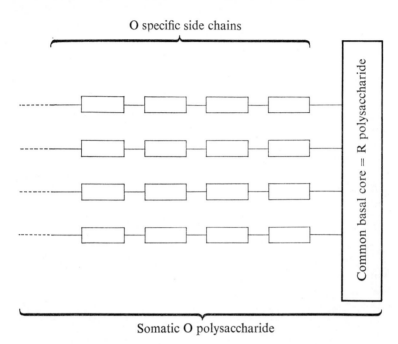

Fig. 14.—Schematic structural diagram of somatic *Salmonella* O polysaccharides.
After Lüderitz, Staub, and Westphal [73].

A number of interesting points arises from this arrangement into
chemotypes. First, it will be noted from *Table XI* that in a number of
cases single chemotypes accommodate more than one serotype. Secondly,
that the converse is not true; a serotype does not belong to more than one
chemotype. This means that identical determinants are built on carbohydrate molecules of identical composition, and in all probability identical
structure too. Thirdly, that three of the unusual 3,6-dideoxyhexoses are
associated with those species most pathogenic for man, and with three of
the most complex chemotypes (XIV, XV, XVI). Although two serogroups
belong to chemotype XIV, no chemotype has more than one of these
sugars; it follows that no serogroup can have more than one either.

We no longer find it surprising that a number of serologically distinct
substances have the same qualitative composition; it simply means that the
constituent parts are arranged differently, sequentially or spatially. For
instance, D-glucose and D-galactose can theoretically form more than fifty

Table XI.—CHEMOTYPES OF *Salmonella*. *After Lüderitz, Staub, and Westphal* [73]

Chemotype	D-Glucosamine	2-Keto-3-deoxy-octonate	L-Glycero-D-manno-heptose	D-Galactose	D-Glucose	D-Mannose	D-Galactosamine	L-Fucose	L-Rhamnose	Ribose	Colitose	Abequose	Paratose	Tyvelose	Serogroup
Re	O														
Rd	O	O													
Rc	O	O	O												
Rb	O	O	O	O											RI
Ra	O	O	O	O	O										RII
I	O	O	O	O	O										J, V, X, Y, 58
II	O	O	O	O	O		Δ								L, P, 51, 55
III	O	O	O	O	O	Δ									C_1, C_4, H, S
IV	O	O	O	O	O	Δ	Δ								K, R
V	O	O	O	O	O			Δ							W
VI	O	O	O	O	O	Δ	Δ								G, N, U
VII	O	O	O	O	O				Δ						T, 59
VIII	O	O	O	O	O	Δ			Δ						M, $(28_1, 28_3)$ 53, 57
XXV	O	O	O	O	O					Δ					52
IX	O	O	O	O	O	Δ			Δ						M, $(28_1, 28_2)$ 56
X	O	O	O	O	O						Δ				O
XI	O	O	O	O	O	Δ					Δ				Z
XII	O	O	O	O	O	Δ	Δ	Δ							I, Q
XIII	O	O	O	O	O	Δ			Δ						E, F, 54
XIV	O	O	O	O	O	Δ			Δ			Δ			B, C_2, C_3
XV	O	O	O	O	O	Δ			Δ				Δ		A
XVI	O	O	O	O	O	Δ			Δ					Δ	D1, D2

Δ = Present in side-chains. O = Present in basal core.

disaccharide structures depending on whether they are in the form of pyranoses or furanoses, α- or β-linked, and whether the link is 1:2, 1:3, 1:4, or 1:6. Which of these structures is actually formed depends on the relevant metabolic processes involved and on the stability of the resulting compound. Thus furanosides are less stable than pyranosides, so that in practice each theoretical possibility is not equally likely.

However this may be, serological cross-reactions between salmonellae and related genera have been noted in cases where the qualitative composition of their respective O polysaccharides is similar. It will be seen in *Table XI*, for instance, that chemotype Ra of R-forms is identical with

Table XII.—CHEMOTYPES OF Escherichia coli. After Lüderitz, Staub, and Westphal [73]

Chemotype	Glucosamine	2-Keto-3-deoxy-octonate	Heptose	Galactose	Glucose	Mannose	Galactosamine	2,6-Dideoxy-2-amino hexose*	Fucose	Rhamnose	6-Deoxy-talose	Colitose
I	O	O	O	O	O							
II	O	O	O	O	O	△						
III	O	O	O	O	O	O	△					
IV	O	O	O	O	O	O	△	△				
V	O	O	O	O	O			△				
VI	O	O	O	O	O		△	△				
VII	O	O	O	O	O				△			
VIII	O	O	O	O	O		△		△			
X	O	O	O	O	O							△
XI	O	O	O	O	O		△					△
XII	O	O	O	O	O	O	△	△		△		
XIII	O	O	O	O	O	O	△			△		
XVII	O	O	O		O		△					
XVIII	O	O	O	O	O		△			△		
XIX	O	O	O		O		△			△		
XX	O	O	O	O	O			△				
XXI	O	O	O	O	O			△		△		
XXII	O	O	O	O	O			△			△	
XXIII	O	O	O	O	O				△			
XXIV	O	O	O	O	O	△				△	△	

Symbols as in Table XI.

* The dideoxyhexosamines in these two columns are distinct.

chemotype I of S-forms and cross-reactions between these two groups do occur. The influence of an uncommon sugar-like colitose would also be expected to have a disproportionately large effect, and though it is found in two serogroups, of chemotypes X and XI, it is of considerable interest to find that Escherichia coli types O 111 and O 55 belong to these same two chemotypes. Indeed, the close relationship between different genera of Enterobacteriaceae is reflected in the fact that 12 out of the first 13 chemotypes of salmonellae are the same as chemotypes of E. coli (Table XII) [73].

When we study the complex serological relationships within a genus like Salmonella we are faced with two possibilities. First, that cross-reactions are due to the presence of the same determinant structure in two distinct species; and, second, that antiserum fails to distinguish between two similar structures. It should therefore be possible to relate serological differences to chemical differences, but the converse is not true since serological identity can mask chemical heterogeneity. In the Kauffmann-White scheme we find that a number of somatic factors is present in more than one serogroup and this is certainly an indication that at least very similar chemical groupings are present in the members of different groups. But, if we are to understand the real implications in chemical terms then we must take account of the fact that the serology of the whole genus has been built on the basis of antisera produced in the rabbit. The use of horse, goat, and hen antisera would probably have resulted in quite a different classification and almost certainly a less useful one from a diagnostic point of view because such antisera frequently react with monosaccharide units, whereas rabbit antibodies are never directed against a unit smaller than a disaccharide.

Thus O factors in the Kauffmann-White scheme always represent determinants of at least this size, but since they may be bigger, anomalies can still arise. As an example we can cite factor 1 which is often found in association with other group factors, such as factor 19 of group E_4. Serological studies with rabbit antisera indicate that the reaction with factor 1 is maximally inhibited by the disaccharide α-glucose-(1$\rightarrow$6)-galactose, whereas the tetrasaccharide α-glucose-(1$\rightarrow$6)-galactose-(1$\rightarrow$6)-mannose-(1$\rightarrow$4)-rhamnose is a much more potent inhibitor of factor 19 [73]. Similar observations have been made in the case of factors 1 and 37 in group G, and in group B where factor 1 can be differentiated into two specificities, 1 and 1_{12}. Like 19, 1_{12} has the terminal structure α-glucose-(1$\rightarrow$6)-galactose to which is linked mannose and possibly rhamnose. That factors 1_{12}, 19, 37, and others that are associated with factor 1 can be distinguished serologically is presumptive evidence that in many cases the determinants of O antigens are at least tetrasaccharides. The main point of interest, however, is that factor 1 is a terminal disaccharide common to a number of other O factors, with which it is therefore found in association, and that it exists as a serological entity to some extent by virtue of the way in which the rabbit responds to antigenic stimuli. The analogy between this situation and the population of antibodies directed against different-sized determinants of dextran is obvious (see p. 48).

Regardless of whether an antideterminant is directed against one, two, or more sugar units, uncommon sugars like the 3,6-dideoxyhexoses can reasonably be expected to have a strong influence on specificity. All the more is this so when it is appreciated that this class of sugars is always terminally placed; a situation in which they would again be expected to exert a maximum effect, although this statement will be qualified later on. Deoxy- and to a greater extent dideoxy-sugars are lipophilic and it is tempting to speculate, as has been done, that this property is associated with increased pathogenicity. So far five out of the eight possible isomers have been found in bacteria, namely: abequose, colitose, paratose, tyvelose, and ascarylose—the last in *Pasteurella pseudotuberculosis*. The structures of these interesting sugars, only recently described in materials of biological origin, are shown in *Fig.* 15, where fucose and rhamnose are included for comparison.

As with the blood-group active substances, the chemical structure of the O-factor determinants has been studied by chemical analysis of poly-saccharide hydrolysates and by serological inhibition tests. The probable structure of some of them is set out in *Table XIII*. Inspection of these and of the table of chemotypes will show that abequose and colitose are each found in more than one serogroup. Once again the distinction is made

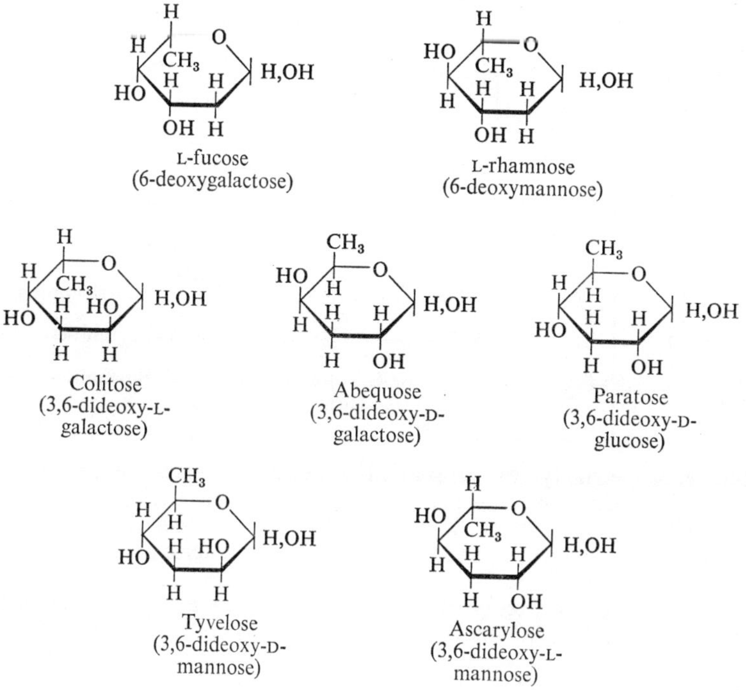

L-fucose
(6-deoxygalactose)

L-rhamnose
(6-deoxymannose)

Colitose
(3,6-dideoxy-L-galactose)

Abequose
(3,6-dideoxy-D-galactose)

Paratose
(3,6-dideoxy-D-glucose)

Tyvelose
(3,6-dideoxy-D-mannose)

Ascarylose
(3,6-dideoxy-L-mannose)

Fig. 15.

with rabbit antisera, whereas strong cross-reactions can be obtained with horse and goat antisera. A remarkable similarity in composition and sequence can also be detected among the serogroups listed in *Table XIII*. In groups B, D, and E the sequence galactose–mannose–rhamnose recurs constantly, indicating that there may be a fairly close relationship between them. Studies of biosynthetic mechanisms leading to the production of these oligosaccharides suggest, however, that there are even closer relation-ships between groups A, B, and D [76].

The similarity of structures of O factors within a single serogroup is even more striking, and in many respects analogies can be found between the oligosaccharides of *Salmonella* O antigens and ABH blood-group substances. In both cases, for instance, several different specificities are carried on each polysaccharide molecule and they cannot be separated from each other either chemically or serologically. A sequential addition of sugars leading to the formation of different specificities is also thought to occur in the case of *Salmonella* oligosaccharides [77], as well as those of blood-group substances. Workers in these two fields have interpreted their results rather differently when it comes to considering the way in which the respective determinants are arranged on oligosaccharide side-chains. In the case of soluble blood-group substances, carrying, for

Table XIII.—Possible Incomplete Structural Formulae of Some *Salmonella* O Factor Determinants. *After Lüderitz, Staub, and Westphal* [73]

O Factors	Serogroup	Oligosaccharide
1	B, E_4, G	α-Glucose-(1→6)-galactose
1_{12}	B	α-Glucose-(1→6)-galactose→mannose→rhamnose
3	$E_{1, 2, 3, 4}$	Mannose→rhamnose→galactose
4	B	Abequose-(1→3)-β-mannose-(1→4)-rhamnose
8	C_2	Abequose→
9	D	Tyvelose→mannose→rhamnose
10	E_1	α-Acetylgalactose→mannose→rhamnose
12_2	D	α-Glucose-(1→4)-α-galactose→mannose→rhamnose
15	E	β-Galactose→mannose→rhamnose
19	E_4	α-Glucose-(1→6)-α-galactose-(1→6)-α-mannose-(1→4)-rhamnose
34	E_3	α-Glucose-(1→4)-β-galactose-(1→6)-α-mannose-(1→4)-rhamnose

instance, A specificity, it is supposed that not all side-chains are completed so that, depending on the genetic pathway involved, H and Lewis specificities may also be present on the shorter chains. Such chains are not necessarily serologically active perhaps because of steric hindrance by the longer A-specific chains.

In the case of O factors of salmonellae there is evidence of a rather different mechanism in which different parts of a complete side-chain are thought to operate as determinants. If we take *Salmonella* group B as an example we find from the table of chemotypes that in addition to the basal sugars three others, D-mannose, L-rhamnose, and abequose, are present; and from the Kauffmann-White table that O factors 1, 4, 5, 12, and 27 are represented in the group. The situation is in fact a good deal more complex even than this would indicate because factor 4 can be subdivided into 4_1 and 4_2, factor 1 into 1 and 1_{12}, and factor 12 into 12_1, 12_2, and 12_3. With the exception of 12_3 all these (and others) are found in group B, though, as we shall see, they cannot all be present on the same oligosaccharide unit. *Fig.* 16 [73] illustrates the way in which different determinants could be related to distinct, but sometimes overlapping, areas of oligosaccharide-repeating units. The thickness of the lines represents the affinity of specific antiserum for the corresponding part of the structure. It is clear from the diagram that abequose plays a dominant role in the specificity of factors 4_1 and 4_2, factor 4 being the group-specific determinant. Factor 5 is at least a trisaccharide with acetylgalactose the dominant sugar, which would account for the absence of this factor in variants of group B in which the acetyl radical is missing. Mild acid hydrolysis removes the acetyl group and also destroys factor 5 specificity. In group E_1 (3, 10), although α-acetyl-galactose is present, it is linked 1→6 to mannose instead of 1→4 as in factor 5. The distinction between the subspecificities of factor 1 is also made apparent in the diagram, a disaccharide constituting factor 1 and at least a tetrasaccharide in the case of

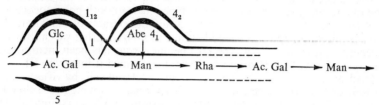

Fig. 16.—Diagrammatic arrangement of immunodominant sugars in group B salmonellae. *After Lüderitz, Staub, and Westphal* [73].

factor 1_{12}. Though abequose does not seem to be part of the determinant of 1_{12}, serologically this factor does not behave in quite the same way in groups B and D, presumably because in the latter tyvelose replaces abequose. It would appear to be impossible to have the specificities of factors 1 and 12_2 on the same oligosaccharide unit since factor 1 is associated with a 1→6 link between glucose and galactose and factor 12_2 with a 1→4 link.

Lüderitz, Staub, and Westphal [73] are insistent that 'the sugar component of O factors best adapted to the specific sites of antibodies . . . is not necessarily a non-reducing terminal sugar'. Here lies the main difference in outlook of workers in the fields of blood-group serology and bacterial polysaccharides. The point is rather well illustrated in the case of bacteria by factor 34 of group E_3 where glucose is the best *mono*saccharide inhibitor of the 34-anti-34 system, but the heptasaccharide

$$Gal→Man→Rha→Gal→Man→Rha$$
$$\uparrow$$
$$Glu$$

inhibits better than the tetrasaccharide

$$Gal→Man→Rha,$$
$$\uparrow$$
$$Glu$$

although glucose is strictly terminal only in the latter. Similar phenomena have been observed with pneumococcal polysaccharides [78]. Lüderitz et al. [73] have coined the term 'immunodominant sugar' to describe those monosaccharides that display the greatest affinity for specific antibody since 'terminal sugar' which used to carry this connotation no longer seems adequate.

Notwithstanding the repeating nature of the side-chains attached to the pentasaccharide core, it is not to be supposed that all identical structures along a side-chain are serologically active because steric hindrance will prevent antibody coming in contact with all of them. This is borne out experimentally by the observation that only a few antibody molecules react with each polysaccharide molecule.

γ. Lysogenic Conversion: The antigenic structure of bacteria is an inherited character and subject to mutational change in just the same way as any other recognizable character. Alteration of the genetic apparatus is not necessarily an endogenous process, however, but may result from the introduction of genetic material from without.

The classic example of this kind of induced variation is the transformation of a rough pneumococcus of one type into a smooth pneumococcus of another type by exposing the former to suitable extracts of the latter. The transforming principle has been identified as DNA, so that we can say that a genetic unit from, say, a type III pneumococcus has been incorporated into one of, say, type II origin and has transformed it into type III.

Nuclear material can also be carried into bacterial cells by viruses. Such viruses, or bacteriophages, may be either virulent, in which case they kill the infected organism, or they may be temperate and have no immediately lethal effect on the host. Under certain conditions temperate phages become virulent and bacteria carrying them are therefore called 'lysogenic'. Some strains of temperate phages that infect salmonellae have been shown to induce antigenic changes in their hosts, and such a process is referred to as 'lysogenic conversion'.

As an example we can take the conversion of *Salmonella uganda* of serotype E_1. Exposure of this organism to autolysates of salmonellae in group E_2 containing the temperate phage ϵ-15 converts *S. uganda* into *S. newington*. The antigenic expression of this change is from somatic factors 3, 10 to factors 3, 15; and chemically the change is from a terminal α-acetylgalactose to β-galactose (*Table XIV*). By a similar process the temperate phage ϵ-34 converts *S. newington*, 3, 15 into *S. illinois*, (3), (15), 34, the chemical equivalent in this case being the addition of a terminal glucose (*Table XIV*).

Table XIV.—MODIFICATION OF ANTIGENIC DETERMINANTS BY LYSOGENIC CONVERSION

Salmonella SPECIES	ANTIGENIC FACTOR	STRUCTURE OF DETERMINANT
S. uganda 3, 10	10	α-Acetylgalactose-$(1\rightarrow6)$-α-mannose-$(1\rightarrow4)$-rhamnose$\rightarrow$
S. newington 3, 15	15	β-Galactose-$(1\rightarrow6)$-α-mannose-$(1\rightarrow4)$-rhamnose$\rightarrow$
S. illinois (3), (15), 34	34	α-Glucose-$(1\rightarrow4)$-β-galactose-$(1\rightarrow6)$-α-mannose-$(1\rightarrow4)$-rhamnose$\rightarrow$

The precise mechanism by which phages induce these alterations is not known. It must be presumed, however, that the action is highly specific and that phage ϵ-34 is not capable of inducing the appearance of factor 34 in members of any serological group; the cell itself must have the capacity to be infected (and changed) by a particular phage. It is all the more interesting then to find that after conversion of members of groups A, B, and D_1 by phage 27 they all acquire a new factor, D 27, and now cross-react with salmonellae of group E. This not only substantiates the close relationship between groups A, B, and D_1, but also indicates a much closer relationship between groups D_1 and E than is apparent from an inspection of the Kauffmann-White scheme, in the sense that the biosynthetic pathway of group E organisms could resemble that of groups A, B, and D. Lysogenic conversion thus not only tells us something about the relationships of factors within a serogroup, but also about relationships between groups.

8. *Classification*: In hierarchical classification systems we are always searching for the most fundamental properties of the members of a group in order that we may arrange them in a systematic fashion. Rather naturally the tendency nowadays is to give greatest weight to properties that are a direct reflection of genetic constitution. For the reasons already advanced a number of times we can regard the Kauffmann-White scheme, based as it is on antigenic characters, as a genetic classification, albeit somewhat incomplete. To what extent it is justifiable to base a classification on the structure of a few molecules remains debatable. The tabulation of salmonellae and escherichiae into chemotypes would seem to be less helpful in the context of classification, especially as in both genera a number of serogroups fall into the same chemotypes. What this arrangement has done is to pinpoint similarities and differences between species and genera, and to indicate areas in which a search might be made for hitherto unsuspected relationships.

Much has been learned of the antigenic structure of Enterobacteriaceae by the study of their serological reactions and by lysogenic conversion, but the ultimate goal in this respect must be the definition of chemical structure and the metabolic pathways by which such structures are formed. Though a formidable task, even considering just the salmonellae, the possibilities of such an approach are already apparent. To what extent the other members of the Enterobacteriaceae could be fitted into the same system of classification remains uncertain. The fact that *Escherichia* and *Salmonella* species have nine chemotypes in common suggests that some members of these two groups of organisms may be more closely related than was thought to be the case. As yet, however, it is only in salmonellae that one important part of polysaccharide molecule, the basal core, has been studied in any detail, and if major differences were discovered here it would suggest that these two genera should still be kept separate.

C. Lipid Antigens

1. NOMENCLATURE AND STRUCTURE

Lipids are either simple or compound. Simple lipids are neutral oils, fats, and waxes of animal and vegetable origin. Oils and fats consist mainly of triglycerides formed from three molecules of fatty acid and one of glycerol. Waxes are fatty-acid esters of the higher alcohols of the methyl alcohol series. We are not much concerned with simple lipids as such since they appear to play little or no part in immunological reactions.

Compound lipids are again subdivided into phospholipids (phosphatides) and glycolipids. The classification and nomenclature of these compounds are rather more confused than those of simple lipids; named substances or classes of substances are frequently composed of bases and fatty acids of different chain length and degree of saturation.

Phospholipids are derivatives of phosphatidic acid and are essential components of vegetable and animal cells. Among the best known are the lecithins, containing two fatty acids, glycerol, and a phosphatidyl choline group (*Fig.* 17). In other closely related compounds the choline base is replaced by ethanolamine or the hydroxy-amino-acid serine $(CH_2OH \cdot CH(NH_2) \cdot COOH)$. Lecithin is of peculiar interest in that it was used in the old experiments on combination immunization (*see* p. 80).

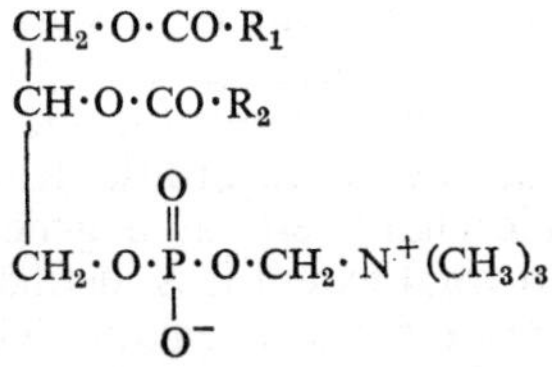

$$CH_2 \cdot O \cdot CO \cdot R_1$$
$$CH \cdot O \cdot CO \cdot R_2$$
$$\overset{\displaystyle O}{\underset{\displaystyle O^-}{CH_2 \cdot O \cdot \overset{\parallel}{P} \cdot O \cdot CH_2 \cdot N^+(CH_3)_3}}$$

Fig. 17.—Lecithin.

A separate category of substances are the so-called 'sphingolipids', a biologically important group of compounds distinguished by their content of sphingosine and numbering among their members both phospholipids and glycolipids. Sphingosine is a long-chain aliphatic hydrocarbon with an amino group at carbon 2, through which it is linked to a fatty acid to form a ceramide. Lignocerylsphingosine is a ceramide of liver (*Fig.* 18). Sphingomyelin, one of the three important sphingolipids, is present in the myelin sheaths of nerves. It is a ceramide (*N*-acyl-sphingosine) to which phosphorylcholine is attached at carbon 1 of sphingosine. An immunological role for sphingomyelin has not been demonstrated as yet.

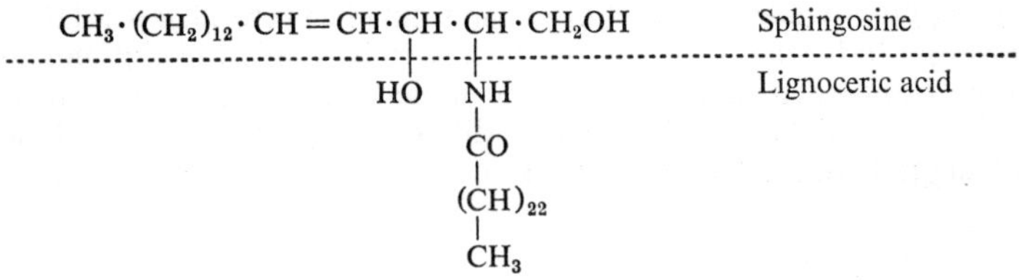

$$CH_3 \cdot (CH_2)_{12} \cdot CH = CH \cdot CH \cdot CH \cdot CH_2OH \qquad \text{Sphingosine}$$
$$\text{HO} \quad \text{NH} \qquad\qquad\qquad\qquad \text{Lignoceric acid}$$
$$\text{CO}$$
$$(CH)_{22}$$
$$CH_3$$

Fig. 18.—Ceramide.

As the name implies, glycolipids contain a carbohydrate moiety. Many of them are ceramides and therefore contain sphingosine. The fatty-acid component is very variable and though this is doubtless biologically important, it has little or no influence on immunological specificity, as we know from Landsteiner's work on fatty acids (q.v.), and as we shall see later.

Glycolipids have been authoritatively reviewed recently [79]. The authors state, 'their nomenclature is both confusing and contradictory'. Before discussing in somewhat more detail the immunologically important glycolipids, we would mention the glycosyl glycerides of plants and algae, which because of their sugar content might be expected to determine specificity; if so, their immunological study could contribute to better understanding of their biochemistry. The same can be said of the unusual phytoglycolipids, also of plants, that combine the structural features of glycolipids and phospholipids. The lipids of mycobacteria too have long excited curiosity and a number have been more or less characterized. The relatively insoluble wax D is apparently a mucolipid (*see later*); the type-specific mycosides are glycolipids, and have a characteristic O-methylated-deoxy hexose terminal sugar; and the almost unique, so-called 'phospho-lipids' of mycobacteria are, like the phytoglycolipids above, both glycolipids and phospholipids. They carry a terminal mannose structure.

Glycolipids of mammalian tissues are based on the ceramide structure and are frequently referred to as glycosphingolipids. The carbohydrate component is attached through carbon 1 of sphingosine (*see Fig.* 18). Hexosamines and sulphate esters of hexose sugars are commonly found in the carbohydrate moiety. So far as we are aware, no immunological work has been done with these sulphate esters, but in view of the strong influence of acid radicals that Landsteiner detected in haptens, one would expect them to play an important role.

Cerebrosides are the simplest of the glycolipids: they consist of ceramide with an additional hexose sugar. Naturally occurring ceramide-mono-hexosides are either gluco- or galactocerebrosides. They are character-istically found in the white matter of brain and in the myelin sheaths of nerves; they also occur in the leaves of plants. The principal fatty-acid components of cerebrosides vary in chain length at least from C_{18} to C_{24}; minor components vary in chain length, hydroxylation, and degree of saturation. An example of an immunologically active cerebroside is kerasin (phrenosin) which is N-lignoceryl-galactosyl-sphingosine.

Ceramide-oligosaccharides have two or more hexose units. Nomen-clature has been complicated by the introduction of the term 'cytoside' for ceramide-disaccharides. Ceramide-trisaccharides have been isolated from blood serum and normal human kidney. Hexosamine and sulphate-ester derivatives could also be included in this group. Cytolipin K, an antigen found in tumour tissues, is a ceramide-trihexoside-galactosamine; and globoside, abundant in red-cell stroma, is chemically N-acetyl-galactos-aminoyl-(1→6)galactosyl-(1→4)galactosyl-(1→4)-glucosyl-ceramide. The wide-ranging function of these glycolipids, and the specificity they display, are suggested by the fact that a red-cell receptor for haemagglutinating enterovirus has been identified as a ceramide-trihexoside-galactosamine.

Gangliosides are still more complex, and besides glucose, galactose, and galactosamine, in varying proportions, contain sialic acid. Sialic acid is the generic name for N-acyl-neuraminic acid; the acyl radical being N-acetyl, diacetyl, or glycolyl. Gangliosides are thus sialic acid containing glyco-sphingolipids. The four major gangliosides isolated from human and bovine brain have a common basic structure: galactosyl-N-acetyl-galactos-aminoyl-galactosyl-glucosyl-ceramide, to which one to three molecules of sialic acid are attached.

Gangliosides are characteristically obtained from ganglion cells of grey matter, but are also found in other organs, e.g., bovine spleen, red blood-cells. There is some evidence that in brain tissue they are present as

macromolecular polymers of the basic unit. It is a matter of pure speculation whether these large structures are necessary for the specialized
functions of ganglion cells.

Finally there are the *mucolipids*, which like the endotoxins of Gram-
negative bacteria contain lipid, carbohydrate, and peptide fractions. They
differ from mucoids (mucoproteins) in having a lipid part, and from
glycolipids in having a polypeptide part. They are soluble in water like the
former and in organic solvents like the latter.

Mucolipids are of interest immunologically since the Forssman antigen
would appear to be such a substance (*see* HETEROPHILE ANTIGENS, p. 86).

Complex lipids thus constitute a series of substances of increasing
complexity and size, beginning with monomeric cerebrosides, through
gangliosides, to mucolipids. In the last category a glyco-lipo-sialo-protein
with enzymic properties has been described in which it is suggested that
the high molecular weight is not a consequence of polymerization but of
true chemical union, linking together sialic acid-rich gangliosides [80].

2. ANTIGENICITY OF LIPIDS

Early work with lipids soon demonstrated that they were neither very
antigenic nor very specific. The latter gave rise to the concept of 'ubiquitous' lipids. It was shown, however, that lipid haptens could be converted
into complete antigens simply by mixing them with proteins *in vitro*.
Stimulation of antibody production by such mixtures has been called
'immunization by combination'; the antibodies produced react with both
lipid and protein moieties.

Immunization by combination differs from other procedures in a
number of ways. (1) The activating protein must be antigenic itself. It
must normally be derived from a donor of different species from the
recipient, which is not the case when haptens are attached to protein
by substitution and conjugation methods. (2) Activation takes place on
simple mixing of protein and lipid *in vitro*, though not if they are injected
separately. (3) Immunization is successful only with alcohol-soluble
substances, e.g., with a Forssman hapten obtained by alcoholic extraction
of horse kidney, or with chemically well-defined substances such as phosphatides. Other kinds of haptens, e.g., polysaccharides, must be conjugated
with proteins in order to become complete antigens.

It was shown many years ago that lipids were activated by adsorption to
particulate matter such as kaolin, charcoal, etc., as well as by combination
with proteins [81]. These experiments were performed with chemically
undefined lipids. Recently it has been demonstrated that the glycolipid of
myelin, in the form of crude extracts of brain, spinal cord, and nerves, can
also be made immunogenic by the addition of Freund's adjuvant, whereas
the chromatographically pure cerebroside needs both Freund's adjuvant
and some other protein to make it strongly immunogenic.

The lipids of serum can be extracted with organic fat solvents without
any loss or change of antigenicity in the serum lipoproteins, which suggests
that their specificity is not influenced by the lipid fraction. The lipid A and
B fractions of Boivin antigens (endotoxins) too are not necessary for their
specificity. It is easy enough to account for specificity in such antigens by
implicating carbohydrate and polypeptide determinants, but in the older

work quoted above neither antigenicity nor specificity can be explained so easily. Admittedly extracts of tissues made with organic solvents contain a wide variety of lipids, perhaps including both glycolipids and mucolipids, but in other cases phosphatides, e.g., lecithin, have been used for immunization by combination. If there is any degree of specificity displayed by such substances it seems unlikely that it would be due to the long-chain fatty-acid moieties, since they have an essentially monotonous structure. In the case of lecithin (*Fig.* 17) the phosphatidyl-choline group could perhaps be implicated in the determinant. However, the outstanding case of specificity associated with a phospholipid is cardiolipin.

Cardiolipin is the active principle in tissue extracts used as 'antigens' in the Wassermann and other reactions for the detection of antibodies in syphilitic sera. It is of interest that the sensitivity of such tests is enhanced by the addition of lecithin and cholesterol to the tissue extracts or to cardiolipin itself. The general formula of cardiolipin is shown in *Fig.* 19, where R indicates the acyl radical of a fatty acid. In ox-heart cardiolipin 80 per cent of the fatty acid is in the form of linoleic acid. In comparative tests with ox-heart and synthetic cardiolipin no significant difference in

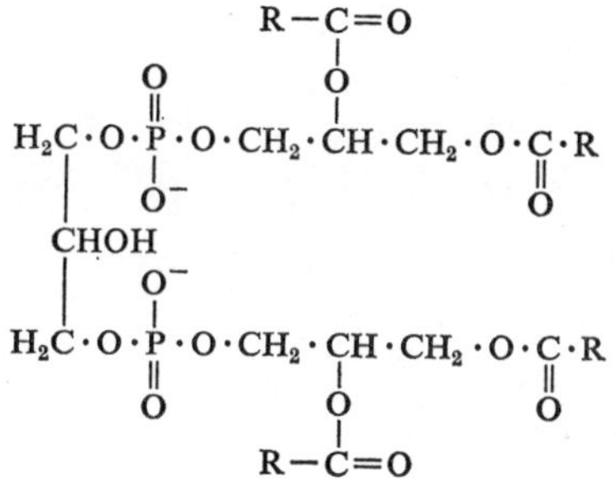

Fig. 19.—Cardiolipin. *After Grey and Macfarlane* [82].

reaction was found, although the latter contained stearic and oleic acids in equimolar amounts instead of linoleic acid [83]. This would seem to indicate that in the phospholipids we have a class of substances in which neither carbohydrate nor oligopeptide structures play any part in deter-mining specificity.

Lipids are widely distributed in tissues, and indeed in living matter as a whole, and since the greater part of the molecule appears to exert no in-fluence on specificity, little room is left in the remainder of the molecule for chemical and immunological variation, and presuming the major biological role of lipids is inherent in their lipidic properties there would be little necessity for variation as well. Perhaps it is for these reasons that antisera to lipids obtained from any one organ display such a broad spectrum of reactivity towards lipids derived from other sources, and which earned lipids the title 'ubiquitous' with an older generation of immunologists.

3. Glycolipids of Tissues

Glycolipids are now an active area of investigation because of an increasing awareness of their biological importance. Though many of their functions remain obscure, their presence in large amounts in central and peripheral nervous tissues indicates that they play a major role in the proper functioning of these structures. In some form, too, they are present in all types of cells, and gangliosides in particular have remarkable properties. They can associate with both hydrophilic and hydrophobic groups, can form micelles at very low concentrations, and are present in relatively high concentrations in mitochondrial and microsomal fractions. There and in cell membranes they may have special functions. There is already some indication that gangliosides are concerned in the active transport of acetylcholine from synaptic vesicles, and that they are involved in the active transport of calcium by serotonin through the cell membrane. In higher mammals the pattern of gangliosides is more complex than in lower ones, though differences in the various anatomical regions of the brain have not so far been found. It is to be hoped that the immunological study of glycolipids, and especially of gangliosides and mucolipids, will contribute to a better understanding of the structure and functioning of the brain.

Cerebrosides, ceramide-oligosaccharides, and gangliosides probably all function as antigens under certain circumstances and more generally as haptens. An immunological background involving glycolipids in the pathogenetic mechanisms of a number of pathological processes is being reported with increasing frequency. For instance, anticerebroside antibodies have been found in the serum and cerebrospinal fluid of rabbits with experimental 'allergic' encephalitis [84, 85]. It has been shown too that kerasin (phrenosin) is one of the organ-specific haptens of brain [86], and that anti-brain serum reacts with natural and synthetic galactocerebrosides providing they are properly combined with auxiliary lipids such as lecithin and cholesterol. Since the simplest ceramide-glycosides can function as haptens, and the role of carbohydrates as antigenic determinants is now well documented, it is not too far fetched perhaps to speculate that all glycosphingolipids are haptenic and that their specificity is determined by the carbohydrate moiety.

That this is so in a number of instances has already been shown. In the case of cerebrosides, distinct serological specificities characterize different ceramide-monosaccharides [86]; also serological activity remains with a sphingosine-galactoside moiety when the fatty acid is split off a cerebroside [85]. Rapport et al. [87] have obtained similar evidence about cytolipin 'H', a ceramide-oligosaccharide derived from human tumours. Serological inhibition tests indicate that the specificity of cytolipin 'H' is due to lactose. This is confirmed by the finding that antiserum to a protein-azophenyl-lactose antigen cross-reacts with cytolipin 'H'; and that synthetic ceramide-lactose, tested with adequate amounts of auxiliary lipids, reacts in essentially the same way as the natural substance. Finally, it would seem that in more complex gangliosides carbohydrates again determine specificity; in this case galactose and N-acetylneuraminic acid are incriminated. It is of interest, however, that NANA is also present in

ABH blood-group substances but has not been identified as part of the determinant in that system.

We are bound to conclude that differences in carbohydrate composition determine the major serological distinctions in this group of organic molecules, and that differences in chain length in the fatty-acid components play relatively little, if any, part as was foreshadowed by Landsteiner's work (*see* p. 42).

4. GLYCOLIPIDS OF RED BLOOD-CELLS

It has been known for some time that blood-group substances are present in human beings in two forms: that is to say, in a water-soluble form in secretions and in an alcohol-soluble form in red blood-cells. Because the water-soluble substances were readily available in large amounts most of the early work on the structure of determinants, etc., was confined to this material. In recent years, however, methods have been devised for extracting blood-group substances from erythrocytes and a start has been made in determining the structure of blood-group antigens on the surface of red cells and elucidating the genetic pathways through which they are elaborated.

All the active extracts contain residues of glucose, galactose, glucosamine, galactosamine, fucose, sialic acid, sphingosine, and fatty acid. Lignoceric ($CH_3(CH_2)_{22}COOH$) and behenic ($CH_3(CH_2)_{20}COOH$) acids are the major fatty-acid components. No amino-acids have been detected. The terminal sugars characteristic of soluble A and B blood-group substances are therefore present in red-cell glycolipids, though it must be admitted that a large part of isolated glycolipids do not possess any ABH specificity: for instance, the globoside mentioned earlier under 'ceramide-oligosaccharides', even though the terminal sugar is GNAc and might be expected to carry A specificity. This can still be explained by invoking structural differences in the two oligosaccharide chains. On the other hand, anti-A_{hel}, a snail extract with anti-A-like specificity, is thought to react with all structures possessing terminal GNAc, but unexpectedly fails to do so with the above globoside. It has been suggested that this is because GNAc, though terminal, is so built into the molecule that it is serologically unavailable [88]. That identical structures are present in red-cell glycolipids and soluble substances is suggested by the following immunological evidence.

a. Antisera prepared against A-specific soluble substance or red-cell antigen give lines of coalescence in gel-diffusion tests when tested with both antigens. The same is true of anti-B sera and B antigens. This is generally regarded as evidence of serological identity, and therefore of a common determinant structure.

b. Precipitation of both A-active glycolipid and A-active mucopolysaccharide by the lectin of *D. biflorus* is inhibited by *N*-acetyl-galactosamine. Similarly rabbit antisera to both substances are inhibited by identical *di*saccharides.

c. The blood-group activity of A-active glycolipid and of A-active mucopolysaccharide is destroyed by the specific enzyme of *Trichomonas foetus*, and in both cases the action of the enzyme is inhibited by *N*-acetylgalactosamine.

d. After treating A substance from both red cells and secretions with enzymes from *T. foetus*, strong cross-reactions are observed with pneumococcus type XIV antigen.

These observations indicate that at least the terminal disaccharide of A-active mucopolysaccharides and glycolipids is identical, and the same is probably true of B substances [47].

The essential difference between blood-group substances in secretions and red cells is thus seen as lying in the fraction to which the carbohydrate portion is bound: ceramide in the case of red cells, and polypeptide in the case of secretions. This arrangement in red cells receives further support from the finding that red-cell stromata from which the glycolipid is extracted concurrently lose most of their blood-group activity. A provisional formula for glycolipid from human red blood-cells is shown in *Fig*. 20. It differs from the formula of tumour glycolipids only in that R represents the carbohydrate structure characteristic of the various blood-group specificities.

Sphingosine-R
|
Lignoceric acid

Fig. 20.—General formula for red-cell glycolipids.

As with mucopolysaccharides the overall chemical composition of glycolipids does not tell us much about blood-group specificity. Presumably here again specificity is due rather to differences in sequence and spatial arrangement. Further, it would seem that even within a single individual the fatty-acid composition of blood-group active glycolipids of red cells may differ: another pointer to the serologically inert nature of this component.

The serological activity of isolated glycolipids in aqueous solutions depends on their state of dispersion. On purification they may become inactive in inhibition tests, though remaining active in precipitation reactions. This can be satisfactorily explained by postulating that the 'avidity' of the glycolipid preparation is insufficient to compete with the more complementary native red-cell antigen in the inhibition reaction.

It is well known that the immunological activity of cardiolipin is greatly enhanced by the addition of lecithin and cholesterol in suitable proportions, and we have seen that the same is true for cerebrosides. A similar situation seems to obtain in the case of red-cell glycolipids [89], and attempts are also being made to produce antibodies against purified blood-group active glycolipids of red cells [90].

Molecular weights of blood-group active glycolipids are still not known, but the state of aggregation is certainly of great importance for serological activity. Red-cell glycolipids have been separated into two fractions, C I and C II [89]. Though serologically inert, fraction C I acts as a 'carrier' for C II: in other words, as an auxiliary lipid. Its action is not specific since carrier from A substance will also activate B substance.

Red-cell glycolipids can also be divided into methanol-soluble and methanol-insoluble fractions. The latter is a hundred times more active in inhibiting haemagglutination by specific antiserum than the former.

The insoluble fraction has a sedimentation coefficient of 64–70S, corresponding to a state of high aggregation. It is equally active serologically with and without the carrier C I. On the other hand, the serological activity of the methanol-soluble fraction is increased by combination with the carrier, and it has a sedimentation constant of only 11·9S. Combination of soluble and insoluble fractions decreases the sedimentation coefficient of the latter to 28·2S and its serological activity is also decreased, presumably as a result of disaggregation. This dependence of serological activity on a high level of aggregation is also shown by the fact that a disaggregated complex is reactivated by the carrier. It is probably also a much more general phenomenon since the dependence of serological activity on degree of aggregation has been noted with Forssman antigens and with various cytolipins.

Blood-group substances from secretions and red cells differ in a number of respects other than those mentioned so far.

a. Glycolipid blood-group substance contains much less fucose than the active mucopolysaccharides of secretions, and indeed no H activity is found in isolated glycolipids of A, B, and O cells when they are tested with animal or human sera, or with lectins. It is possible that in red cells H antigen is a mucopolysaccharide; alternatively, it is a glycolipid not extractable by the methods in use at the moment. It is also possible that in red cells A and B substances are formed directly from precursor substance, in contrast to the postulated sequence of events in secretions. If this is so, it will not prove possible to unmask H substance in A and B glycolipids by enzymatic action. There can be no doubt that H antigen is present, to a greater or lesser degree, in A, B, AB, and O red cells. However, it has not appeared as a serological entity in the red-cell extracts that have been studied so far.

b. The somewhat lower serological activity of red-cell glycolipids compared with mucopolysaccharides of secretions is perhaps due to some of the determinants in the former being buried within the micelles.

c. Delayed hypersensitivity reactions have not been obtained with blood-group glycolipids, presumably because the antibodies responsible for this type of reaction are mainly directed against the polypeptide moiety of blood-group active mucopolysaccharides.

d. Water-soluble blood-group substance of individuals of group AB is precipitated by either anti-A or anti-B sera, i.e., both A and B reactive sites are present on the same molecule. It has been suggested that the A and B activities of purified glycolipids of AB red cells can be separated. If confirmed, this would imply that the antigenic sites on human blood-cells, which are governed by alleles at the same locus, are on different molecules. This is probably also the situation in the serum gamma-globulin groups of rabbit and man.

e. Some enzymes that inactivate water-soluble ABH blood-group substances by splitting off certain sugars do not attack blood-group specific glycolipids in the intact cell.

5. Genetic Control of Red-cell Glycolipids

If it is true, as suggested above, that A and B substances of red cells are not formed through the intermediary of H substance, then an element of uncertainty is introduced if we try to apply the proposed genetic pathways of blood-group substances in secretions to red cells. Along these lines Wiener [91] suggests that H substance is not a precursor for A and B substances, and that all three compete in parallel for a common precursor. On the other hand, Krüpe [92] has modified the current hypothesis of sequential addition of sugars to accommodate the formation of A and B red-cell glycolipids with the previous formation of H. He assumes the production of an H determinant in red cells, governed by an O gene, that differs from the H of secretions in possessing additional structures characteristic of O specificity.

It is evident that until the discrepancy between the presence of H antigen on red cells and its absence in red-cell extracts is resolved a definitive account of genetic pathways cannot be given. Nevertheless, because so much is already known about blood-group substances, both chemically and immunologically, and because their hereditary transmission can be studied so easily, it can be readily appreciated that they provide an exceptionally useful tool for the study of human genetics, and that this usefulness will be enhanced when the genetic pathways through which these substances are governed are fully known.

D. Heterophile Antigens

Cross-reactions between phylogenetically unrelated antigens have frequently been observed. Initially, therefore, they have the appearance of being non-specific reactions. The antigens involved are known as heterophile antigens, of which the best known example is the Forssman antigen. The presence of this antigen is inferred when antisera to unrelated antigens are shown capable of lysing sheep red cells in the presence of complement. We would not nowadays accept that such reactions were non-specific, but rather that they were manifestations of the presence of the same, or nearly the same, determinants on otherwise unrelated antigens.

The somatic antigen, O 5, is apparently responsible for the Forssman specificity exhibited by some salmonellae. This is just one link in the long chain of evidence that suggests that the determinant of the Forssman antigen is a carbohydrate structure. However, the search for a single Forssman antigen may well be doomed to failure since it is not to be supposed that the surface of the sheep red cell carries a single antigenic specificity [93].

A number of heterophile antigens, of quite different specificities, are widely distributed in nature and it is probably better to eschew the term 'Forssman antigen' in the generic sense altogether, and simply include this early example in the general category of heterophile antigens.

The presence of Forssman antigen in human tissues has been widely reported. Cross-reactions between this antigen and human blood-group A substance is said to be due to sharing a common disaccharide, α-N-acetyl-galactosaminoyl-$(1\rightarrow3)$-D-galactose [94]. It is small wonder then that a 'purified' Forssman hapten derived from pooled sheep red blood-cells was found to contain, as the principal ingredients, galactose, galactosamine, lignoceric acid, and sphingosine [95].

REFERENCES

1. KOLECKI, B. J., and SPRINGER, G. F. (1965), 'Monosaccharide Structures precipitating Anti-human Blood Group H(O) Antibody', *Fedn Proc. Fedn Am. Socs exp. Biol.*, **24**, 631.
2. UHLENBRUCK, G. (1965), 'Immunchemie zellulärer und sezernierter ABH- und Lewis-Blutgruppensubstanzen', *Medsche Welt, Stuttg.*, 906.
3. WILSON, G. S., and MILES, A. A., ed. (1964), *Topley and Wilson's Principles of Bacteriology and Immunity*, 5th ed. London: Arnold.
4. SELA, M., and ARNON, R. (1960), 'Studies on the Chemical Basis of the Antigenicity of Proteins. III, The Role of Rigidity in the Antigenicity of Polypeptidyl Gelatins', *Biochem. J.*, **77**, 394.
5. CINADER, B. (1963), 'Dependence of Antibody Responses on Structure and Polymorphism of Autologous Macromolecules', *Br. med. Bull.*, **19**, 219.
6. DOWNE, A. E. R. (1955), 'Inhibition of the Production of Precipitating Antibody in Young Rabbits', *Nature, Lond.*, **176**, 740.
7. MAURER, P. H. (1964), 'Use of Synthetic Polymers of Aminoacids to study the Basis of Antigenicity', *Prog. Allergy*, **8**, 1.
8. MAURER, P. H., GERALAT, B. F., and PINCOCK, P. (1964), 'Antigenicity of Polypeptides. XII, Immunological Studies with a New Group of Synthetic Copolymers', *J. exp. Med.*, **119**, 1005.
9. SELA, M. (1966), 'Immunological Studies with Synthetic Polypeptides', *Adv. Immun.*, **5**, 29.
10. MAURER, P. H. (1954), 'The Cross Reactions between Albumins of Different Species and Gammaglobulins of Different Species', *J. Immun.*, **72**, 119.
11. LANDSTEINER, K. (1962), *The Specificity of Serological Reactions*. New York: Dover.
12. BRYSON, V., and VOGEL, H. J. (1965), *Evolving Genes and Proteins*. New York: Academic.
13. FURTH, J. (1925), 'Antigenic Character of Heated Protein', *J. Immun.*, **10**, 777.
14. HALBERT, S. P., and FITZGERALD, P. L. (1958), 'Studies on the Immunological Organ Specificity of Ocular Lens', *Am. J. Ophthal.*, **46**, 187.
15. HALBERT, S. P., MANSKI, W., and AUERBACH, I. (1961), 'Lens Antigen and Evolution', in *The Structure of the Eye* (ed. SMELZER, G. K.). New York: Academic.
16. FRANCOIS, J. R. M., WIEM, R. J., and KAMINSKI, M. (1956), 'Study of the Antigens of the Crystalline Lens', *Am. J. Ophthal.*, **42**, 577.
17. MILGROM, F., TUGGAC, M., and WITEBSKY, E. (1963), 'Immunological Studies on Adrenal Glands. III, Interspecies Relations of Thermostable Adrenal-specific Antigens', *Immunology*, **6**, 105.
18. ROSE, N. R., METZGAR, R. S., and WITEBSKY, E. (1960), 'Studies on Organ Specificity. XI, Isoantigens of Rabbit Pancreas', *J. Immun.*, **85**, 575.
19. CARPENTER, P. L. (1956), *Immunology and Serology*. Philadelphia: Saunders.
20. KARUSH, F., and EISEN, H. N. (1962), 'A Theory of Delayed Hypersensitivity', *Science, N.Y.*, **136**, 1032.
21. SPRINGER, G. F., and WILLIAMSON, P. (1962), 'Immunochemical Significance of L- and D-Fucose Derivatives', *Biochem. J.*, **85**, 282.
22. KABAT, E. A. (1962), 'Structural Similarities of Methylated D- and L-Fucose Derivatives as seen in Three Dimensional Models', *Biochem. J.*, **85**, 291.
23. POLLOCK, M. R. (1963), 'Penicillinase-antipenicillinase', *Ann. N.Y. Acad. Sci.*, **103**, 989.
24. MILLS, J. A., and HABER, E. (1963), 'The Effect on Antigenic Specificity of Changes in the Molecular Structure of Ribonuclease', *J. Immun.*, **91**, 536.
25. BERSON, S. A., and YALOW, R. S. (1961), 'Immunochemical Distinction between Insulins with Identical Amino-acid Sequences', *Nature, Lond.*, **191**, 1392.
26. CINADER, B. (1963), 'Introduction: Immunochemistry of Enzymes', *Ann. N.Y. Acad. Sci.*, **103**, 495.
27. CARTER, B. G., CINADER, B., and ROSS, C. A. (1961), 'Immunochemical Analysis of the Multiple Forms of Bovine Ribonuclease', *Ann. N.Y. Acad. Sci.*, **94**, 1004.
28. INGRAM and HUNT, quoted by LEHMANN, H. (1962), 'The Pathology of Globin Synthesis', *Triangle*, **5**, 335.
29. GOODMAN, M., and CAMPBELL, D. H. (1953), 'Differences in Antigenic Specificity of Human Normal Adult, Fetal and Sickle-cell Anaemia Hemoglobins', *Blood*, **8**, 422.

30. KAMINSKI, M. (1965), 'The Analysis of the Antigenic Structure of Protein Molecules', *Prog. Allergy*, **9**, 79.
31. STEWART, J. M., and WOOLLEY, D. W. (1965), 'Importance of the Carboxyl End of Bradykinin and Other Peptides', *Nature, Lond.*, **207**, 1160.
32. PAGE, L., HABER, E., and LAGG, S. (1965), 'Quantitative Immunochemical Determination of Angiotensin', *J. clin. Invest.*, **44**, 1083.
33. UCHIDA, T., ROBBINS, P. W., and LURIA, S. E. (1963), 'Analysis of the Serologic Determinant Groups of the *Salmonella* E-group O-antigens', *Biochemistry*, **2**, 663.
34. PRESS, E. M., and PORTER, R. R. (1962), 'Isolation and Characterisation of Fragments of Human Serum Albumin containing some of the Antigenic Sites of the Whole Molecule', *Biochem. J.*, **83**, 172.
35. CEBRA, J. J. (1961), 'Studies on the Combining Sites of the Protein Antigen Silk Fibroin. III, Inhibition of the Silk Fibroin Antifibrin System by Peptides derived from the Antigen', *J. Immun.*, **86**, 205.
36. KARUSH, F. (1963), 'Immunologic Specificity and Molecular Structure', *Adv. Immun.*, **2**, 1.
37. RAPPAPORT, J. (1965), 'The Antigenic Structure of the Tobacco Mosaic Virus', *Adv. Virus Res.*, **11**, 223.
38. FELTON, L. D. (1949), 'The Significance of Antigen in Animal Tissues', *J. Immun.*, **61**, 107.
39. LANDSTEINER, K., and VAN DER SCHEER, J. (1938), 'On Cross-reactions of Immune Sera to Azoproteins. II, Antigens with Azocomponents containing Two Determinant Groups', *J. exp. Med.*, **67**, 709.
40. KABAT, E. A., and MAYER, M. M. (1961), *Experimental Immunochemistry*, 2nd ed. Springfield, Ill.: Thomas.
41. LANDSTEINER, K. (1900), 'Zur Kenntnis der antifermentativen, lytischen und agglutinierenden Wirkungen des Blutserums und der Lymphe', *Zentbl. Bakt. ParasitKde*, Abt. I, **27**, 357.
42. LANDSTEINER, K. (1901), 'Über Agglutinationserscheinungen normalen menschlichen Blutes', *Wien klin. Wschr.*, **14**, 1132.
43. DECASTELLO, A. V., and STURLI, A. (1902), 'Über die Isoagglutinine im Serum gesunder und kranker Menschen', *Münch. med. Wschr.*, **49**, 1090.
44. WATKINS, W. M. (1965), 'Relationship between Structure, Specificity and Genes within the ABO and Lewis Blood Group Systems', *Int. Congr. Blood Transf.* Basel: Karger.
45. UHLENBRUCK, G. (1965), 'Immunochemical Studies on Erythrocyte Mucoids. The Nature of the M and N Specific Substances', *Int. Congr. Blood Transf.* Basel: Karger.
46. MORGAN, W. T. J. (1965), 'Human Blood-group Specific Substances', *Antigene und Spezifität*, p. 73 (15*tes Kolloquium Ges. phys. Chemie*). Berlin: Springer-Verlag.
47. MORGAN, W. T. J. (1964), 'Some Aspects of Immunological Specificity in Terms of Carbohydrate Structure', *Bull. Soc. chim. Biol.*, **46**, 1627.
48. KABAT, E. A., BASSET, E. W., PRYZWANSKY, K., LLOYD, K. O., KAPLAN, M. E., and LAYUG, E. J. (1965), 'Immunochemical Studies on Blood Groups. XXXIII, The Effects of Alkaline Borohydride and of Alkali on Blood Group A, B and H Substances', *Biochemistry*, **4**, 1632.
49. WATKINS, W. M., and MORGAN, W. T. J. (1957), 'Specific Inhibition Studies relating to the Lewis Blood-group System', *Nature, Lond.*, **180**, 1038.
50. SPRINGER, G. F. (1965), 'Die Beziehung blutgruppenaktiver Substanzen zu Bakterien, höheren Pflanzen und Viren', *Antigene und Spezifität*, p. 90 (15*tes Kolloquium Ges. phys. Chemie*). Berlin: Springer-Verlag.
51. SCHIFFMAN, G., KABAT, E. A., and THOMPSON, W. (1964), 'Immunochemical Studies on Blood Groups. XXX, Cleavage of A, B and H Blood Group Substances by Alkali', *Biochemistry*, **3**, 113.
52. SCHIFFMAN, G., KABAT, E. A., and THOMPSON, W. (1964), 'Immunochemical Studies on Blood Groups. XXXII, Immunochemical Properties of and Possible Structures for the Blood Group A, B and H Antigen Determinants', *Biochemistry*, **3**, 587.
53. LLOYD, K. O., and KABAT, E. A. (1964), 'Some Products of the Degradation of Blood Group Substances by Alkaline Borohydride', *Biochem. biophys. Res. Commun.*, **16**, 385.

54. PAINTER, T. T., WATKINS, W. M., and MORGAN, W. T. J. (1965), 'Serologically Active Fucose-containing Oligosaccharides isolated from Human Blood Group A and B Substances', *Nature, Lond.*, **206**, 594.

55. MARCUS, D. M., KABAT, E. A., and SCHIFFMAN, G. (1964), 'Immunochemical Studies on Blood Groups. XXXI, Destruction of Blood Group Activity by an Enzyme from *Clostridium tertium* which deacetylates *N*-acetyl-galactosamine in Intact Blood Group Substances', *Biochemistry*, **3**, 437.

56. WIENER, A. S. (1965), 'Blood Groups of Chimpanzees and Other Non-human Primates. Their Implications for the Human Blood Groups', *Trans. N.Y. Acad. Sci.*, **27**, 488.

57. MORGAN, W. T. J. (1965), personal communication.

58. HUMMEL, K. (1965), 'Über A-Untergruppen und schwache A-Eigenschaften', *Das ärztliche Laboratorium*, **11**, 221.

59. PUSZTAI, A., and MORGAN, W. T. J. (1964), 'Studies in Immunochemistry. XXIII, Some Observations on the Heterogeneity of Preparations of Human Blood-group-specific Substances', *Biochem. J.*, **93**, 363.

60. RACE, R. R. (1965), 'Modern Concepts of the Blood Group Systems', *Ann. N.Y. Acad. Sci.*, **127**, 877.

61. PROKOP, O., and UHLENBRUCK, G. (1963), *Lehrbuch der menschlichen Blut- und Serumgruppen*. Stuttgart: Thieme.

62. UHLENBRUCK, G., and KRÜPE, M. (1965), 'Cryptantigenic N_{Vg} Receptor in Mucoids from Mu/Mu Cells', *Vox Sang.*, **10**, 326.

63. ROMANOWSKA, E. (1964), 'Reactions of M and N Blood-group Substances Natural and Degraded with Specific Reagents of Human and Plant Origin', *Vox Sang.*, **9**, 578.

64. RULE, A. H., and BOYD, W. C. (1964), 'Relationship between Blood Group Agglutinogens: Role of Sialic Acids', *Transfusion, Philad.*, **4**, 449.

65. COSTEA, N., YAKULIS, V., and HELLER, P. (1965), 'An Antibody with Anti-I Characteristics produced in Rabbits', *Fedn Proc. Fedn Am. Socs exp. Biol.*, **24**, 630.

66. MORGAN, W. T. J., and WATKINS, W. M. (1964), 'Blood Group P_1 Substance. I, Chemical Properties', *Int. Congr. Blood Transf.* Basel: Karger.

67. WATKINS, W. M., and MORGAN, W. T. J. (1964), 'Blood Group P_1 Substance. II, Immunological Properties', *Int. Congr. Blood Transf.* Basel: Karger.

68. BARKER, S. A., SOMERS, P. J., STACEY, M., and HOPTON, J. W. (1965), 'Arrangement of the L-Rhamnose Units in *Diplococcus pneumoniae* Type II Polysaccharide', *Carbohydrate Res.*, **1**, 106.

69. HEIDELBERGER, M., and ADAMS, J. (1956), 'The Immunological Specificity of Type II *Pneumococcus* and its Separation into Partial Specificities', *J. exp. Med.*, **103**, 189.

70. HOW, M. J., BRIMACOMBE, J. S., and STACEY, M. (1964), 'The Pneumococcal Polysaccharides', *Adv. Carbohyd. Chem.*, **19**, 303.

71. BARKER, S. A., HEIDELBERGER, M., STACEY, M., and TIPPER, D. J. (1958), 'Immuno-polysaccharides. The Structure of the Immunologically Specific Polysaccharide of Pneumococcus Type XIV', *J. chem. Soc.*, Part III, 3468.

72. KAUFFMANN, F. (1966), *The Bacteriology of Enterobacteriaceae*. Copenhagen: Munksgaard.

73. LÜDERITZ, O., STAUB, A. M., and WESTPHAL, O. (1966), 'Immunochemistry of O and R Antigens of *Salmonella* and Related Enterobacteriaceae', *Bact. Rev.*, **30**, 192.

74. KAUFFMANN, F., LÜDERITZ, O., STIERLIN, H., and WESTPHAL, O. (1960), 'Zur Chemie der O-Antigene von Enterobacteriaceae. I, Analyse der Zuckerbausteine von Salmonella-O-Antigenen', *Zentbl. Bakt. ParasitKde*, Abt. I, **178**, 442.

75. KAUFFMANN, F., JANN, B., KRUGER, L., LÜDERITZ, O., and WESTPHAL, O. (1962), 'Zur Immunchemie der O-Antigene von Enterobacteriaceae. VIII, Analyse der Zuckerbausteine von Polysacchariden weiterer *Salmonella*- und *Arizona*-O-Gruppen', *Zentbl. Bakt. ParasitKde*, Abt. I, **186**, 509.

76. MATSUHASHI, M., and STROMINGER, J. L. (1965), 'Reversible 2-Epimerization of CDP-paratose and CDP-tyvelose', *Biochem. biophys. Res. Commun.*, **20**, 169.

77. OSBORN, M. J., ROSEN, S. M., ROTHFIELD, L., ZELEZNICK, D, and HOERECKER, B. L. (1964), 'Lipopolysaccharide of the Gram Negative Cell Wall: Biosynthesis of a Complex Heteropolysaccharide occurs by Successive Addition of Specific Sugar Residues', *Science, N.Y.*, **145**, 783.

78. MAGE, R. G., and KABAT, E. A. (1963), 'The Combining Regions of the Type III *Pneumococcus* Polysaccharide and Homologous Antibody', *Biochemistry*, **2**, 1278.

79. CARTER, E. C., JOHNSON, P., and WEBER, E. J. (1965), 'Glycolipids', *Ann. Rev. Biochem.*, **34**, 109.
80. KUHN, R., and MULDNER, H. (1964), 'Über Glyko-lipo-sialo-proteide des Gehirns', *Naturwissenschaften*, **51**, 635.
81. LANDSTEINER, K., and SIMMS, S. (1923), 'Production of Heterogenetic Antibodies with Mixtures of the Binding Part of the Antigen and Protein', *J. exp. Med.*, **38**, 127.
82. GREY, G. M., and MACFARLANE, M. G. (1958), 'Separation and Composition of the Phospholipids of Ox Heart', *Biochem. J.*, **70**, 409.
83. BRUJN, J. H. DE (1966), 'Chemical Structure and Serological Activity of Natural and Synthetic Cardiolipin and Related Components', *Br. J. ven. Dis.*, **42**, 125.
84. KUWERT, E., and NIEDIECK, B. (1965), 'Anti-cerebroside Antibodies in Cerebrospinal Fluid of Rabbits with Experimental "Allergic" Encephalomyelitis', *Nature, Lond.*, **207**, 991.
85. NIEDIECK, B., KUWERT, R., PALACIOS, O., and DRESS, O. (1965), 'Immunochemical and Serological Studies on the Lipid Hapten of Myelin with Relationship to Experimental Allergic Encephalomyelitis (EAE)', *Ann. N.Y. Acad. Sci.*, **122**, 266.
86. JOFFE, S., RAPPORT, M. M., and GRAF, L. (1963), 'Identification of Organ-specific Lipid Haptens in Brain', *Nature, Lond.*, **197**, 60.
87. RAPPORT, M. M., GRAF, L., and YARIV, J. (1961), 'Immunochemical Studies of Organ and Tumour Lipids. IX, Configuration of the Carbohydrate Residues in Cytolipin H', *Archs Biochem. Biophys.*, **92**, 438.
88. KIM, Z., and UHLENBRUCK, G. (1966), 'Über die Natur des A_{hel} Rezeptors', *Jap. J. legal. Med.*, **20**, 246.
89. KOSCIELAK, J. (1965), 'ABO Blood Group Substances from Erythrocytes as "Lipid" Antigens', *Int. Congr. Blood Transf.* Basel: Karger.
90. KOSCIELAK, J. (1965), personal communication.
91. WIENER, A. S. (1966), 'The Relationship of the H Substance to the A-B-O Blood Groups', *Int. Archs Allergy appl. Immun.*, **29**, 82.
92. KRÜPE, M. (1966), personal communication.
93. JENKIN, C. R. (1963), 'Heterophile Antigens and their Significance in the Host–parasite Relationship', *Adv. Immun.*, **3**, 351.
94. CHEESE, I. A. F., and MORGAN, W. T. J. (1961), 'Two Serologically Active Trisaccharides isolated from Human Blood Group A Substance', *Nature, Lond.*, **191**, 149.
95. DIEHL, J. E., and MALLETTE, M. F. (1964), 'Nature of the Forssman Hapten from Sheep Erythrocytes', *J. Immun.*, **93**, 965.

CHAPTER 3

IMMUNOGLOBULINS

By E. R. Gold and D. B. Peacock

I. Introduction

In the past serum proteins associated with antibody activity have been grouped together under the general heading of 'gamma-globulins'. This expression arose as a result of the electrophoretic separation of serum proteins into fractions of varying mobility (*Fig.* 21). In a hyperimmune serum antibody activity is located mainly in the gamma-globulin peak. Though electrophoresis is a highly sensitive technique for the separation of proteins, it is to some extent inappropriate for separating antibody molecules. With the advent of immuno-electrophoresis a different order of resolution became available. The gamma-globulins could now be distinguished on the basis of their antigenic structure as well as their electrophoretic mobility (*Fig.* 22). It immediately became apparent that old boundaries were crossed and that the principal antibody component of hyperimmune sera formed a homogeneous whole that ran right through the gamma-globulin peak and into the beta-globulin region, as judged by the appearance of a continuous line of precipitation. As the properties of antibody molecules became better known, a nomenclature that separated

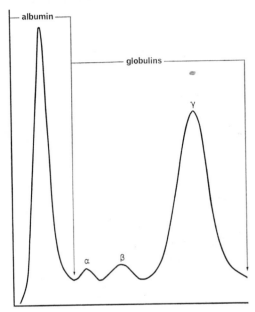

Fig. 21.—Outline of the electrophoretic pattern of serum proteins in a hyperimmune serum.

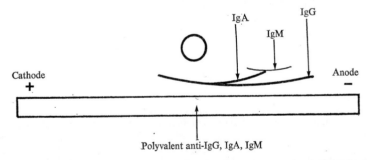

Fig. 22.—Illustration of the resolving power of immuno-electrophoresis for immunoglobulins.

them on the basis of a single character, namely the electric charge they carried, became less and less acceptable. The expression 'immunoglobulin' was coined and is now in general use. It is a term born, one might say, of the 'immuno-chemical' approach, and under such a heading we can accommodate not only antibody molecules of all classes but also those chemical substances belonging to the same general category which do not necessarily display antibody activity. Since a great deal of what is known about the structure of antibody molecules is inferred from a study of myeloma proteins, and it was not certain initially that these proteins may possess antibody activity, it can be seen that discussion was greatly facilitated by a generic term that carried no special meaning in some allied discipline.

Examination of the serum of animals by electrophoresis during the course of immunization sometimes reveals an increasing proportion of a component, variously termed β_2M or γ_1, that migrates rather faster than the gamma-globulins. The M of β_2M stands for 'macroglobulin', and molecules with a sedimentation constant $19S$ and molecular weight 900,000 are associated with this fraction. The principal antibody fraction of hyperimmune sera associated with gamma-globulin mobility has a sedimentation constant of $7S$ and molecular weight of 160,000.

Following the introduction of immuno-electrophoresis [1] a third still faster, but antigenically related, immunoglobulin was detected and labelled γ_{1A} or β_{2A}. Though this immunoglobulin tends slightly to polymerize in serum and occurs in quite a different form in the secretions of exocrine glands, the basic unit is scarcely different from the gamma-globulins.

Consequent upon the general adoption of the term 'immunoglobulin' a new nomenclature was proposed in which the prefix γ or Ig stood for immunoglobulin and a suffix denoted the particular class of immunoglobulin. Thus the $7S$, 160,000 M.W., gamma-globulins became IgG or γG, the macroglobulins became IgM or γM, and the third class of immunoglobulins, IgA or γA [2]. Synonyms of the old and new nomenclatures are set out in *Table XV* which has been adapted from the proposals of the W.H.O. committee on the nomenclature of immunoglobulins [2]. Apart from the three classes of immunoglobulin already mentioned, two other classes of human immunoglobulin, IgD [3] and IgE [4], are now known.

Some of the main characteristics of immunoglobulins of the five known classes are shown in *Table XVI*. The values given for IgA are appropriate to serum immunoglobulin only. The form found in seromucous secretions has a sedimentation coefficient of $11S$ and consists of two $7S$ units associated with another fragment called transport or T piece [5]. The greater size of IgE (IgND) is provisionally attributed to a longer heavy chain [6]. It is worth noting at this juncture the considerable similarity in size of four out of five immunoglobulins; only IgM differs strikingly and, as we shall see later, is itself made of units with the same basic structure as the other members of this group. By contrast, the carbohydrate content differs markedly between classes, and even within classes [7], though the significance of these variations is by no means clear as yet. In other situations we have remarked on the great contribution that oligosaccharides make to determining the specificity of even protein antigens; in the case of immunoglobulins there is no evidence yet that they play any such role.

The concentration of individual immunoglobulins in serum is subject to considerable fluctuations, since they will be perpetually altering in the face of infections, and probably for other reasons as well. On this basis the

Table XV.—NOMENCLATURE OF IMMUNOGLOBULINS AND THEIR CONSTITUENT PARTS. *After W.H.O.* [2]

NEW	OLD
Classes	
γG or IgG	7*S*γ, γ_2, γ_{ss}
γA or IgA	γ1A, β_2A
γM or IgM	19Sγ, γ_1M, β_2M, γ macroglobulin
γD or IgD	
γE or IgE	
Types	
Light chain	
Type K κ	Type I, 1, B
Type L λ	Type II, 2, A
Heavy chains	
of IgG γ	
of IgA α	
of IgM μ	
of IgD δ	
of IgE ε	
Fragments	
Fab fragment (antigen binding)	Fragment A, C, S, I, II
Fc fragment (crystallizable)	Fragment B, F, III
Fd fragment	A piece

Table XVI.—PROPERTIES OF HUMAN IMMUNOGLOBULINS. *After Cohen and Milstein* [5]

	IgG	IgM	IgA	IgD	IgE
Sedimentation coefficient (S_{W}^{20})	7	19	7*	7	7·9†
Molecular weight‡	150,000	900,000	140,000	—	196,000†
Carbohydrate (per cent)	2·9	11·8	7·5	—	10·7§
Serum concentration (mg. per cent)	800–1680	50–190	140–420	0·3–40	5–50§
Percentage of total in intravascular pool	55	100	40	75	—
M.W. of heavy chain	53,000	70,000	64,000	—	75,500†

* Monomeric serum IgA only.
† Bennich and Johansson [6].
‡ Approximate values.
§ Johansson, Mellbin, and Vahlquist [8].

three classes discovered first, IgG, IgM, and IgA, would appear to be the major constituents, though it must be admitted that very much higher levels of IgE have been reported in Ethiopian children suffering from round-worm infestations [8]. It is not easy to define what is normal when dealing with the response to infection and infestation, since none of us is reared in an environment free from parasitic invasions. Nevertheless, mean levels in adult serum of 3 mg. per 100 ml. for IgD [3], and in children of 16 mg. per 100 ml. for IgE [8] have been recorded in countries of high economic development, and suggest that these two immuno-globulins are ordinarily present in concentrations well below that of the three major classes.

II. PATHOLOGICAL IMMUNOGLOBULINS: PROTOTYPES OF IMMUNOGLOBULIN STRUCTURE

We have already noted that immunoglobulin levels alter as a result of infection; but although this is a consequence of a pathological process it is properly termed a physiological response. At the same time there are also pathological states of the immune system itself in which immunoglobulin patterns are again disturbed. Such states may have an immensely varied aetiology ranging from disorders of the immune process associated with immunoglobulin production to inborn or acquired disorders of immuno-globulin metabolism.

In many conditions with a chronic infectious element or of a presumed auto-immune aetiology there is a hyperglobulinaemia, but the normal ratios of immunoglobulin classes are not preserved. Tomasi records IgG:IgA ratios as low as 2·8 in Laennec's cirrhosis and as high as 26·3 in lupoid hepatitis, against his normal figure of 6·4 [9].

The hyperglobulinaemias resulting from a pathological proliferation of lymphoid tissues have been divided into so-called monoclonal and polyclonal gammopathies [10]. In the former over-production by one (perhaps a few in practice), and in the latter by many, clones is assumed. Already most of the possible combinations of defects have been observed, at least in connexion with the three main classes of immunoglobulins [11]. The same also holds for those diseases of the immunological system that lead to deficiencies of antibody production, hypogamma-globulinaemias having been observed with one, two, or all three major classes absent or depressed [11]. The proliferative lymphoid disorder, multiple myeloma-tosis, is of particular interest since it has provided the biochemist with a naturally occurring source of relatively pure immunoglobulins of a single class. It has also led directly to the discovery of IgD and IgE, which otherwise are present in serum in too low a concentration to be readily detectable.

The deficiency diseases have been important for defining the role of humoral antibodies as such in infectious disease. The remarkable recovery of children with severe immunoglobulin-deficiency disease from virus infections—children who, without antibiotics, were doomed to die at an early age from bacterial infection—has constituted one of the main pieces of evidence that an alternative mechanism of immunity, cell-mediated immunity, exists.

Certain of these dysgamma-globulinaemias are sex-linked or bear other evidence of heritable characteristics. This has led in its turn to considerable speculation on the genetic control of immunoglobulin synthesis and the precise point of breakdown. At this juncture it is probably sufficient to say that the immune response is immensely complicated, with respect both to cellular differentiation and protein synthesis, and that interruptions must be possible at a number of points in a long chain of events, all of which will be under some form of genetic control.

III. ANIMAL IMMUNOGLOBULINS

Although we have dealt exclusively with human immunoglobulins up to this point, what has been said applies equally well to animals, and different classes of immunoglobulin have been found in a number of species. The pressure for investigation has come in general from two directions, for defining the chemistry of complex proteins and for defining the biological properties of different immunoglobulins. In other words, animal immunoglobulins have been studied from the point of view of both structure and function. Enough has already been said for the reader to be aware that even within the single animal immunoglobulins form a very heterogeneous population without taking into account different combining specificities for antigens. One of the first steps in understanding behaviour of such molecules must therefore be to identify groups within this population. This is the fundamental meaning of classes of antibody, such classes being based primarily on physical and antigenic characters. Still finer antigenic distinctions within classes lead on to the definition of subclasses, and serum groups in man and to allotypes in the rabbit. In a number of instances the final goal of the molecular biologist has been almost reached in that antigenic distinctions have been correlated with chemical differences of amino-acid sequence.

In those animal species principally studied the immunoglobulin classes follow very much the general pattern found in man, at least in so far as 7S and 19S antibodies or their broad equivalents are found in all forms of life above the primitive elasmobranchs, such as the smooth dogfish, *Mustelus canis*. In the mouse five classes of immunoglobulin have been described: IgG (γ2a), IgH (γ2b), IgM, IgA, and IgF [12]. IgM and IgA appear to be the functional equivalents of the same classes in man. The remaining three classes all have a sedimentation coefficient of 7S, but to what extent they correspond to IgG and other classes in man remains to be determined. In a number of animal species work has progressed only to the point of recognizing broad distinctions and without detailed comparisons having been made with the immunoglobulins of other species. This rather confused state is reflected in the six named classes or subclasses of horse immunoglobulin: IgM, IgA, IgGa, IgGb, IgGc, and 10$S$$\gamma$1-globulin [13, 14]. The first two probably correspond again to the so-named classes of man. The IgG's are 7S immunoglobulins and the last-named, as its name implies, is intermediate in size between 7S and 19S immunoglobulins. Investigation of bovine and ovine classes is more incomplete, but in sheep four classes, 7S γ1, 7S γ2, γ1M, and γ1A, similar to those in mice, have been described [15]. Bovine immunoglobulins, like those of the horse, include a class of intermediate size, 12S [16]. Heterogeneity of immunoglobulins has also been noted in a number of other animal species [17].

IV. GENERAL STRUCTURE

It is only within the past decade that the immunochemist has recognized that the potentialities for unravelling the very complicated structure of large proteins such as globulins lie within his grasp. It was methods applied to the analysis of other large proteins such as polypeptide chain separation by reduction–alkylation, and assays of N-terminal and C-terminal amino-acids that ultimately led Porter to propose his now famous four-chain model of rabbit IgG in 1962 [18]. The model showed two pairs of chains, one long and one short, arranged symmetrically with the chains linked covalently by disulphide bonds. The interpretation arrived at then has since been modified only in detail and in *Fig.* 23 is a diagrammatic illustration of our present concept of the IgG molecule. It differs from Porter's model chiefly in the positioning and number of disulphide bonds.

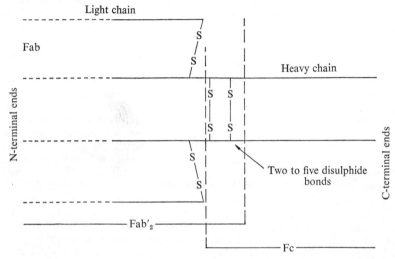

Fig. 23.—Model of human IgG.

The IgG molecule possesses two antideterminants (combining sites for antigen) and these are located at the N-terminal ends of the long or heavy chains. It is possible that the N-terminal end of short or light chains also takes part in the formation of the antideterminant.

It is widely accepted that this four-chain model describes the basic structure of all immunoglobulins, not only the IgG molecule, and in all species of animal that have been investigated as well. This is a striking concept and needs substantiation, especially in view of the fact that there are differences in size between even the three major classes of immunoglobulin. Assuming the basic structure is present in all classes there are three possibilities: (1) That the individual chains are longer and therefore heavier; (2) That polymers are formed; (3) That additional material is present.

In the case of the IgM macroglobulin disruption is relatively easily effected by mild reduction with 2-mercapto-ethanol; the breaking of these interchain disulphide bonds yields five smaller units per molecule [19, 20] and further disruption of the units reveals that they are built on the same general principle as IgG molecules. Nevertheless, the molecular weight of the heavy chain of IgM is 70,000 [21], which is considerably in excess of that of IgG (*see Table XVI*).

It will not have escaped attention that the molecular weights of the heavy chains in the different classes vary considerably (*Table XVI*). In the case of IgE this has been calculated on the difference between the combined weight of light chains subtracted from the estimated whole-molecule weight. What is not shown in *Table XVI* is that exocrine IgA may have molecular weights ranging from 370,000 (rabbit colostrum) to 510,000 (human colostrum), so that here we must invoke some other reasons. The explanation of these wide departures in size from serum IgA and from IgG lies in the composition of such molecules from two or three basic four-chain units [22, 23] together with an antigenically distinct protein known as 'T' or 'transport piece', which has a molecular weight of 40,000 [23].

The three possibilities envisaged above are thus all seen to have been invoked. IgM and possibly IgA and IgE have heavy chains larger than IgG; IgM and serum IgA occur or may occur in polymeric forms of the basic structure; and in IgA of seromucous secretions there is an additional protein. Indeed, this may also be the case in IgM, where a five-chain structure has been postulated [24]. It is, of course, early days yet and we can safely assume that there are some surprises in store for us still, even with regard to the gross structure of immunoglobulins. It is true to say, however, that the four-chain structure is found consistently in all classes of immunoglobulin and all species of animal, and that it probably represents a basic form from which all immunoglobulins were further evolved.

The foregoing is simply an explanation of how apparent dissimilarities of gross structure can be reconciled with a basic unity of structure. The four-chain model was, of course, based on a much firmer foundation of fact than this. The early evidence comprises, among other things, the reduction of rabbit IgG in urea solution with the resultant yield of a number of smaller units, suggesting a multichain structure for immunoglobulin [25, 26]. Overcoming a number of experimental difficulties, Fleischman, Pain, and Porter [27] went on to separate reduced alkylated human IgG on Sephadex columns with the demonstration of two peaks of elution representing polypeptides of two distinct sizes—evidence for the light and heavy chains. Taken with C-terminal and N-terminal assays the balance of evidence was thought to favour the four-chain hypothesis; later studies that provided confirmation are summarized by Cohen and Porter [28].

A further step in correlating function of antibodies with chemical structure was made possible by techniques involving enzymatic cleavage of the immunoglobulin molecule. First used thirty years ago to reduce the antigenicity of horse antitoxin in man, the method has been extensively applied to the study of immunoglobulin structure. Hydrolysis by papain separates the IgG molecule into three roughly equal portions [29]. Two of the fragments are identical and carry the antibody sites (Fab). The third fragment is composed of the two C-terminal halves of the heavy chains still joined by a disulphide bond. Derived from rabbit or guinea-pig immunoglobulin, this fragment (Fc) crystallizes readily [28]. From this property it can be inferred that Fc has a very constant composition, even though it is derived from a population of antibodies carrying specificities directed towards many different antigens; and this inference is amply borne out on investigation, as we shall see later.

Hydrolysis by pepsin at pH 5 splits the H chains of IgG on the C-terminal side of the inter-heavy-chain disulphide bonds (*Fig.* 23), with the production of a large divalent antibody fragment $(Fab')_2$ which is capable of precipitating antigen [30]. The molecular weight of this large fragment is about 100,000 and the remainder of the heavy chains is split into a number of smaller peptides. Treatment with a number of mild reducing agents will disrupt $(Fab')_2$ into two fragments, Fab', each slightly larger than Fab resulting from papain hydrolysis.

The reason for the susceptibility of the region around the disulphide bonds linking the two heavy chains to attack by enzymes was something of a puzzle. The answer may be found in the studies on sedimentation and viscosity in which it was observed that the whole molecule was less compact than the enzymatically separated fragments [31]. The conclusion reached was that the fragments were linked by a relatively extended portion of peptide chain. Other arguments can be brought forward in support which indicate an area of flexibility in this region consistent with the extended chain hypothesis. For instance, the analytical data already presented do not support the concept of antibody sites placed at opposite poles of an ellipsoid molecule, as some authors have contended, and yet the biological properties of antibody molecules do not readily admit of explanations in which the antideterminants are placed side by side in the manner shown in *Fig.* 23. The suggestion has therefore been made that in the uncombined state IgG immunoglobulin is a fairly compact structure with dimensions of $120 \times 80 \times 34$ Å; that it retains this form when combined with a single antigenic site; but in order to combine with a second site the molecule can 'click open' [32] to reach across gaps as wide as 200 Å.

The exquisite electron-micrographs taken by Valentine and Green [33] indicate that the IgG molecule is not quite as versatile as this since the 'hinge' is in the region of the inter-heavy-chain bonds; all the same they record a maximum distance between ferritin conjugated molecules of 140 Å. The alternative use of a small dinitrophenyl (DNP) hapten was particularly advantageous in allowing the authors to examine the shape of complexes formed with purified anti-DNP IgG, since such complexes were formed in the plane of the supporting membrane of the specimen. The hapten itself was too small to be recognized. In the electron-micrographs, appearances indicative of dimers, trimers, tetramers, pentamers, and some larger figures are seen. These forms take on linear, triangular, square, and pentagonal shapes respectively. The principle is shown in *Fig.* 24, where the angle between the Fab arms is 60°. In the case of a dimer the arms can be extended to the maximum of 180°. Also in *Fig.* 24 the Fc components are shown as projecting at the apices of the triangle and this appearance is easily recognizable in the electron-micrographs. Even more striking, however, is their disappearance after the aggregates have been treated with pepsin. The evidence presented by Valentine and Green is therefore quite compatible with the view of an extended and flexible region in the heavy chains of the molecule.

Of equal interest, though in a different context, are the electron-micrographs of IgM presented by Chesebro, Bloth, and Svehag [34]. The 'spidery' appearance the authors describe is due to a central core from which protrude five misshapen legs. According to our present concepts, the central core would represent five Fc portions of the 7S subunits, each with two half-cysteines through which it is linked to the adjacent subunits. The distorted legs represent the flexible part terminating in a compact portion of the molecule containing the antibody combining site(s).

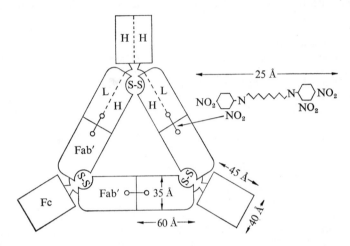

Fig. 24.—Diagram of a hapten-linked trimer of IgG molecules. *By kind permission of Valentine and Green* [33].

Two points of particular interest remain to be answered. The first is: How big is the interdeterminant gap that the IgM molecule can span? And the second: How many valencies has the IgM molecule got? Chesebro et al. [34] attempt to answer only the first of these, and according to their observations free-lying IgM molecules have a central ring structure of 100 Å diameter, with projecting legs 125 Å in length. Thus the maximum span would be approximately 350 Å. This figure correlates well with previous observations by the same authors [34] of the distance bridged by IgM between enterovirus particles. In general these observations also conform to the appearance of earlier electron-micrographs in which agglutinating IgM in moderate excess was 'stapled' along bacterial flagella, with an interdeterminant distance of 140 Å [35].

The second point regarding the number of valencies in the IgM molecule has aroused, and still does, a good deal of speculation and controversy. If one accepts the postulate that the parent molecule is constructed from five units built on the same model as the IgG molecule, and there is a considerable body of evidence to support this view now, then the maximum number of combining sites in such a molecule could be ten, a value that has been found experimentally [36]. Other workers have concluded that their evidence is more consistent with five valencies per molecule in the case of pathological human IgM [37] and rabbit IgM antibody [38]. Also that in the former case only 50 per cent of the isolated Fab fragments bound antigen [37]. Unless the process of separating the fragments is responsible, it appears from this evidence that we are faced with a very tricky situation in attempting to explain the synthesis of such asymmetrical proteins.

V. DETAILED STRUCTURE AND ANTIGENIC COMPOSITION

Although knowledge of the detailed structure of immunoglobulins is not pursued simply for the sake of defining antigenic structure in physicochemical terms, the fact remains that these two areas of study are to some extent complementary. Thus differences in amino-acid sequence can sometimes be correlated with known differences in antigenic specificity; equally antigenic specificities and other biological properties of immunoglobulin molecules can indicate profitable areas for chemical study.

It is now very generally accepted that the amino-acid sequence of polypeptide chains largely, and sometimes entirely, determines secondary, tertiary, and even quaternary structure of proteins. Indeed, analysis of the primary sequence of the light and heavy chains could in theory tell us all we need to know about the structure and behaviour of immunoglobulins in general and antibodies in particular. There are, however, one or two difficulties to be overcome before this ideal state of affairs can be attained.

We now know that immunoglobulins are constructed on the principle of two identical pairs of chains, light and heavy, arranged as two light–heavy complexes joined together by disulphide bridges between the heavy chains. Reduction–alkylation methods are used, followed by gel filtration, to separate light and heavy chains in order to provide starting material for investigation. From here, conventional methods of peptide mapping, involving the separation and identification of peptide fragments by resolving them chromatographically in two directions, are used in conjunction with sequential amino-acid analyses of the peptide fragments. Overlapping peptides are sought so as to establish their order and ultimately the amino-acid sequence throughout the whole chain. The peptide fragments themselves are obtained by controlled hydrolysis with proteolytic enzymes, such as trypsin, which act on a wide variety of peptide bonds, or with more selective reagents, such as cyanogen bromide, which disrupt bonds between certain residues.

In order that identifiable peptides may be obtained in these ways, a certain purity of starting material is essential. The degree of purity required is perhaps not as great as was originally thought. Nevertheless, unless a good proportion of the fragments obtained fall into definable groups no advance can be made. If our starting material is purified serum globulin, then we will be dealing with a mixture containing substantial quantities of all three major classes of immunoglobulins. In addition, there would be those heterogeneities due to antibodies of different specificity being present, as well as those differences of structure among immunoglobulins that serve to distinguish subclasses, allotypes, and so on. The separation of IgG from other immunoglobulins is not a difficult procedure, however, and pooled IgG would represent a considerable scaling down of the problem. A further improvement could be immediately effected if a single individual is accepted as the donor. Even then, a single class of immunoglobulin obtained from a single donor provides an unwanted degree of diversity of molecular structure, and it is here that Nature has provided suitable material in the form of myeloma proteins.

Two pathological conditions of the lymphoid tissues, multiple myeloma and Waldenström's macroglobulinaemia, particularly of man and mouse, lead to the overproduction of immunoglobulins. These conditions arise as a result of uncontrolled proliferation of lymphoid cells, and the proliferating cells are clones derived from a single, or sometimes a few, parent cells. It is now well established that the hypergamma-globulinaemias that result are frequently monoclonal and occasionally oligoclonal. So far, proliferative conditions of this sort have been associated with all five of the known human immunoglobulin classes. It is evident that such a source will provide a homogeneous immunoglobulin population, and this has proved to be of inordinate benefit in the chemical analysis of immunoglobulins.

In addition, in multiple myelomatosis, the metabolism of immunoglobulin-producing cells is so disordered that excessive amounts of certain components are produced and excreted in large amounts as Bence Jones protein in the urine of patients. The demonstration that Bence Jones proteins were identical with the light chains of the corresponding myeloma protein [39] proved an enormous step forward in the availability of investigative material. At much the same time, it was also observed that half the length of the polypeptide chains of Bence Jones proteins was of constant amino-acid sequence while the other half was variable [40]. Subsequently it has become apparent that the light chain, of all immunoglobulins, is divisible into almost exactly equal halves, of which the C-terminal half of approximately 107 residues is the constant section. The N-terminal half varies from one Bence Jones protein to another, and in normal serum, of course, from one molecule to another. It is this variable region which constitutes the most characteristic feature of immunoglobulins, serving to distinguish them, as far as is known, from all other proteins.

Since whole sequences of a number of light chains [5, 41] and a few heavy chains [42] are now becoming known it is also becoming possible to correlate details of amino-acid sequence with other properties of immunoglobulins. Ultimately, of course, it is hoped that the basis for serological specificity of antibody molecules will be determined, and already we are justified in predicting that it will be determined largely by amino-acid sequence. But if this is so, then it already brings problems of its own in train, namely, How are we to account for the genetic basis of the very large number of peptide chains that represent antibody specificity? First, however, we can turn to the structure of the polypeptide chains themselves and to the simpler problems of correlating chemical structure with antigenic structure.

A. Structure of Light Chains

Before any details of amino-acid or, indeed, grosser structure were known, Bence Jones proteins had already been separated into two distinct antigenic classes [43], which were subsequently designated type K and type L (*Table XV*). The same specificities can be recognized in immunoglobulins of normal serum [40], and indeed, the immunoglobulins of all classes, subclasses, etc., and probably of all animal species, can be divided into the same two types. The implication here, of course, is that though classes of immunoglobulin may differ in other respects they all have light chains in common. That this is actually so is indicated by the fact that absorption of antisera to human immunoglobulins with light chains from any class will remove all cross-reacting antibodies between classes [44]. It follows that immunoglobulins can be divided into the same two groups; the light chains derived from them are referred to as κ and λ respectively (*Table XV*). The same specificities are found in the light chains of mouse immunoglobulins and in Bence Jones protein of mice [12].

The complete amino-acid sequences of a number of human κ and λ chains derived from myelomata have now been established [41, 45, 46]. The length of the chain is variously put at 213–221 residues, and within these limits the amino-acid sequence of the C-terminal half of all chains is virtually constant. A similar invariable structure has been noted in the C-terminal half of λ chains. The only well-established variation in this section of κ chains, according to Cohen and Milstein [5], is in position 191 (numbered from the N-terminal end) where the allotypic specificities of Inv(2) and Inv(3) are associated with leucine and valine residues respectively. Inv antigens are associated with κ chains only. The corresponding antigen in λ chains is probably Oz, and the report that Oz+ and Oz− involve arginine/lysine alternatives at position 190 in λ chains is of extreme interest [47]. The numbers assigned to any position remain somewhat arbitrary, since insertions and deletions, particularly in the N-terminal half, have so far prevented any general system being adopted. It should be stated at once that Inv and Oz specificities do not form the basis on which κ and λ chains are distinguished; they form subdivisions of these two chain types.

Comparison of human and mouse κ chains shows a very striking similarity in the C-terminal section. Nearly 60 per cent of the 107 residues are identical, and this compares with only 39 per cent identity between human κ and λ [5].

The structural features that determine type K and type L specificities appear to reside in the variable region of light chains, and if this is so one is forced to conclude that stable antigenic differences must be reflected in constant sequences in the variable region. Since complete sequences of a number of Bence Jones proteins of type K are known, opportunities for comparison of the variable region in κ chains of different origin have already arisen. It is quickly apparent that the N-terminal half is not arranged in an entirely random fashion and that comparison with the C-terminal half reveals that there are very considerable areas of homology where residues match exactly, even in Bence Jones proteins from different individuals and probably of different Inv subtype. Homology becomes even more apparent when allowances are made for insertions and deletions of residues in the chains; in other words, when gaps are left in one or other chain so that they can be arranged for maximum matching. Such methods may smack of chicanery to the uninitiated, but they are perfectly proper provided that they are exercised with caution and insight, and concepts dealing with insertions and deletions have a sound experimental basis in the genetic control of protein synthesis.

Apart from any questions of antigenicity, certain residues must also be essential to the basic structure of immunoglobulins. Thus the light chain is a double-looped structure in which the loops are formed primarily as a result of intra-chain disulphide bonds. There are two of these bonds in

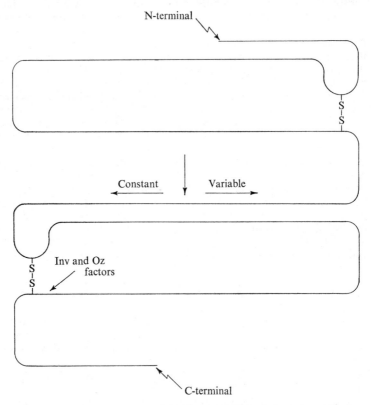

Fig. 25.—Double-loop structure of the immunoglobulin light chain. *After Putnam* [41] *and Hill, Lebovitz, Fellows, and Delaney* [48].

each light chain (*Fig.* 25) formed between invariant half-cystine resi-dues [41, 48]. There is a further half-cystine residue in light chains that forms the bond between light–heavy chain pairs. In κ chains it is the C-terminal residues, and in λ chains the subterminal residue. A number of other amino-acids are particularly, if not always necessarily, associated with imposing configurational restraints on polypeptide chains. Proline, for instance, occurring singly, as a pair or a triplet, in all probability induces a kink in the chain; at the other extreme glycine, with no side-chain, cannot easily be replaced without affecting spatial considerations;

alternatively, such residues may have been retained because they impart flexibility to the variable region.

It came as something of a surprise to immunochemists to find extreme variability in one half of the light chain of immunoglobulins. At that time evidence weighed heavily in favour of placing the combining site of antibodies on the heavy chain, and variation in that chain would have been consistent with such a view. Of course, to find a variable region in the light chain does not mean that we must now consider the combining site to be contained there, but rather that we can visualize the light chain as playing a more particular part in the formation of the antideterminant, perhaps by influencing the configuration of the heavy chain.

The degree of variation already observed in the N-terminal section is considerable. Cohen has collected evidence of variation in 40 positions in κ chains [45]. He points out that in some positions the number of variations is greater than two, but even if only two the number of different chains would be 2^{40} or 10^{10}. This implies, of course, that there is no restriction on alternatives. The possibilities, in terms of specificity of combining sites, are obvious.

So far, then, we have considered the light chains of immunoglobulins as polypeptides with a characteristic two-loop structure. The N-terminal half is further characterized as having a very labile primary structure which it would seem must be associated in some way with the specificity of the antideterminant. Although 40 positions where variations can occur are already known in the N-terminal half, and no doubt this number will increase, this figure should still be set against the background of some 108 residues that comprise the whole variable region. It is then clear that there is still scope for a considerable element of constancy here. Perhaps in the final tally there will still be more constant positions than variable ones. This aspect of structure is of considerable significance when we come to consider the evolution of light chains. In addition, the variable region sets very special problems when it comes to understanding how the synthesis of such polypeptide chains might be controlled. Before we turn our attention to problems of this sort, however, we must first look at the structure of immunoglobulin heavy chains and see how they compare with what we have discovered about light chains.

B. Structure of Heavy Chains

The problems connected with unravelling the primary structure of heavy chains of immunoglobulins can be expected to be greater than those associated with light chains for a number of reasons. First, heavy chains, even of the simplest immunoglobulin, IgG, are approximately twice as long as light chains. Second, they differ quite markedly from one immunoglobulin class to another, both in length and antigenic structure. Third, there are a number of antigenic differences within classes which subdivide them still further. All this adds up to a massive heterogeneity of structure which could render attempts at sequential amino-acid analysis very unrewarding. In addition, there is no readily available source of heavy chains comparable to Bence Jones proteins and, although 'heavy-chain disease' has now been described [49], it is very much rarer than Bence Jones proteinuria. Heavy chains can, of course, be isolated from myeloma proteins. A surprising feature of the work in this field, however, is the success that has attended sequence studies of normal rabbit IgG. This success has been largely due to the recognition that the ability to crystallize the Fc fragment of heavy chains reflected a high degree of homogeneity in that part of the chain [29], and that a situation analogous to that of the constant region in light chains in all probability existed. Confirmation came with the identification of a C-terminal peptide of 18 residues from rabbit IgG [50], and the extension of this work to 120 residues [51], and ultimately to the entire Fc fragment of some 216 residues [48].

The general structure of the rabbit Fc fragment bears a remarkable resemblance to the light-chain structure, with half-cystines at positions 37 and 91, and at 138 and 195, forming the two loops in the chain [48]. The

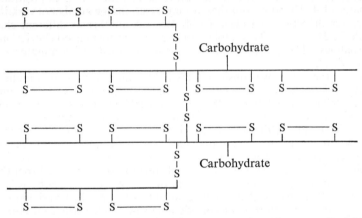

Fig. 26.—The possibilities of symmetry in the arrangement of intrachain dilsulphide bonds in the immunoglobulin molecule. *After Edelman* [52].

same general pattern is observed in human IgG. Edelman and his colleagues have carried out a concentrated attack on a single human myeloma protein, Eu. Some of their preliminary results have been reported by Edelman [52]. By comparing amino-acid sequences of fragments of Eu protein obtained by various disruptive procedures, they placed the seven cyanogen bromide fragments in an unequivocal order. From these data Edelman derives a model that illustrates strikingly the similarity between the four quarters of the heavy chain and the two halves of the light chain (*Fig.* 26).

As for more detailed structural homogeneity, two human myeloma IgG's, Daw and Cor, of identical subclass and allelic character, show also an identical amino-acid sequence in their Fc fragments [53]; and with regard to the N-terminal end Porter states that 'the variant section runs at least as far as . . . position 110' [54]. In other words, the possibility of a variable N-terminal quarter and a constant C-terminal three-quarters in the γ chain can be credibly envisaged. As we shall see, the division of the heavy chain into comparable quarters has an important bearing on theories of the evolution of immunoglobulins.

It has been said before that the various immunoglobulin classes differ in antigenic structure as well as physically. These differences must be confined to the heavy chains, since light chains are common to all classes. So far, insufficient is known about amino-acid sequences of heavy chains from different classes to be able to correlate such details of chemical structure with antigenic distinctions. Indeed, the same is very largely still true of antigenic differences within the most highly studied IgG class, and the complete sequence of too few γ chains is known for comparisons to reveal the basis of antigenic specificities with certainty.

VI. Subdivisions of Immunoglobulin Classes

Just as myeloma proteins represent the product of a single, or a few, clones of immunoglobulin-producing cells, so normal serum immunoglobulins are derived from multiple clones. We therefore expect and find a great diversity of antigenic structure among immunoglobulin molecules in normal serum. Although there is great diversity, it is nevertheless ordered and subject naturally to the strict laws of inheritance.

Human IgG has been divided primarily into four subclasses. Their new and old nomenclatures are given in *Table XVII*, together with the types of heavy chain that these specificities define. All four subclasses are found in all normal sera, but the amount of each subclass that is present is not the same. The actual relationships are given in *Table XVIII*.

The subclasses themselves can be further divided into serum groups or allotypes on the basis of still subtler antigenic differences. Such isospecificities have been described in man and monkey, as well as in a number of lower mammals and the domestic fowl. In the rabbit these groups are termed 'allotypes' [55], a word that is being increasingly applied to serum groups in man, although there is by no means a full understanding of the genetic factors involved in the distribution of these antigenic specificities.

Allotypes in the rabbit appear to have received rather more than their fair share of attention considering that myeloma proteins are not found in this species of animal. The reason for this is that they can be studied by the relatively simple technique of precipitation, using antisera prepared in other rabbits. A genetic system governing rabbit IgG antigenic specificities has been worked out on the basis of three alleles at either of two loci, a and b, although a number of other specificities are now known [5] and may necessitate modifications. The whole subject has been extensively reviewed by Kelus and Gell [55].

The number of serum group factors in man is still increasing. Two categories, Inv and Oz, we have already met in connexion with light chains. A third category, Gm, is exclusively associated with heavy chains of IgG, as is ISf(1), the first antigen of a newly discovered serum group independent of the Gm system. Well over twenty Gm factors have now been described (*Table XVII*), though some of them are not distinct entities. In view of what has been said above about the use of myeloma proteins and isolated heavy chains for the detection of Gm specificities, it is worth noting that some specificities behave quite differently in the whole molecule and in isolated chains. Thus the antigenic activity of Gm(1) is preserved and even enhanced in the isolated form, whereas that of Gm(4) is almost entirely lost. Reference to *Fig.* 27 shows that Gm(1) is located in the Fc fragment and Gm(4) in Fd. The interesting speculation then arises that just as the configuration of the antibody combining site is influenced by the light chain so may that part of the heavy chain that expresses Gm(4) specificity, in spite of the fact that an heritable character must represent a 'constant' amino-acid sequence.

Table XVII.—NOTATION FOR THE HEREDITARY Gm AND Inv FACTORS OF IMMUNOGLOBULINS

ORIGINAL	NEW	AUTHORS AND YEARS OF REPORT
Gm(a)	Gm(1)	Grubb and Laurell (1956)
Gm(x)	Gm(2)	Harboe and Lundevall (1959)
Gm(b$^\omega$) or Gm(b^2)	Gm(3)	Steinberg and Wilson (1963)
Gm(f)	Gm(4)	Gold, Martensson, Ropartz, Rivat, and Rousseau (1965)
Gm(b) or Gm(b^1) or Gm(bγ)	Gm(5) or Gm(12)	Harboe (1959)
Gm(c) or Gm(like) or Gm(c^3)	Gm(6)	Steinberg, Giles, and Stauffer (1960)
Gm(r)	Gm(7)	Brandtzaeg, Fudenberg, and Mohr (1961)
Gm(e)	Gm(8)	Ropartz, Rivat, and Rousseau (1965)
Gm(p)	Gm(9)	Waller, Hughes, Townsend, Franklin, and Fudenberg (1963)
Gm(bα) or Gm(b^3)	Gm(10) or Gm(13)	Ropartz, Rivat, and Rousseau (1963)
Gm(bβ)	Gm(11)	
Gm(b^4)	Gm(14)	Steinberg and Goldblum (1965)
Gm(s)	Gm(15)	Martensson, van Loghem, Matsumoto, and Neilson (1966)
Gm(t)	Gm(16)	
Gm(z)	Gm(17)	Litwin and Kunkel (1966)
RO$_2$	Gm(18)	Ropartz, Rivat, Rousseau, Fudenberg, Molter, and Salmon (1966)
RO$_3$	Gm(19)	
Gm(z)	Gm(20)	Klemperer, Holbrook, and Fudenberg (1966)
Gm(g)	Gm(21)	Natvig (1966)
Gm(y)	Gm(22)	Litwin and Kunkel (1966)
Gm(n)	Gm(23)	Kunkel, Young, and Litwin (1966)
Gm(c^5)	Gm(24)	van Loghem and Martensson (1966)
Inv(l)	Inv(1)	Ropartz, Rivat, and Rousseau (1961)
Inv(a)	Inv(2)	Ropartz, Lenoir, and Rivat (1961)
Inv(b)	Inv(3)	Steinberg and Wilson (1962)
San Francisco 1	ISf(1)	Ropartz, Fudenberg, Rivat, Rousseau, and Lebreton (1967)

It should be stressed that each Gm factor is associated with a single subclass of γ chain. So far, however, these factors have been found in only three out of the four, namely IgG1, IgG2, and IgG3. In addition, the factors are distributed very unevenly among these three (*Table XVIII*) [56], especially bearing in mind that IgG3 accounts for only 9 per cent of all IgG (*Table XVIII*). In *Fig.* 27 is shown the distribution of Gm factors in IgG1 molecules. First, it will be noticed that Gm factors occur in both Fc and Fd fragments; second, that allelic pairs are, of course, located in the same part of the chain.

As indicated above, it is early days yet to correlate amino-acid sequence data with antigenic specificities of heavy chains since comparisons between sufficiently large fragments of heavy chains of different allotype are only just beginning to appear. Porter reports that an N-terminal peptide of Fd

Table XVIII.—NOMENCLATURE, PERCENTAGE OF TOTAL IgG, AND DISTRI-BUTION OF KNOWN SERUM GROUP FACTORS IN THE SUBCLASSES OF HUMAN IgG. After Natvig, Kunkel, and Gedde-Dahl [56]

IgG1 (We)* (γ2b)* (70 per cent)	IgG2 (Ne)* (γ2a)* (18 per cent)	IgG3 (Vi)* (γ2c)* (8 per cent)	IgG4 (Ge)* (γ2d)* (3 per cent)
Gm(1)	Gm(23)	Gm(5)	None
Gm(2)		Gm(6)	
Gm(3)		Gm(10)	
Gm(4)		Gm(11)	
Gm(7)		Gm(12)	
Gm(8)		Gm(13)	
Gm(9)		Gm(14)	
Gm(17)		Gm(15)	
Gm(18)		Gm(16)	
Gm(20)		Gm(21)	
Gm(22)		Gm(b⁰)	
ISf(1)		Gm(b⁵)	
		Gm(c³)	
		Gm(c⁵)	

* Old nomenclatures.

of rabbit IgG has arginine at position 9 in allotypes Aa1 and Aa2, but that it is absent in Aa3 [54]. Cohen and Milstein [5] have compared sequences of the C-terminal octadecapeptide of IgG derived from a number of different sources. In the case of human IgG1, IgG2, and IgG3 chains these sequences are the same except for a difference of one or two adjacent residues in IgG3 [5]. The difference of one residue between the IgG3 chains could represent the difference between Gm factors 5 and 21. From the appearance of Table XVIII and Fig. 27 it would seem likely that there remain to be discovered a fair number of Gm factors.

Antiglobulins defining allotypic specificities were first found in patients with rheumatoid arthritis [57]. Later it was found that such antibodies were also present in normal sera, though much more rarely. Sera containing the former have been called 'Raggs', are of high titre, and may possess more than one specificity; those containing the latter have been called 'SNaggs', and are of low titre and monospecific. Antiglobulins can also be classified according to their 'inhibitability'. This term derives from the serological methods used to detect and define serum group specificities in human immunoglobulins. Inhibitable antiglobulins are prevented from agglutinating antibody-coated cells by native immuno-globulin. Therefore, their homologous antigenic determinants are accessible in both the native and denatured forms of the immunoglobulin molecule. With non-inhibitable antiglobulins the specificity is directed towards determinants exposed only when antibody is immunologically denatured, i.e., when 'new' determinants are exposed after an antibody has combined with its specific antigen. Intermediate forms also exist [58].

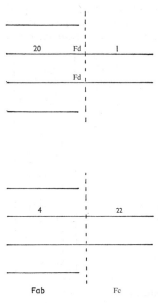

Fig. 27.—Distribution of some allelic Gm factors in the Fab (Fd) and Fc fragments of the IgG1 molecule.

The way in which SNaggs and Raggs arise in human sera is still a matter for conjecture. If we assume an antigenic stimulus at least three kinds could be associated with SNaggs: first, there are the antigens trans-fused with whole blood or its products; second, foetal blood leaking across the placenta, only in this case we are concerned with serum protein in-compatibilities rather than red-cell incompatibilities; and third, the normal placental transfer of maternal IgG to the foetus. Raggs could result from the stimulation of the immunological system by auto-antigens, in which case proof would simply rest on the demonstration that their specificity is directed towards autologous native or autologous denatured immunoglobulin. The issue is quite clear-cut. Unfortunately, the evidence is contradictory, so that no conclusion can yet be reached.

So far, we have described a wide range of antigenic specificities that are or may be present in immunoglobulins. Such antigens may be present in all individuals of a species, in groups of individuals, or only in individuals. No account would be complete without mention being made of idiotypic antigens, i.e., antigens unique to the individual. The question may be asked whether such antigens really exist. In answer, it can be said that some myeloma and macroglobulin proteins possess antigens of individual specificity, and that antisera directed towards them cannot be shown to react with immunoglobulins in normal sera. By the very nature of the problem, however, all normal sera in which these specificities might exist cannot be tested. Also the reduction in titre noted when antisera to such 'idiotypic' antigens are repeatedly absorbed with pooled immunoglobulins might indicate that these antigens are just very rare, and that these antigens cannot be detected in normal sera simply because these antigens are present in very low concentration.

It will be noted that in this argument the tacit assumption is once again made that myeloma proteins, though arising as a result of a pathological process, represent normal immunoglobulins even if they are abnormally homogeneous in molecular structure. The evidence of molecular structure presented here is consistent with the view that they do not differ from normal immunoglobulins, and the growing body of evidence that these paraproteins also possess the same biological properties as their normal counterparts supports this contention.

VII. Evolution and Control of Immunoglobulin Structure

Determination of the amino-acid sequences of light and heavy chains is principally directed towards two targets: first, to defining the nature of antibody specificity and, second, to understanding the biosynthetic mechanisms that lead to the expression of specificity.

To some extent the first goal has already been achieved in that it is generally anticipated that the variable region of the heavy chain, alone or in combination with the variable region of the light chain, will prove to be responsible for antibody specificity. However, attempts to define further the amino-acid composition of antibodies of particular specificity have met with unexpected setbacks. In particular, the amino-acid composition of 'cold anti-I agglutinin' shows differences between the variable section of its light chains that are greater on the whole than those of type K chains of Bence Jones protein chosen at random [59]. Cold agglutinins of anti-I specificity have been chosen for this type of work because they form in any one person a homogeneous population comparable to a myeloma protein. They are usually IgM molecules of type K. Analysis of rabbit IgG has led Koshland to the essentially similar conclusion that 'the light chain from any one antibody was heterogeneous with respect to its amino-acid content despite its average characteristic composition' [60].

Reaching the second target depends to some extent on attaining the first, but there are two related though distinct aspects that must be considered together. These are concerned with the control of the constant and variable sections of immunoglobulin polypeptide chains.

One of the most striking features to emerge from studies on the amino-acid sequences of immunoglobulins has been the repetitive nature of long stretches of the constituent chains. These regions are referred to as internal homologies, have been noted in other proteins, and are thought to arise by a process of gene duplication.

In immunoglobulins, external homology was first detected between the constant regions of light chains, and, as we have seen, this even extended across the species barrier, so that κ chains of man and mouse were more alike than κ and λ chains of man. As more evidence has come to light so this concept of homology has been strengthened. It has also been extended to the N-terminal half, where from Cohen's figure of 40 variable positions [45] we can argue that there remain some 60 invariable. No doubt this figure will be reduced as more sequences are detailed. In comparisons that Hilschmann [46] makes of five partial sequences it looks as if this ratio of 40 : 60 could be reversed, nevertheless still leaving a substantial degree of homology. Putnam [41] and his colleagues have extended this work to the variable region of λ chains from three myelomas. Variation between any two is recorded at 54 positions in the N-terminal half, a ratio of exactly 50 : 50. Still more striking is the apparent concentration of variability in certain sections, so that there are sequences of four or five residues where a different amino-acid is present in each of the three chains. Conversely, there are four sequences of four, one of five, and even one of seven where all the amino-acids are the same in all three chains, so that up to now regions of homology are rather more in evidence than regions of variability. We are inevitably led to conclude, therefore, that there may well be regions in the variable part of light chains that are highly variable, and other regions that are truly constant.

On the basis of much more fragmentary evidence of similarities between light and heavy chains in the region of the combining site, Singer and Doolittle [61] postulated a common genetic origin for the two polypeptide chains of immunoglobulins. They went on to look for and find sequence homologies in the constant parts of light and heavy chains. Subsequently Hill, Delaney, Fellows, and Lebovitz [62] were able to compare sequences of the whole of the human light chain with large parts of the rabbit Fc fragment, comparisons that fully corroborated the hypothesis of Singer and Doolittle that heavy and light chains shared a common genetic heritage. Since this time, evidence has steadily accumulated of sequence homologies between the two halves of the light chain, and between the halves of the Fc fragment, as well as between heavy and light chains [48]. It is on this basis that an ancestral gene coding for one half of the light chain is postulated, with successive gene duplications resulting in the appearance of light and heavy chains.

The phylogenetic approach to the evolution of immunoglobulins has been reviewed by Good and Papermaster [63], and it is clear that this kind of approach is not entirely consistent with the molecular approach that we have employed above. One obvious stumbling block is that we have perforce taken the IgG molecule as our model, whereas it is not the first immunoglobulin to develop, either phylogenetically or ontogenetically.

Immunoglobulins appear to be confined to vertebrate species and to have evolved at roughly the same time, since neither they nor their possible precursors, such as light chains, have been recognized in invertebrates. In the lowest vertebrates IgM and not IgG is found, and, although 7S immunoglobulins may also be present, they are related immunologically to the 19S IgM, and are thought to be monomeric units of the polymeric IgM [64].

One of the difficulties in the way of accepting theories of gene duplication of immunoglobulins is the very different sizes of heavy chain in the various classes. A number of explanations is possible. One is that the higher molecular weight assigned to the μ chain is in fact due to the presence of a fifth polypeptide, as is the case in some immunoglobulins of other animal species, as is the case in human exocrine IgA in a sense, and as has been postulated, as stated earlier, in the case of IgM. A second possibility is that the different classes of immunoglobulins evolved separately, but by roughly the same mechanism. This is simply one of many areas of uncertainty that remain to be resolved.

It is frequently held that the phylogenetic development of immuno-globulins is repeated in ontogeny, and in the immune response as well. It would indeed be surprising if this were not the case in embryological development, since this type of repetition is one of the central tenets of evolutionary hypotheses. As far as the immune response to antigenic stimulus is concerned, the relative sensitivity of methods for detecting IgM compared with those for IgG has tended to place undue emphasis on the early production of IgM, and we are no longer so certain that IgM production precedes IgG. On the other hand, it does seem fairly certain that IgA is the last of these three to develop ontogenetically and phylo-genetically [65]. IgM and IgG have been detected in lymphoid cells of the human foetus at 140 days' gestation [66], whereas no IgA was found up to the time of parturition.

The absence of recognizable adaptive immunity and immunoglobulin precursors in species lower than vertebrates constitutes a hindrance to the determination of evolutionary aspects of specific immunity. However, this is not the only approach to evolution and parallel investigations into control mechanisms of immunoglobulin synthesis are under way. An understanding of the genetic factors involved in the control of the manu-facture of antibodies of different specificity could well lead to a better appreciation of how these mechanisms evolved. The hard central core of this problem is how variability of amino-acid sequence is built into segments of both chains.

If we accept the current dogma that DNA→RNA→protein, then it is evident that there must be a concomitant variation in DNA base pairs. Such possibilities for variation must either be inherited through the germ line, or must arise by somatic events leading to differences of phenotypic expression between cells.

To many people the idea that the germ line carries all the information required to produce antibodies of all the specificities which we know an animal to be capable of lacks credibility. It is interesting to recall that it was precisely on this rock that Ehrlich's side-chain theory of immunity foundered, since it was supposed that all antigens found preformed specific receptors awaiting them at the cell surface. Following Land-steiner's demonstration that antibodies could be produced that were specific for chemical groupings not found in biological materials, the template theories of the 1930's were developed. Since that time, intelligent guesswork would seem to put the required number of specificities at around 10^5, by no means an astronomical figure. Germ-line mutation to account for all the possible variations of the N-terminal regions of light and heavy chains would still seem to be a clumsy process for controlling such variation, implying, as it does, regions of hypermutability in chromosomes, a situation which admittedly is not unknown in bacteria. In general it would seem that, since there is an immense proliferation of lymphoid tissue throughout life anyway, explanations involving somatic mutation or rearrangements of chromosomal material at the same level are inherently more likely, and at the same time less potentially hazardous for the perpetuation of a species.

The large number of hypotheses put forward in recent years [61, 67–72] is indicative of the interest generated by the accumulating knowledge of immunoglobulin chemistry, and also, of course, of the incompleteness of that knowledge. It can at least be said that any speculations about genetic control must take account of the variability of some sections and the stability of others, both of them within the variable region as a whole. Some authors attempt to do this principally on the basis of somatic mutation, some on the basis of the rearrangement of nucleotides already present in the gene. A major difficulty at the moment is that attempts to explain a unique situation are being made in terms of genetic principles evolved for other situations. Further, we are not certain yet just how unique the immunoglobulin situation is, and until a good many more complete determinations of amino-acid sequences are available we shall be in no position to define the pattern of variability in these polypeptide chains, nor, therefore, to understand the mechanism by which their synthesis is controlled.

It is interesting to note that the general acceptance that protein synthesis is directly under genetic control also implies that cells may have a very restricted capacity to produce antibody of different specificities. That this is so is indicated by the fact that although whole serum from a single individual will contain IgG antibodies of all four subclasses, and there will be serum group antigens present within these subclasses, nevertheless antibody of one specificity will be restricted in a number of respects. The classic example, already mentioned, does not fall into any of the above categories; it is the anti-I cold agglutinin of human red cells that is almost invariably IgM of type K. One further implication of far-reaching significance is that, if at any stage in antibody production certain cells are committed genetically to producing antibody of certain specificity, then the antigenic stimulus must exert a measure of selectivity, and we are right back with the concepts that Ehrlich propounded in his side-chain theory. (*See* Chapter 4.)

VIII. BIOLOGICAL PROPERTIES OF IMMUNOGLOBULINS

The characteristic and striking diversity of structure among the proteins that we group together under the title of 'immunoglobulins' is expressed in a number of ways. We recognize those chemical differences between the heavy chains that serve to distinguish between classes antigenically; physical differences of molecular weight and electric charge; structural differences in the form of monomers and polymers; and compositional differences in that polypeptide chains additional to the basic four-chain model may be present, as in the case of secretory IgA, and perhaps of IgM and IgE as well.

Diversity of structure is, of course, also inherent in the chief biological property of immunoglobulins, i.e., in their antibody activity. That specificity of antibody for antigen should prove to be of survival value to the host is scarcely surprising; nor, therefore, that this type of diversity should persist evolutionarily. But we might justifiably ask why there should be as many as five classes of immunoglobulin, and whether they have separate functions. These are questions directed towards the properties of the molecule as a whole. We can ask questions about the biological properties of parts of the molecule as well, such as: Is the combining site part of the heavy or the light chain, or both? Are all combining sites on antibody molecules produced in response to a single stimulus the same? Do constant regions of the antibody molecule serve any biological function? We shall try to deal with each of these questions, and some others, in the following pages.

A. The Whole Molecule

In *Table XVI* (p. 94) is shown the intravascular concentration of the five immunoglobulin classes in healthy adult human beings. What it does not reveal is that, whereas 80 per cent of the IgM remains intravascular, more than half, 60 per cent, of IgG is outside the vascular system [11]. Furthermore, although IgA is present in serum, there is a very considerable, but as yet unmeasurable, outpouring of secretory IgA onto mucous surfaces of the respiratory and alimentary tracts, and elsewhere. Bearing this distribution in mind, we can look more closely at the immunological properties and functions of the different classes of antibody.

IgG is a small molecule compared with IgM and is generally present in much higher concentration in both tissues and circulation than the other immunoglobulins. It enters the picture very early in life, since it is the only immunoglobulin that can cross the placental barrier in humans to reach the foetal circulation. This is not so in all animals, and defence against pathogenic micro-organisms in newborn pigs and calves, for instance, is mediated through antibody, principally IgA, secreted in the colostrum. In man, serum IgG levels in the newborn are as high as, or even slightly higher, than those in maternal circulations. Maternal antibodies are important for guarding the infant life from bacterial and other microorganismal invasion. They are gradually lost from the baby's circulation during the course of the first 4–6 months, being replaced with the infant's own antibodies. The half-life of IgG is 23 days [11] and maternal antibody can be expected to be lost by the infant at least at this rate. If the infant mounts an immune attack against the 'foreign' protein then it could well be quicker.

Transport across the placenta is not simply a function of the size of the molecule of IgG, but is due to a property of the Fc fragment. Digestion with pepsin leaves the combining sites of IgG intact, but the antibody is now unable to cross the placental barrier.

On the basis of its high relative concentration and widespread distribution, it is reasonable to conclude that IgG plays a major role among antibodies in defence against infectious disease. Tested experimentally, IgG is particularly effective in neutralizing bacterial toxins, possibly because its combining site is comparatively large. In terms of combination with oligosaccharide haptens, it reacts with at least the pentasaccharide [73]. Parameters of antigen–antibody interactions that may be affected by the size of the reactive sites are avidity and affinity. By avidity we mean the speed of a reaction; and by affinity the strength of the forces that hold antigen and antibody together. A firm union could be important in the neutralization of toxins, which will themselves have affinities for tissue receptors. The size of antideterminants could therefore have an important bearing on the effectiveness of the immune response and its resultant survival value for the host.

IgM antibody differs markedly from the other immunoglobulins, most obviously in respect of size. With its five basic units, it might be supposed to possess 10 combining sites per molecule. The evidence on this point is somewhat conflicting, however, with some authors subscribing to a valency of 5 or 6 [5, 31], and others to a valency of 10 [29]. It may be, too, that the combining site of IgM for carbohydrate determinants is very much smaller than that of IgG, since it has been reported that the terminal galactosamine of A blood-group substance is as effective in inhibiting the action of an IgM anti-A as the tri- and pentasaccharides [73].

From its mainly intravascular position it must be supposed that IgM functions effectively in this milieu. The capacity of single molecules to fix the serum factors, known collectively as 'complement', is well attested, but, as we shall see later (Chapters 5 and 6), the protective action of complement is not well understood as yet, though it is gradually becoming clearer. It is probable that IgM with, and to some extent without, complement enhances the uptake of bacteria by phagocytes, and might therefore be considered a powerful weapon in the prevention of persisting bacteriaemia. There can be no doubt as to the potential danger to the host posed by bacterial invasion of the blood-stream, so perhaps it is no accident that low levels of IgM, with specificities directed towards the Gram-negative bacteria that commonly inhabit the gut, are persistently found in human serum. The presence of such a defence mechanism was probably also an early requirement in the evolution of higher forms of animal life. IgM is also an efficient agglutinator of bacterial and other cells, whether by virtue of its size, its multiple valencies, its effect on surface charge, or other physico-chemical parameters, is not known; but this property too could limit the dissemination of micro-organisms mechanically, as well as lead to their more efficient phagocytosis.

The separate function of IgA in serum is by no means clear as yet. We have already noted that IgA arises late in the development cycle [65] and probably after birth [66]. By contrast with our uncertainty about its role in serum, its function on the surface of mucous membranes is easily explained in teleological terms. Here it could obviously exert a protective effect at the very site where quick action against potential invaders would be most effective. By way of example, we see a kind of local immunity developing when live poliomyelitis virus vaccine is given orally. The immunity conferred is specific and prevents any significant multiplication of the same virus type in cells of the alimentary tract. Conversely, this type of immunity does not develop when killed vaccine is given by the usual parenteral route, although both vaccines are effective immunizing agents in the clinical sense. One inference that can be drawn is that infection of the alimentary-tract cells with a vaccine strain stimulates an initial immune response that leads, on subsequent contact with a wild or vaccine strain of virus, to a rapid 'secondary response' (Chapter 4) or outflowing of IgA produced locally [65], so that virus is rapidly neutralized and eliminated. Injected vaccine, although it gives rise to protective levels of antibody in the serum, does not act until an initial phase of virus replication in the epithelial tissues of the gut has occurred and deeper invasion begins.

The association of exocrine IgA with an additional protein naturally led to speculation regarding its role. Originally thought to be involved in the transport of the molecule through the epithelial cells lining the lumen, it now appears just as likely that it can penetrate through the inter-cellular spaces [74]. The so-called 'T' or 'transport piece' is now generally referred to as the 'secretory piece' or 'SP' [75]. Whether the polymeric structure of exocrine IgA is associated with or necessary for its immunological function is not yet clear.

IgD was first recognized in 1965 in the form of a myeloma protein [76]. Although undoubtedly an immunoglobulin, because the antigenic specificity of light chains can be demonstrated, antibody activity has not yet been established beyond doubt. Studies in European and African communities suggest that it may be particularly associated with chronic infections [77]. At one time it was thought that IgD might be reaginic antibody, i.e., antibody associated with immediate hypersensitivity reactions (Chapter 6), and physicochemically it is similar [80]. However, serum levels of IgD do not correlate with hypersensitive states or with the capacity of such sera to transfer hypersensitivity passively.

In a remarkable series of studies on immediate hypersensitivity, the team of workers led by Ishizaka demonstrated that reaginic antibody to ragweed pollen was not associated with any of the immunoglobulin fractions precipitated with antisera to IgG, IgM, IgA, and IgD [78]. They defined another globulin, referred to as γ-E-globulin, and showed that, as it was precipitated by a specific antiserum from the serum of patients sensitive to ragweed pollen, so the reaginic activity of serum disappeared. Subsequently a myeloma protein, IgND, was described [79]. It shares antigenic determinants with the E-globulin of Ishizaka and at a meeting held under the auspices of the W.H.O. it was characterized as IgE, the fifth class of immunoglobulins. The identification of IgE with reaginic antibody is currently under investigation [80].

As is the case with many of the other biological properties of immunoglobulins, such as the placental transfer site, complement fixation, and capacity to resist catabolism, the skin-fixing site of IgE appears to be associated with the Fc part of the molecule. The Fc fragment is not therefore simply an inert platform to which the antideterminants are attached, but actually possesses biological properties of its own that are important for the proper functioning of antibody activity, in addition to any antigenic characteristics that may be located in that part of the heavy chain.

B. The Combining Site

Long before the chemistry of proteins was sufficiently advanced for it to be stated unequivocally that the primary sequence in polypeptide chains determines secondary and tertiary structures of proteins, it had been recognized that specificity of antibodies must imply a quality of uniqueness in their configuration. One interesting question that arose from this interpretation was whether this provision of unique structures within the immunological system itself gave rise to antigenic stimuli. In other words, can antisera be raised to antideterminants? Many attempts to do this have been made, but one difficulty has been to obtain undoubtedly homogeneous preparations of antideterminants. The discovery of antigenic activity in the combining site of antibodies has been claimed from time to time, but such claims have to withstand scrutiny on two counts before they can be regarded as substantiated: first, the possibility of an idiotypic specificity must be excluded, i.e., of an antigenic specificity unique to that antibody but not associated with the combining site, and, second, the more serious objection of defining 'uniqueness', without first testing all other antibody molecules, assuming such a project to be remotely feasible. However, if the antideterminant is antigenically active it should be possible to approach the question from the angle of antigenic similarity between antibodies with the same specificity but raised in genotypically different animals. Nevertheless, what evidence there is suggests that even using what are thought to be highly homogeneous sources of antibody, namely the IgM cold agglutinins of type K, differences of composition can still be detected both chemically and immunologically [59, 81]. However, before we turn our attention to the way in which antideterminants to the same antigen might differ from each other, let us consider briefly how these specific configurations are achieved in the immunoglobulin molecule.

It is commonly assumed nowadays that the combining site derives its unique property of specific interaction with antigen from a unique arrangement of amino-acids in the variable regions of the heavy or light chains, or both. There are not many who would maintain that the light chain was solely responsible for the specificity of antibody. The evidence that the combining site is formed by the heavy chain is reviewed by Cohen and Milstein [5], and includes the observed capacity of isolated heavy chains to combine with homologous antigen. The recovery of antibody activity after the removal of reducing and denaturing agents also constitutes the very strongest evidence that the primary structure of proteins determines their three-dimensional structure. The role of the light chain is particularly apparent in the greatly increased combining affinity exhibited when homologous light and heavy chains are allowed to recombine [5]. The light chain may participate by forming part of the combining site, or it may exert its effect through the heavy chain. Recombination of separated chains also shows an element of specificity, or at least a mutual preference, for the original pairing.

If we exclude antigenic specificity attributable to the antideterminant, we are still left with two other attributes of this part of the molecule that reflect its heterogeneity, namely avidity and affinity. These terms have already been defined as rate and strength of union respectively, and these concepts receive further attention in Chapter 6, 'Antigen–antibody Reactions'. For the moment we are concerned only with the effect of heterogeneity of the combining site on the immunological behaviour of antibody and its implication in terms of antibody production.

The first place to look for evidence of heterogeneity among antibodies of the same specificity is perhaps among the different classes of immunoglobulin, particularly IgM and IgG. The first detailed study using modern techniques was into the haemolytic efficiency of $7S$ and $19S$ antibodies by Talmage, Freter, and Talioferro [82]. Although we may no longer subscribe in precise terms to these early findings, the general inference that IgM antibody is a more effective haemolysin than IgG, on a molar basis, has been amply confirmed. The reasons for this increased effectiveness of IgM are rather complex and not entirely due to the combining site, but they are not relevant at the moment and are further discussed in Chapter 5. Differences between rabbit IgM and IgG are also noted in their agglutinating capacity for human red cells [83]. IgM is several hundred times more effective on a molar basis, even though only one-fifth as many IgM molecules are taken up per red cell as IgG. Again, it is possible that parts of the molecule other than the combining site play some role in the process of agglutination. Other workers have used a hapten–antihapten system in order to avoid any ambiguity in the determinant site, as usually occurs when whole cells are used. With the hapten p-azobenzenearsonate attached to red blood-cells, comparisons on a molecular basis showed IgM to have 60–180 times the agglutinating capacity of IgG [84]. It has been pointed out, of course, that affinity of antibody for antigen as measured by determination of the combining constant will reflect the number of combining sites involved, and that IgM has an advantage of at least 5 to 2 over IgG in this respect [85].

Since Landsteiner first laid the foundations of immunochemistry, it has been recognized that antigen–antibody reactions are reversible chemical processes. In the above context, the transfer of antibody from cell to cell is well documented [86], but the meaning in terms of biological activity is less clear. Particularly does this seem to be the case with immune haemolysis where single molecules of IgM are probably sufficient to initiate haemolysis, but a number of IgG molecules acting in concert, and adjacent to each other, may be necessary. Under these circumstances, and providing the antigenic determinants on a red cell are less than saturated, it may be a positive advantage for IgG molecules to have a low affinity, in order that they may dissociate and recombine in a more favourable position to fix complement. It is of interest, therefore, that antisera of different haemolytic efficiency, i.e., causing lysis at different rates, can be produced by altering the immunization schedule, and, of course, by the time of collection [87].

Configurational variations in the combining sites of antibodies may affect the rate and strength of union between antigen and antibody. Yet another aspect of heterogeneity that may well influence the nature of this union is the actual size of the antideterminant. The likelihood of the IgM antideterminant being relatively small has already been noted. On the face of it, this might suggest that IgM would have a lower affinity and higher dissociation constant than IgG, and though this is in agreement with some data it does rather conflict with what has been said above regarding the mechanism of complement fixation. However, although IgM antibody is effective for fixing complement, it is not as efficient as IgG when it comes to sensitizing red blood-cells to the lytic action of complement, possibly because the attachment of IgM to the cell surface lacks permanence. It is still necessary to bear in mind the greater number of valencies of IgM, and indeed it is by no means impossible to conceive of situations where the distribution of antigenic sites, or the relative proportions of antigen and antibody, or the manner in which they are brought together, is such that agglutination or any other serological reaction might be favoured by a low affinity rather than the reverse. It must, indeed, always be borne in mind that even *in vitro* we are usually dealing with immensely complicated situations, and that forces quite separate from those acting between determinant and antideterminant may be operating.

So far, we have been speaking mainly about the heterogeneity of combining site between different classes of immunoglobulins. It must also be recognized that heterogeneity may be just as extreme within classes, and may take on the same forms that we have been discussing. The element of selection exerted by antigen has also been mentioned before; and in a biological situation the expectation is that the selected cells not only differ among themselves, but that this difference is reflected in the kind of antibody they produce. In this sense, antigenic stimulation will result in a population of antibodies which differ among themselves in a number of important particulars, such as avidity, affinity, and specificity. Selection by antigen operating at this level may have two important consequences. First, it may be that only certain clones of cells are selected for producing antibody of a certain specificity. This in turn means that, although serum as a whole contains a great range of immunoglobulins of all classes and subclasses, and those allotypic specificities inherited by that individual, antibody directed towards a particular antigenic determinant is usually of more restricted antigenic specificity. The classic example of anti-I cold agglutinins has been mentioned.

The second consequence is perhaps more far-reaching and stems from the possibility that different cell clones will produce antibodies with slightly different combining sites, not simply from the point of view of size but of actual configuration. Thus, out of the whole range of antibodies produced in response to a single stimulus, may arise certain molecules that react more weakly, as strongly, or more strongly with heterologous antigens. This is one way in which cross-reactions can arise; the whole question of cross-reactions will be dealt with more fully in Chapter 6. It is sufficient to say here that the heterogeneity of the antibody response can be one cause of the lack of specificity sometimes displayed by serological reactions, as well as for their specificity.

REFERENCES

1. GRABAR, P., and WILLIAMS, C. A. (1953), 'Méthode permettant l'Étude conjugée des Propriétés électrophorétiques et immunochimiques d'un Mélange de Protéines. Application au Sérum sanguin', *Biochim. biophys. Acta*, **10**, 193.
2. WORLD HEALTH ORGANIZATION (1964), 'Nomenclature for Human Immunoglobulins', *Bull. Wld Hlth Org.*, **30**, 447.
3. ROWE, D. S., and FAHEY, J. L. (1965), 'A New Class of Human Immunoglobulins. II, Normal Serum IgD', *J. exp. Med.*, **121**, 185.
4. WORLD HEALTH ORGANIZATION (1968), 'Immunoglobulin E, a New Class of Human Immunoglobulin', *Bull. Wld Hlth Org.*, **38**, 151.

5. COHEN, S., and MILSTEIN, C. (1967), 'Structure and Biological Properties of Immunoglobulins', *Adv. Immun.*, **7**, 1.
6. BENNICH, H., and JOHANSSON, S. G. O. (1967), 'Studies on a New Class of Immunoglobulins. II, Chemical and Physical Properties', in *Nobel Symposium 3. Gamma Globulins* (ed. KILLANDER, J.). New York: Interscience.
7. CLAMP, J. R., DAWSON, G., and HOUGH, L. (1966), 'Heterogeneity of Glycopeptides from a Homogeneous Immunoglobulin', *Biochem. J.*, **100**, 35C.
8. JOHANSSON, S. G. O., MELLBIN, T., and VAHLQUIST, B. (1968), 'Immunoglobin Levels in Ethiopian Preschool Children with Special Reference to High Concentrations of Immunoglobulin E (IgND)', *Lancet*, **1**, 1118.
9. TOMASI, T. B. (1965), 'Analytical Review; Human Gammaglobulin', *Blood*, **25**, 382.
10. WALDENSTRÖM, J. (1962), 'Monoclonal and Polyclonal Gammopathies and the Biological System of Gammaglobulins', *Prog. Allergy*, **6**, 320.
11. FAHEY, J. L. (1965), 'Antibodies and Immunoglobulins. II, Normal Development and Changes in Disease', *J. Am. med. Ass.*, **194**, 255.
12. POTTER, M., and LIEBERMAN, R. (1967), 'Genetics of Immunoglobulins in the Mouse', *Adv. Immun.*, **7**, 91.
13. ROCKEY, J. H., KLINMAN, N. R., and KARUSH, F. (1964), 'Equine Antihapten Antibody. I, 7S β2A and 10S γ1 Globulin Components of Purified Anti-β-lactoside Antibody', *J. exp. Med.*, **120**, 589.
14. ROCKEY, J. H., KLINMAN, N. R., and KARUSH, F. (1965), 'Antigenic Heterogeneity of the Subunits of Equine Anti-β-lactoside Antibody', *Fedn Proc. Fedn Am. Socs exp. Biol.*, **24**, 332.
15. OSEBOLD, J. W., AALUND, O., and MURPHY, F. A. (1965), 'The Gammaglobulins of Sheep', *Fedn Proc. Fedn Am. Socs exp. Biol.*, **24**, 503.
16. JENNESS, R., ANDERSON, R. K., and GOUGH, P. M. (1965), 'Fractionation of Bovine Milk and Blood Agglutinins for Brucella by Gel Filtration and Specific Adsorption Techniques', *Fedn Proc. Fedn Am. Socs exp. Biol.*, **24**, 503.
17. FUDENBERG, H. H. (1965), 'The Immune Globulins', *Ann. Rev. Microbiol.*, **19**, 301.
18. PORTER, R. R. (1963), 'Chemical Structure of Gamma Globulin and Antibodies', *Br. med. Bull.*, **19**, 197.
19. LAMM, M. E., and SMALL, P. A. (1966), 'Polypeptide Chain Structure of Rabbit Immunoglobulins. II, γM-immunoglobulin', *Biochemistry*, **5**, 267.
20. MILLER, F., and METZGER, H. (1965), 'Characterization of a Human Macroglobulin. I, Molecular Weight of its Subunit', *J. biol. Chem.*, **240**, 3325.
21. COHEN, S., and FREEMAN, T. (1960), 'Metabolic Heterogeneity of Human γ-globulin', *Biochem. J.*, **76**, 475.
22. CEBRA, J. J., and SMALL, P. A. (1967), 'Polypeptide Chain Structure of Rabbit Immunoglobulins. III, Secretory γA-immunoglobulin from Colostrum', *Biochemistry*, **6**, 503.
23. HONG, R., POLLARA, B., and GOOD, R. A. (1966), 'A Model for Colostral IgA', *Proc. natn. Acad. Sci. U.S.A.*, **56**, 602.
24. DEUTSCH, H. F. (1967), 'Subunit Structure of Gamma-M Globulins', in *Nobel Symposium 3. Gamma Globulins* (ed. KILLANDER, J.). New York: Interscience.
25. EDELMAN, G. M. (1959), 'Dissociation of γ-globulin', *J. Am. chem. Soc.*, **81**, 3155.
26. EDELMAN, G. M., and POULIK, M. D. (1961), 'Studies in Structural Units of γ-Globulin', *J. exp. Med.*, **113**, 861.
27. FLEISCHMAN, J. B., PAIN, R. H., and PORTER, R. R. (1962), 'Reduction of γ-Globulins', *Archs Biochem. Biophys.*, Suppl. **1**, 174.
28. COHEN, S., and PORTER, R. R. (1964), 'Structure and Biological Activity of Immunoglobulins', *Adv. Immun.*, **4**, 287.
29. PORTER, R. R. (1958), 'Separation and Isolation of Fractions of Rabbit Gammaglobulin containing the Antibody and Antigenic Combining Sites', *Nature, Lond.*, **182**, 670.
30. NISONOFF, A., WISSLER, F. C., LIPMAN, L. N., and WOERNLEY, D. L. (1960), 'Separation of Univalent Fragments from Bivalent Rabbit Antibody Molecule by Reduction of Disulphide Bonds', *Archs Biochem. Biophys.*, **89**, 230.
31. NOELKEN, M. E., NELSON, C. A., BUCKLEY, C. E., and TANFORD, C. (1965), 'Cross Conformation of Rabbit 7S γ-Immunoglobulin and its Papain-cleaved Fragments', *J. biol. Chem.*, **240**, 218.
32. FEINSTEIN, A., and ROWE, A. J. (1965), 'Molecular Mechanism of Formation of an Antigen–antibody Complex', *Nature, Lond.*, **205**, 147.

33. VALENTINE, R. C., and GREEN, N. M. (1967), 'Electron Microscopy of an Antibody-hapten Complex', *J. molec. Biol.*, **27**, 615.
34. CHESEBRO, B., BLOTH, B., and SVEHAG, S.-E. (1968), 'The Ultrastructure of Normal and Pathological IgM Immunoglobulins', *J. exp. Med.*, **127**, 399.
35. FEINSTEIN, A., and MUNN, E. A. (1966) 'An Electron Microscopic Study of the Interaction of Macroglobulin (IgM) Antibodies with Bacterial Flagella and of the Binding of Complement', *J. Physiol., Lond.*, **186**, 64P.
36. MERLER, E., KARLIN, L., and MATSUMOTO, S. (1968), 'The Valency of Human γM Immunoglobulin Antibody', *J. biol. Chem.*, **243**, 386.
37. STONE, M. J., and METZGER, H. (1967), 'The Valence of a Waldenström Macroglobulin Antibody and Further Thoughts on the Significance of Paraprotein Antibodies', *Cold Spring Harb. Symp. quant. Biol.*, **32**, 83.
38. ONOUE, K., YAGI, Y., GROSSBERG, A. L., and PRESSMAN, D. (1965), 'Number of Binding Sites of Rabbit Macroglobulin Antibody and its Subunits', *Immunochemistry*, **2**, 401.
39. EDELMAN, G. M., and GALLY, J. A. (1962), 'The Nature of Bence Jones Proteins. Chemical Similarities to Polypeptide Chains of Myeloma Globulins and Normal γ-Globulins', *J. exp. Med.*, **116**, 207.
40. PUTNAM, F. W. (1962), 'Structural Relationships among Normal Human γ-Globulin, Myeloma Globulin, and Bence Jones Proteins', *Biochim. biophys. Acta*, **63**, 539.
41. PUTNAM, F. W. (1967), 'Structural Evolution of Kappa and Lambda Light Chains', in *Nobel Symposium 3. Gamma Globulins* (ed. KILLANDER, J.). New York: Interscience.
42. EDELMAN, G. M., CUNNINGHAM, B. A., GALL, W. E., GOTTLIEB, P. D., RUTISHAUSER, U., and WAXDAL, M. J. (1969), 'The Covalent Structure of an Entire γG Immunoglobulin Molecule', *Proc. natn. Acad. Sci. U.S.A.*, **63**, 78.
43. KORNGOLD, L., and LIPARI, R. (1956), 'Multiple-myeloma Proteins. III, The Antigenic Relationship of Bence Jones Proteins to Normal Gamma-globulin and Multiple-myeloma Serum Proteins', *Cancer, N.Y.*, **9**, 262.
44. PORTER, R. R. (1967), 'The Structure of Immunoglobulins', *Biochem. J.*, **105**, 417.
45. COHEN, S. (1967), 'Heterogeneity of Immunoglobulin Light Chains', in *Nobel Symposium 3. Gamma Globulins* (ed. KILLANDER, J.). New York: Interscience.
46. HILSCHMANN, N. (1967), 'The Structure of the Immunoglobulins (L-chains) and the Antibody Problem', in *Nobel Symposium 3. Gamma Globulins* (ed. KILLANDER, J.). New York: Interscience.
47. APELLA, E., and EIN, D. (1967), 'Two Types of Lambda Polypeptide Chains in Human Immunoglobulins based on an Amino Acid Substitution at Position 190', *Proc. natn. Acad. Sci. U.S.A.*, **57**, 1449.
48. HILL, R. L., LEBOVITZ, H. E., FELLOWS, R. E., and DELANEY, R. (1967), 'The Evolution of Immunoglobulins as reflected by the Amino Acid Sequence Studies of Rabbit Fc Fragment', in *Nobel Symposium 3. Gamma Globulins* (ed. KILLANDER, J.). New York: Interscience.
49. FRANKLIN, E. C., LÖWENSTEIN, J., BIGELOW, B., and MELTZER, M. (1964), 'Heavy Chain Disease—A New Disorder of Serum γ-globulins', *Am. J. Med.*, **37**, 332.
50. GIVOL, D., and PORTER, R. R. (1965), 'The C-terminal Peptide of the Heavy Chain of the Rabbit Immunoglobulin IgG', *Biochem. J.*, **97**, 32C.
51. HILL, R. L., DELANEY, R., LEBOVITZ, H. E., and FELLOWS, R. E. (1966), 'Studies on the Amino Acid Sequence of Heavy Chains from Rabbit Immunoglobulin G', *Proc. R. Soc., B*, **166**, 159.
52. EDELMAN, G. M. (1967), 'Studies on the Primary and Tertiary Structure of γG Immunoglobulins', in *Nobel Symposium 3. Gamma Globulins* (ed. KILLANDER, J.). New York: Interscience.
53. PRESS, E. M., and PIGGOT, P. J. (1967), 'The Chemical Structure of the Heavy Chains of Human Immunoglobulin G', *Cold Spring Harb. Symp. quant. Biol.*, **32**, 45.
54. PORTER, R. R. (1967), 'The Chemical Structure of the Heavy Chain of Immunoglobulins', in *Nobel Symposium 3. Gamma Globulins* (ed. KILLANDER, J.). New York: Interscience.
55. KELUS, A. S., and GELL, P. G. H. (1967), 'Immunoglobulin Allotypes of Experimental Animals', *Prog. Allergy*, **11**, 141.

56. NATVIG, J. B., KUNKEL, H. G., and GEDDE-DAHL, T. (1967), 'Genetic Studies of the Heavy Chain Subgroups of γG Globulin', in *Nobel Symposium* 3. *Gamma Globulins* (ed. KILLANDER, J.). New York: Interscience.
57. GRUBB, R., and LAURELL, A. B. (1956), 'Hereditary Serological Human Serum Groups', *Acta path. microbiol. scand.*, **39**, 390.
58. GOLD, E. R., and FUDENBERG, H. H. (1969), 'Simultaneous Agglutination Tests with Human Antiglobulins', *Vox Sang.*, **16**, 57.
59. COHEN, S., and COOPER, A. G. (1968), 'Chemical Differences between Individual Human Cold Agglutinins', *Immunology*, **15**, 93.
60. KOSHLAND, M. E. (1966), 'Primary Structure of Immunoglobulins and its Relationship to Antibody Specificity', *J. cell. Physiol.*, **67**, Suppl. 1, 33.
61. SINGER, S. J., and DOOLITTLE, R. F. (1966), 'Antibody Active Sites and Immunoglobulin Molecules', *Science* N.Y., **153**, 13.
62. HILL, R. L., DELANEY, R., FELLOWS, R. E., and LEBOVITZ, H. E. (1966), 'The Evolutionary Origin of the Immunoglobulins', *Proc. natn. Acad. Sci. U.S.A.*, **56**, 1762.
63. GOOD, R. A., and PAPERMASTER, B. W. (1964), 'Ontogeny and Phylogeny of Adaptive Immunity', *Adv. Immun.*, **4**, 1.
64. CLEM, L. W., and SMALL, P. A. (1967), 'Phylogeny of Immunoglobulin Structure and Function. I, Immunoglobulins of the Lemon Shark', *J. exp. Med.*, **125**, 893.
65. SOUTH, M. A., COOPER, M. D., HONG, R., and GOOD, R. A. (1967), 'The IgA Antibody System', in *Current Topics in Developmental Biology*, vol. 2 (ed. MONROY, A., and MOSCONA, A. A.). New York: Academic.
66. VAN FURTH R., SCHUTT, H. R. E., and HIJMANS, W. (1965), 'The Immunological Development of the Human Fetus', *J. exp. Med.*, **122**, 1173.
67. DREYER, W. J., and BENNETT, J. C. (1965), 'The Molecular Basis of Antibody Formation: A Paradox', *Proc. natn. Acad. Sci. U.S.A.*, **54**, 864.
68. BRENNER, S., and MILSTEIN, C. (1966), 'Origin of Antibody Variation', *Nature, Lond.*, **211**, 242.
69. EDELMAN, G. M., and GALLY, J. A. (1967), 'Somatic Recombination of Duplicated Genes: An Hypothesis on the Origin of Antibody Diversity', *Proc. natn. Acad. Sci. U.S.A.*, **57**, 353.
70. WHITEHOUSE, H. L. K. (1967), 'Crossover Model of Antibody Variability', *Nature, Lond.*, **215**, 371.
71. SMITHIES, D. (1967), 'Antibody Variability', *Science, N.Y.*, **157**, 267.
72. MILSTEIN, C. (1967), 'Linked Groups of Residues in Immunoglobulin κ Chains', *Nature, Lond.*, **216**, 330.
73. KAPLAN, M. E., and KABAT, E. A. (1966), 'Studies on Human Antibodies. IV, Purification and Properties of Anti-A and Anti-B obtained by Absorption and Elution from Insoluble Blood Group Substances', *J. exp. Med.*, **123**, 1061.
74. HEREMANS, J. F., and CRABBÉ, P. A. (1967), 'Immunohistochemical Studies on Exocrine IgA', in *Nobel Symposium* 3. *Gamma Globulins* (ed. KILLANDER, J.). New York: Interscience.
75. HANSON, L. Å., and JOHANSSON, B. G. (1967), 'Studies on Secretory IgA', in *Nobel Symposium* 3. *Gamma Globulins* (ed. KILLANDER, J.). New York: Interscience.
76. ROWE, D. S., and FAHEY, J. L. (1965), 'A New Class of Immunoglobulins. I, A Unique Myeloma Protein', *J. exp. Med.*, **121**, 171.
77. ROWE, D. S., CRABBÉ, P. A., and TURNER, M. W. (1968), 'Immunoglobulin D in Serum, Body Fluids and Lymphoid Tissues', *Clin. exp. Immun.*, **3**, 477.
78. ISHIZAKA, K., ISHIZAKA, T., and HORNBROOK, M. M. (1966), 'Physicochemical Properties of Reaginic Antibody. V, Correlation of Reaginic Activity with γE-globulin Antibody', *J. Immun.*, **97**, 840.
79. JOHANSSON, S. G. O., and BENNICH, H. (1967), 'Immunological Studies of an Atypical (Myeloma) Immunoglobulin', *Immunology*, **13**, 381.
80. COOMBS, R. R. A., HUNTER, A., JONAS, W. E., BENNICH, H., JOHANSSON, S. G. O., and PANZANI, R. (1968), 'Detection of IgE (IgND) Specific Antibody (probably Reagin) to Castor-bean Allergen by the Red-cell-linked Antigen–antiglobulin Reaction', *Lancet*, **1**, 1115.
81. WILLIAMS, R. C., KUNKEL, H. G., and CAPRA, J. D. (1968), 'Antigenic Specificities related to the Cold Agglutinin Activity of Gamma M Globulins', *Science, N.Y.*, **161**, 379.

82. TALMAGE, D. W., FRETER, G. G., and TALIOFERRO, W. H. (1956), 'Two Antibodies of Related Specificity but Different Haemolytic Efficiency separated by Centrifugation', *J. infect. Dis.*, **98**, 300.
83. GREENBURY, C. L., MOORE, D. H., and NUNN, L. A. C. (1963), 'Reaction of 7*S* and 19*S* Components of Immune Rabbit Antisera with Human Group A and AB Red Cells', *Immunology*, **6**, 421.
84. ONOUE, K., TANIGAKI, N., YAGI, Y., and PRESSMAN, D. (1965), 'IgM and IgG Anti-hapten Antibody; Haemolytic, Haemagglutinating and Precipitating Activity', *Proc. Soc. exp. Biol. N.Y.*, **120**, 340.
85. GREENBURY, C. L., MOORE, D. H., and NUNN, L. A. C. (1965), 'The Reaction with Red Cells of 7*S* Rabbit Antibody, its Sub-units and their Recombinants', *Immunology*, **8**, 420.
86. BOWMAN, W. M., MAYER, M. M., and RAPP, H. J. (1951), 'Kinetic Studies on Immune Haemolysis. II, The Reversibility of Red Cell-antibody Combination and the Resultant Transfer of Antibody from Cell to Cell during Haemolysis', *J. exp. Med.*, **94**, 87.
87. NELSON, R. A. (1965), 'The Role of Complement in Immune Phenomena', in *The Inflammatory Process* (ed. ZWEIFACH, B. W., GRANT, L., and MCCLUSKEY, R. T.). New York: Academic.

CHAPTER 4

THE PRODUCTION OF ANTIBODY

By J. Verrier Jones

I. The fate of antigen

II. Production of antibody
    A. Natural antibody
    B. The primary response
        1. The lag phase
        2. The log phase
    C. The secondary response
        1. The specificity of the secondary response
    D. Quantitative aspects of antibody production
        1. Sequential production of $19S$ and $7S$ antibodies
        2. Change in affinity of antibody during the immune response
        3. Immunological memory
    E. Cellular aspects of antibody production
        1. Cells which form antibody
            a. Plasma cells
            b. Lymphocytes
        2. How many antibodies from one cell?
        3. The role of the macrophage
        4. Cellular proliferation and antibody production
            a. Cellular events during the lag phase
            b. Cellular events during the log phase
            c. Cellular events during the plateau and decline phases
            d. Cellular basis of memory
            e. Theoretical implications of cellular studies

III. Factors which increase the immune response
    A. Adjuvants
        1. Non-antigenic adjuvants
        2. Antigenic adjuvants
            Immune deviation

IV. Factors which depress the immune response
    A. X-irradiation and immunosuppressive drugs

    B. Immunological paralysis
         Cellular basis of paralysis
    C. Desensitization
    D. Passively administered antibody
    E. Antigenic competition

V. Summary and conclusions

ATTENTION was first drawn by Glenny and Südmersen [1] to the fact that antibody production in an animal which is exposed to an antigen for the first time differs strikingly from that seen on subsequent exposures. They investigated the antibodies produced after injecting diphtheria toxin in guinea-pigs, rabbits, goats, horses, and humans (*Fig.* 28). After the first injection the rise in level of antitoxins, which was often barely detectable,

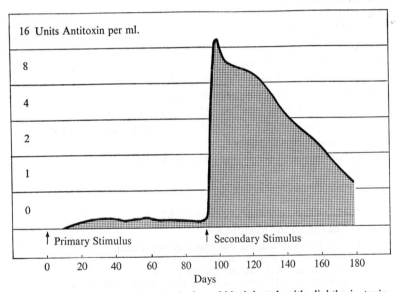

Fig. 28.—Production of antitoxin by rabbit injected with diphtheria toxin–antitoxin at Day 0. The primary response is weak and delayed, the secondary response is accelerated, greater, and more sustained. *After Glenny and Südmersen* [1].

began after a latent period of about 2 weeks. After the second injection of toxin the difference was dramatic. Antitoxin production began after only 4 days and was at a maximum in 10 days. The peak levels reached were often a hundredfold greater than after the first injection. They suggested the term 'primary stimulus' for the first injection and 'secondary stimulus' for the subsequent one. The first and second periods of antibody production are now known as the 'primary' and 'secondary' responses.

Subsequent investigations have shown that a primary and a secondary response, differing in the rate and total amount of antibody production, are found in the immune response of many animals to many antigens. In considering the cellular and biochemical events which underlie antibody production, it will be convenient to discuss in turn the fate of administered antigen, the primary response, and the secondary response.

I. THE FATE OF ANTIGEN

Following the administration of an antigen, the lymphoreticular system becomes modified in such a way that it produces antibody of great specificity, and in increasing amounts, directed against the antigen. One of the main problems of immunology is to determine the nature of this change and how it is brought about.

A logical first step is to consider the fate of an antigen after its administration to an animal. The rate at which antigen disappears from the blood after intravenous administration was studied by Glenny and Hopkins [2], who found a curve consisting of two components (*Fig. 29*). The initial,

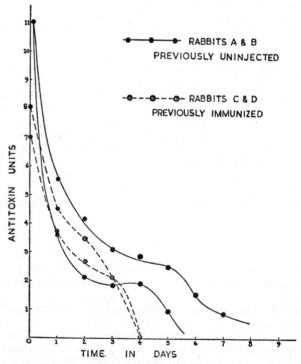

Fig. 29.—Disappearance of horse diphtheria antitoxin from blood of two previously uninjected rabbits (A and B) after intravenous injection. Disappearance of horse diphtheria antitoxin from blood of two rabbits (C and D) previously sensitized to horse serum by intravenous injection. *Data from Glenny and Hopkins* [2]. *Reproduced from Humphrey and White* [171].

slow component which lasts for 4–6 days is followed by a second, more rapid fall which continues exponentially until the antigen is exhausted. Readministration of the same antigen later gives a rapid disappearance curve. This type of curve is associated with the development of immunity to the antigen and is referred to as 'immune elimination'.

In what tissues does antigen accumulate and what changes accompany its arrival? Two groups of workers have published detailed studies on this. White and his co-workers have studied changes in the spleen of chickens following the administration of protein antigens [3, 4]. Human serum albumin (HSA) 1–10 mg. was injected intravenously into 6–10-week-old chickens. Four days after injection clusters of dividing cells appeared in the white pulp of the spleen. These germinal centres contained numerous cells in mitosis, and by 7 days had developed into rounded collections of medium and large lymphocytes. Antigen could be identified in these centres by staining with a HSA antibody conjugated to a fluorescent dye. A group of branching cells was outlined by the dye: they were scattered throughout the germinal centre, and White termed them 'dendritic cells'. He suggested that antigen localization on the dendritic cells depends on the presence of circulating antibody and that the antigen is present in the form of antigen–antibody complexes. Germinal centres did not appear before 3 days and antigen could not be detected on dendritic cells before 24 hours.

Ada, Nossal, and their co-workers [5] have also studied the localization of administered antigen. As antigens they used flagella from *Salmonella adelaide*, or a protein, flagellin, prepared by acid digestion, which has a molecular weight of about 38,000 and is highly immunogenic in rats. Flagellin was labelled with ^{125}I and injected intravenously or into the hindfoot pad of rats. Intravenous antigens are localized mainly in the spleen, while those administered into the foot pad accumulate in the draining lymph-nodes. Localization of antigen in these organs can be studied by autoradiography.

After foot-pad injection, antigen appeared within 3 minutes in the circular sinus of the draining lymph-nodes. Within 30 minutes it was found in macrophages in the medulla of the node. The antigen in particles and pinocytic vesicles became surrounded with protolysosomes, and phagolysosomes were formed which persisted for several months. Plasma cells also accumulated in increasing numbers in the medullary cords. These cells are known to secrete antibody. There was no evidence in this work to suggest that antigen passes from macrophages to plasma cells, and none of the plasma cells or lymphoid cells contained labelled antigen.

At the same time as antigen is appearing in macrophages in the medulla it is also spreading from the circular sinus into the cortex of the lymph-node, where, at 4 hours, it forms an annular pattern surrounding the primary lymphoid follicles (*Fig.* 30). After 24 hours it is spread throughout all the follicles in the cortex [6]. In the cortex the antigen appears to be mainly extracellular. In some areas it seems to be associated with long, dendritic processes arising from the reticular cells (cf. p. 128).

The arrival of antigen in the lymphoid follicles is followed by a burst of mitotic activity. A study of lymph drained from glands at this stage [7] showed rising titres of antibody and increasing numbers of lymphoblastic cells containing numerous free ribosomes.

The dendritic cells and macrophages make up a specialized system for trapping and retaining antigen. The rapid burst of mitotic activity in germinal centres may be associated with the development of antibody-secreting plasma cells which do not appear to leave the node in which

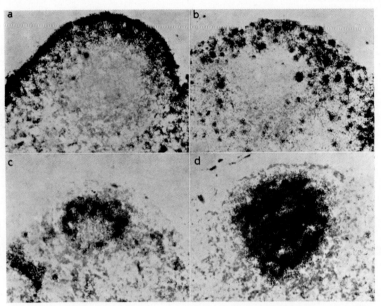

Fig. 30.—A series of radio-autographs showing the accumulation of flagella labelled with radioactive iodine in germinal centres in the lymph-node of an unimmunized rat: (a) 30 minutes after injection, antigen is entering the follicle from the circular sinus, (b) 12 hours, (c) 4 hours, (d) 24 hours after injection. Antigen is gradually penetrating the primary follicle. *Reproduced from G. J. V. Nossal et al.* (1965), '*Immunology*', vol. 9, p. 349, by kind permission of Blackwell Scientific Publications, Oxford.

they are formed. The lymphoblastic cells in the efferent lymph may be messenger cells, disseminating the antibody response to other centres.

II. PRODUCTION OF ANTIBODY

A. Natural Antibody

Antibody can be demonstrated in the serum of animals which have never been deliberately stimulated by antigen, and this antibody has been referred to as 'natural antibody'. The origin of natural antibody and its role in the immune response have been discussed by Boyden [8].

Adult mice which have never been immunized against sheep red-cells show some circulating antibody [9] and have antibody-producing cells in the spleen. However, no animal in its natural environment can strictly be

5

regarded as immunologically unstimulated, since from the moment of birth it is exposed to bacterial and viral antigens in the gut and the respiratory tract, and to immunogenic substances in the food. These natural antigens undoubtedly cross-react with antigens of experimental interest. Is this sufficient to account for the production of natural antibodies? Šterzl [10] has reviewed the evidence from gnotobiotic experiments. If piglets are taken by Caesarean section into isolator chambers and reared in germ-free conditions on a non-antigenic diet consisting of hydrolysed proteins, they are clearly, for practical purposes, unstimulated. Such animals have a lower level of gamma-globulin than normal animals (though it is interesting that gamma-globulin is not completely absent). No natural antibodies can be detected, even after concentrating the serum, and no antibody-producing cells can be detected in the spleen. Šterzl concludes that natural antibody is the result of early exposure to natural antigen, and that in newborns not stimulated with antigen, cells producing antibodies do not occur, and molecules with antibody specificity are not found.

On this view, natural antibodies differ only quantitatively from antibodies produced by direct antigenic challenge. There are, however, two curious points of difference between natural antibodies and immune antibodies, which are so far unexplained. (1) The level of immune antibodies in the serum can be depressed by giving preformed antibody at the same time as the antigen. Natural antibodies are not depressed by passively administered antibody [9]. (2) Doses of anti-lymphocyte serum sufficient to depress the formation of antibodies against *Salmonella typhi* in dogs have no effect on the level of natural antibody [11].

Natural antibodies have been found against a wide range of bacterial and viral antigens [8], and against red-cell antigens (*see* p. 50) and this raises the question of whether experimental challenge with an antigen can ever be regarded as strictly a 'primary' stimulus in conventionally reared animals. Kim, Bradley, and Watson [12], studying the 'true primary' response in colostrum-deprived gnotobiotic piglets, found a number of features which appear strikingly different from those usually described in the primary response. One of the most remarkable findings was that the first antibody produced was a 19S globulin which was antigenically identical with IgG. It is an extreme but arguable view that all work on the primary response will eventually need to be repeated in gnotobiotic animals.

B. The Primary Response*

Since Glenny and Südmersen [1] first described the primary and secondary antibody responses a great deal of information has accumulated on the

---

* The classification and nomenclature of the immunoglobulins has been discussed in Chapter 3, IMMUNOGLOBULINS (p. 93). The terms IgG and IgM have not been used in the following section for two reasons: (1) Much of the work discussed has been in animals, often with immunoglobulins of differing antigenic specificity. (2) If the work of Kim, Bradley, and Watson [12] is confirmed in other animals, we may need to think again before accepting that 19S immunoglobulins are IgM. For these reasons, I shall refer to 19S and 7S antibodies in the following sections.

kinetics of antibody formation. Uhr and Finkelstein [13] have recently reviewed the subject. The early work emphasized the striking differences between primary and secondary responses. The primary response was sluggish, weak, short-lived, and composed mainly of 19S antibodies. The secondary response was swift, powerful, prolonged, and composed mainly of 7S antibodies. The idea grew that there was a qualitative difference between primary and secondary responses.

More recent work has emphasized the similarity between the two responses: if the dose of antigen is adjusted, primary and secondary responses can be made to resemble each other quantitatively [14].

It has also been shown [15] that experimental artefacts may often be responsible for the impression that 19S antibodies are produced first, followed after a considerable lag by 7S antibodies (see p. 135). Nossal, Austin, and Ada [14] have shown that by varying the dose of flagellin the amount of 19S antibody in the secondary response can be varied at will.

1. THE LAG PHASE

After the intravenous injection of an antigen there is a delay before antibody can be detected in the serum. This has been referred to as the 'latent period' or 'lag phase'. Its duration is variable. Glenny and Südmersen [1] found a delay of 3 weeks before the appearance of antibodies to diphtheria toxin. The latent period is shorter for particulate antigens than for soluble antigens, and has been found to be as low as 20 hours for the bacteriophage ϕX 174 [16]. The duration of the latent interval is, of course, an experimental artefact. It depends in part on the dose of antigen, since the first antibody to be produced will combine with circulating antigen and will therefore not be detected by most tests. It is also affected by the sensitivity of the method used to detect antibody: the more sensitive the method, the shorter is the latent period. Jerne [17] points out that the most sensitive methods available leave undetected 10^{10} molecules of antibody per ml. of serum, and Svehag and Mandel [18] found that the curve for early antibody production would extrapolate almost to zero.

The latent period has recently undergone further drastic reductions. Baker and Landy [19] and Sercarz and Modabber [20], using a technique capable of detecting 225 molecules of antibody on a single cell, described antigen-reactive spleen cells produced in unimmunized mice within 4 hours by pneumococcal polysaccharide. However, in 1967, Litt [21] swept the board with the sensational claim that he had detected primary antibody in guinea-pig lymph-nodes within $7\frac{1}{2}$ minutes of the injection of avian erythrocytes into the foot pad. He argued persuasively that he was observing genuine immune haemolysis: further evidence on this point will be keenly awaited. Clearly, if it can be shown that the primary latent period is measured in minutes rather than days, this is of great theoretical importance and will affect theories of the mechanism of antibody production. However, it is important to bear in mind that no response in a conventionally reared animal can strictly be regarded as primary (see p. 130), and there is a strong possibility that Litt was describing the destruction of red cells by antibody which developed originally against a natural, crossreacting antigen.

2. The Log Phase

At the end of the latent period antibody appears in the serum in increasing amounts. The rate and extent of antibody formation depend on the nature and quantity of the antigen administered. The kinetics of this response are discussed by Uhr and Finkelstein [13]. The first antibody to be detected is usually a 19S globulin. Provided the dose of antigen is sufficient, the increase in antibody concentration in the serum is such that the logarithm of the concentration plotted against time gives a straight line, until the fourth or fifth day. This is known as the 'log phase' or exponential phase of antibody production (*Fig.* 31).

A useful measurement during this phase is the length of time taken for the antibody concentration to increase twofold. This is the 'doubling time'. For guinea-pigs given ϕX 174 intravenously the shortest doubling time is 6 hours. The same figure was obtained by Svehag and Mandel [18] for the doubling time of rabbit antibody against poliovirus. Smaller doses of antigen give a longer doubling time.

Soluble antigen produces 19S antibody after a longer latent period [22, 23]. The rate of formation of 19S antibody is probably still exponential [24].

From about the fifth day to the tenth day of the response the rate of 19S antibody synthesis falls and then stops completely. From about the tenth day the rate of decay of 19S antibody in the serum is similar to that of passively administered antibody.

In the primary response, 7S antibody is usually detected after 19S antibody. When ϕX 174 is injected into guinea-pigs the latent period for 7S antibody is 4–7 days (compared with 20 hours for 19S). The latent period for 7S antibodies to poliovirus in rabbits is shorter (36–48 hours) [18]. Although the rate of formation of 7S antibody is slower than that of 19S there is again an exponential phase of antibody production, lasting for 4 days. For antibodies to ϕX in guinea-pigs the doubling time is 10 hours or more.

At the end of the log phase of 7S antibody production the serum concentration falls much more slowly than that of 19S, and, in fact, slow rates of 7S antibody formation may continue for years.

There is some evidence to suggest that, unlike 19S antibodies, 7S antibodies against soluble antigens are produced at the same rate, and in the same amounts, as those against particulate antigens [25, 26].

C. The Secondary Response

A second injection of an antigen, following the first after an interval, provokes an earlier rise in antibody titre which reaches a higher level than the primary response. This is the secondary or anamnestic response.

The latent period in Litt's [21] sensational system (avian erythrocytes in guinea-pig lymph-nodes) is reduced from $7\frac{1}{2}$ minutes to 30 seconds. For salmonella flagella in rats [14] the latent period is reduced from 4 days to 2 days. A similar reduction in the latent period is seen in the response of rabbits to a second injection of sheep erythrocytes [27] and to bovine serum albumin [28].

The antibody formed in the secondary response is usually 7S, though under some circumstances 19S antibody can also be detected [13, 14].

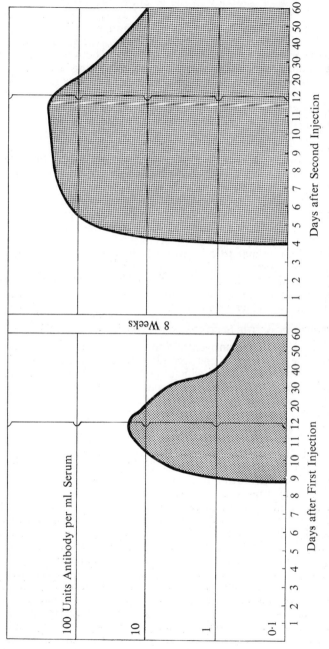

Fig. 31.—Antibody production in rabbit in response to injection of bovine serum albumin. Note the striking difference between primary and secondary response. *After F. J. Dixon et al.* [24].

5*

The rate of rise of antibody in the serum is again exponential, and the doubling time (for ϕX antibody) is about 7 hours. This is faster than the doubling times observed for primary $7S$ antibody (10 hours) [13] and comparable to those for primary $19S$ antibody. The exponential phase of antibody synthesis continues for about 8 days. Between 10 and 17 days after secondary stimulation there is a period during which antibody is produced at slower rates. After 2 weeks serum antibody levels fall off to a plateau.

Subsequent injections of antigen may produce some further increase in antibody production. After a variable number of further injections (depending on the dose and type of antigen) antibody production reaches an absolute ceiling, and the animal is said to be 'hyperimmunized'. Eventually, further doses of antigen may produce a state of immunological desensitization when antibody production may actually be suppressed by the antigen (see p. 152).

It is convenient for experimental purposes to give single, discrete injections of antigen to an animal, and to distinguish primary, secondary, tertiary, and subsequent responses; but it is important to bear in mind that these responses are a laboratory artefact. In most cases the natural exposure of an animal to an antigen is by way of a bacterial or viral infection, and immunity will develop as a result of prolonged and continuous antigenic stimulation. There will be no distinct primary or secondary response; antibody production will move gradually from a less efficient to a more efficient phase.

THE SPECIFICITY OF THE SECONDARY RESPONSE

The specificity of the antigen–antibody reaction is discussed elsewhere (p. 184). The specificity of the secondary response is strikingly similar in many respects. If an animal which has been stimulated once by a single antigen is later stimulated with a second, quite unrelated antigen, it will develop a second primary response. If the second antigen is identical with the first one, the animal will develop a secondary response. However, if the second antigen is similar to, but not identical with, the first antigen a number of interesting cross-reactions can be observed, and these throw considerable light on the nature of the secondary response.

Davenport, Hennessy, and Francis [29, 30] observed that adult humans who were vaccinated with influenza virus reacted by producing antibodies not to the vaccinating strain but to the first strain of influenza virus they had encountered naturally in childhood, sometimes as much as 60 years earlier. This phenomenon was referred to as 'Original Antigenic Sin' by Francis [31], who implied that the taint carried by a human after his first encounter with antigen was as ineradicable as that acquired by Adam after his first encounter with Sin. The topic has since been extensively discussed by Fazekas de St. Groth and Webster [32, 33]. After the first response to antigen, primed cells are produced with a wide variety of specificities. In the normal secondary response all of these will be restimulated, producing a heterogeneous population of antibody molecules. When the animal is restimulated with a cross-reacting antigen, a much smaller population of cells will be stimulated, producing only those antibodies directed against antigens common to the primary and secondary stimulus. The antibody produced will have a limited heterogeneity and every antibody molecule produced can be absorbed by both the primary and the secondary antigen. In the words of Fazekas de St. Groth: 'Original Antigenic Sin acts as a narrow-pass filter on an anamnestic response.'

It has recently been shown in an experimental situation [34] that a single molecule can act as a primary and secondary stimulus simultaneously. Guinea-pigs were sensitized to either the benzyl-penicilloyl group conjugated to poly-L-lysine as a carrier or to dinitrophenyl-poly-L-lysine. The animals were then tested with a compound in which the benzyl-penicilloyl groups and the dinitrophenyl groups were both conjugated to the same molecule of poly-L-lysine. The animals produced simultaneously a secondary response to the priming hapten, and a primary response to the new hapten! The situation of original antigenic sin is analogous in the sense that the virus strain used for restimulation shares some determinants with the primary strain and evokes a secondary response to these. Other antigenic determinants are unique to it; to these it evokes a primary response.

It has already been demonstrated (p. 39) that the specificity of antigen–antibody reactions is such that small alterations in the antigen molecule will modify or abolish its reaction with its antibody. In general, it has been found that the specificity of the secondary response is similar but rather broader [35]. Alterations to the antigen molecule which abolish its binding to antibody will reduce or abolish its ability to stimulate a secondary response. This observation is of great importance to theories of antibody production and will be discussed in this context later.

D. Quantitative Aspects of Antibody Production

1. SEQUENTIAL PRODUCTION OF 19S AND 7S ANTIBODIES

Most workers have agreed that during the primary response 19S antibody is detected in the serum before 7S antibody. However, the sensitivity of most methods for determining antibodies depends on the affinity (see p. 174) between the antigens and the antibody produced. It is known that 19S antibodies have a greater affinity than 7S antibodies for bacteriophage particles [33], and greater efficiency in producing haemolysis and haemagglutination [15]. This means that in a haemagglutinating system, for instance, a molecule of 19S antibody may be 750 times more efficient than a molecule of 7S antibody [15]. Conversely, a given haemagglutinating titre of 7S antibody may represent 750 times more molecules than the same titre of 19S antibodies. If 19S and 7S antibodies are produced simultaneously, the lower affinity of the 7S antibodies will cause them to be detected later. There will therefore appear to be a sequence of antibody production, starting with 19S antibody and followed by 7S antibody. Wei and Stavitsky [15] and Finkelstein and Uhr [40] both conclude that in the systems they studied, 19S and 7S antibodies are produced simultaneously in the primary response, and that the apparent sequence from 19S to 7S is an experimental artefact. There is also no evidence for a 19S–7S sequence in the production of rabbit antibodies to diphtheria toxin, bovine gamma-globulin, or Salmonella O antigen, or of chick antibodies to human serum albumin or bovine serum albumin [15].

Finkelstein and Uhr [40] point out the biological advantages of early production of 19S antibodies. They are of high affinity and extremely efficient in the agglutination of bacterial and virus particles. Because of their high molecular weight, they are retained intravascularly and therefore build up to a high concentration rapidly.

Although there is doubt about the sequential appearance of 19S and 7S antibodies initially, there is no doubt that later in the immune response 19S synthesis stops, while 7S synthesis continues at increased rates. A possible explanation for this is considered later (p. 158).

2. CHANGE IN AFFINITY OF ANTIBODY DURING THE IMMUNE RESPONSE

The affinity of antibody will be defined later (p. 174). It has generally been observed that antibody produced early in the immune response is of lower affinity than antibody produced later. Glenny and Barr [36] first demonstrated differences in the affinity of diphtheria antitoxin and Jerne [37] showed that primary antibody was of lower affinity than secondary antibody. That affinity increases as the immune response proceeds has now been demonstrated for most of the species of animal and types of antigen that have been studied. So far the turtle seems to be the laggard [38]: despite the most vigorous stimulation with bovine serum albumin and haemocyanin, it seems incapable of producing antibodies with increasing affinity.

The clearest evidence for increasing affinity is for 7S antibodies. Eisen and Siskind [39] found that 7S antibody formed to 2,4-dinitrophenol in rabbits increased in affinity by a factor of 10,000 during the immune response. Finkelstein and Uhr [40] studied the affinity of antibodies formed in guinea-pigs to the bacteriophage ϕX 174, and similarly found a progressive increase in affinity of 7S antibodies during the primary response. Taliaferro, Taliaferro, and Pizzi [41] showed that rabbit haemolysins increase in affinity during the secondary response. The affinity of 19S antibodies to ϕX 174 also increases between days 4 and 10 of the immune response [40]. The comparative affinity of 19S and 7S antibody molecules has already been mentioned (p. 135).

3. IMMUNOLOGICAL MEMORY

If equal doses of antigen are given to an animal on two occasions the second will often lead to the production of more molecules of antibody. This excess of secondary over primary antibody production gives a useful measure for 'immunological memory'. In guinea-pigs, immunological memory can be detected within a month of the primary injection, and continues to increase until the interval between the primary and secondary stimuli is increased to a year. When the primary dose is reduced, the length of time during which memory increases is shortened to 6 months. Similar observations have been made in man, where immunological memory has been detected over 20 years after the primary stimulus [42].

Nossal, Austin, and Ada [14] studied the factors related to the development of memory in rats by using a computer to analyse the results of primary and secondary immunization with flagella from *Salmonella adelaide* or with flagellin. They studied some 10,000 titrations on 2000 rats:

the doses of antigen varied in tenfold steps from 10 pg. to 100 μg. They found that to elicit memory in this system, the secondary dose should be as great as or greater than the primary dose. Under these conditions memory was shown to increase steadily with an increasing primary stimulus up to 10μg. of flagella. The increase of memory was remarkably constant over a scale in which the antigen dose was increased a millionfold. Primary doses of less than 10 ng. produced a measurable memory, although too small to produce a detectable antibody response. The combination of a small, sub-immunogenic primary dose (1 ng.) with a large secondary dose was found to favour the demonstration of memory in the 19S response. In many other systems memory can be evoked by a much smaller dose of antigen than the primary response. The immune system, in effect, is a highly efficient biological amplifier.

E. Cellular Aspects of Antibody Production

1. CELLS WHICH FORM ANTIBODY

a. Plasma Cells

In 1898, Pfeiffer and Marx [43] examined the organs of animals injected subcutaneously with cholera vaccine and found that the highest concentration of antibodies was produced in the spleen. Huebschmann, in 1913 [44], studied the cellular content of the spleen in a number of infections and concluded: 'The cells which are most numerous in the sites where defensive reaction of the organism is strongest, and where the highest concentration of antibodies accumulates, are the plasma cells.'

The plasma cell, which was first named by Waldeyer in 1875, was defined by Cajal [45], Unna [46], and von Marschalko [47] as a round or oval cell with strongly basophilic cytoplasm, often containing a light zone adjacent to the nucleus. The nucleus itself is eccentrically placed with 'clotted' chromatin, sometimes wheel-shaped (*Fig. 32 A*). In 1937, Bing and Plum [48] drew attention to the increased number of plasma cells found in conditions associated with an increase in serum gamma-globulin, and suggested that gamma-globulin is in fact produced by plasma cells. Fagraeus in 1948 [49], in an extensive experimental study, confirmed that antibody production in tissues was closely associated with the presence of plasma cells and their precursors, and showed that plasma cells *in vitro* are capable of producing antibody. Coons and his co-workers, who had developed the method of conjugating fluorescent compounds to antibody molecules (*see* p. 195), showed, in an important series of papers in 1955 [50, 51, 52], that antibody against a specific antigen could be identified in plasma cells in the spleen and lymph-nodes.

De Petris, Karlsbad, and Pernis [53] studied under the electron microscope plasma cells from rabbits which had been hyperimmunized with ferritin. They used ferritin as a label to demonstrate the site of antibody production within the cell and showed that the antibody accumulated within the endoplasmic reticulum (*Fig. 32 B*).

There is no doubt, then, that mature plasma cells produce antibody. There is, however, evidence that they are not the only antibody-producing cells.

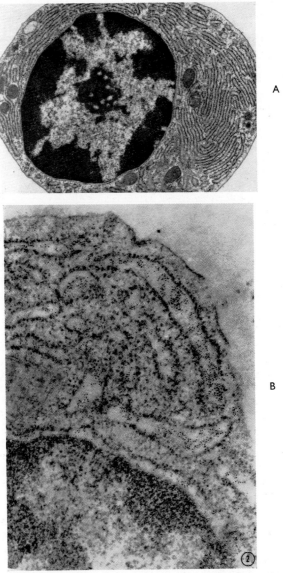

A

B

Fig. 32.—A, Plasma cell. Electron micrograph of a guinea-pig plasma cell, showing coarse pattern of chromatin and extensive endoplasmic reticulum. (×8000.) (*Reproduced from W. Bloom and D. W. Fawcett (1968), 'A Textbook of Histology', by kind permission of the Authors and of Saunders, Philadelphia.*) B, Electron micrograph of plasma cell showing ferritin granules attached to antibody in endoplasmic reticulum. *Reproduced from S. de Petris et al. (1963), 'Journal of Experimental Medicine', vol. 117, p. 849, by kind permission of the Authors and of the Rockefeller University Press, New York.*

b. Lymphocytes

When rabbits are stimulated to form antibody against sheep red blood-cells, the efferent lymph from the stimulated gland contains a variety of cells, ranging from small lymphocytes, through medium and large lymphocytes to plasma cells. Harris and his co-workers [54] showed that the plasma cells were not the only cells producing antibody. Using a modification of the Jerne plaque technique (*see* p. 224), he showed that some of the antibody-forming cells were lymphocytes containing a few strands of endoplasmic reticulum. He suggested that these cells are precursors of plasma cells, and that antibody can be produced in a variety of cells ranging from medium lymphocytes to mature plasma cells. Whether these cells represent stages in the formation of the mature plasma cell, or whether every cell in the spectrum, from the small lymphocyte with a few strands of endoplasmic reticulum in its cytoplasm through the medium and large lymphocytes to the mature plasma cell with a dense tightly packed endoplasmic reticulum, is a fully mature and specialized end-product we do not yet know. Van Furth et al. [55, 56, 57, 58] have, however, studied the production of immunoglobulins by normal human cells *in vitro*, and found that while plasma cells and large and medium lymphocytes all produce IgG, IgA, and IgM, small lymphocytes produce only IgM. This may, perhaps, suggest a specialized function for each type of cell. Sell and Asofsky [59] have reviewed the role of lymphocytes in the production of antibodies.

2. How Many Antibodies from One Cell?

It is of great importance in considering theories of antibody production to know how flexible the equipment of an individual plasma cell can be. Can a single plasma cell produce more than one class of immunoglobulin? Is it capable of producing more than one type of antibody? A considerable amount of recent work has thrown light on these questions.

It has been widely found that individual plasma cells produce only immunoglobulins of a single class, and probably of a single subclass and allotype (*see* Pernis [60] for discussion and references). There seem to be a few exceptions. Costea et al. [61] have described myeloma cells in a human which appear to produce both IgG and IgA. Nossal et al. [62] found that in immunized rabbits when antibody production is shifting from predominantly IgM to IgG molecules, individual cells may appear to contain antibodies in both classes.

Until recently, the question of whether a single plasma cell could produce more than one type of antibody was ground for heated controversy. On the one hand, Attardi et al. [63, 64] examined cells from rabbit lymph-nodes after stimulation with two types of bacteriophage which are antigenically distinct. Single cells were cultured in micro-drops and antibody was measured by phage inactivation. It was found that nearly a quarter of the antibody-producing cells were forming antibody against both antigens. Hiramoto and Hamlin [65], using an immunofluorescent technique, also found plasma cells producing two antibodies simultaneously. However, Green et al. [66], who studied rabbits forming antibodies against the dinitrophenol group conjugated to bovine serum albumin or bovine gamma-globulin, found that single cells produced antibodies either against the hapten (DNP) or against the carrier protein, but never against both. They sharply criticized the earlier work. In 1967, Mäkelä [67], who had previously [68] found evidence for single cells producing antibodies against two types of *Salmonella*, repeated the experiments of Attardi with more stringent precautions, and found, out of 112 cells producing antibody, none which was producing antibody of more than one type. Earlier results were probably due to artefacts.

In an even more extensive series of experiments Sela and his co-workers [69] examined 17,000 cells from mice producing antibodies to rabbit and camel erythrocytes and 28,000 cells from rabbits producing antibodies to two synthetic haptens, and found no instance of a cell producing more than one antibody.

The current view, then, is that a single plasma cell or lymphocyte will almost always produce gamma-globulin of only one class, subclass, or allotype, and that a single antibody-producing cell is committed to producing antibody of one specificity only. There is no currently acceptable evidence of cells producing more than one type of antibody.

3. THE ROLE OF THE MACROPHAGE

Macrophages are mononuclear phagocytic cells which are found in large numbers in inflammatory exudates and are also present in lymph-nodes (*Fig.* 33). Van Furth [70], by labelling mononuclear cells in mice with ^{3}H-thymidine, showed that the macrophages which arise in peritoneal exudates in response to a chemical irritant are derived from mononuclear cells in the blood, which arise in turn from pro-monocytes in the bone-marrow.

The role of macrophages in trapping antigen has been discussed earlier (p. 129). The relationship between delayed hypersensitivity and the inhibition of macrophage migration *in vitro* is considered elsewhere (p. 256).

The main question to be considered here is the relationship of macrophages to antibody-producing cells. It is known that phagocytosis of antigen by macrophages is an essential preliminary to antibody production [71]. It is known that particulate antigens are more strongly antigenic than soluble antigens, and also that they are more readily phagocytosed. Dresser [72] showed that if bovine gamma-globulin (BGG) was subjected to high-speed centrifugation to remove aggregated particles, the soluble BGG which remained was no longer immunogenic. Frei, Benacerraf, and Thorbecke [71] first suggested that a soluble antigen gaining direct access to a lymphocyte would produce immunological paralysis, while a particulate antigen, after being processed by macrophages, would be presented to the lymphocytes in an immunogenic form. This hypothesis is supported by Dresser and Mitchison [73].

It is widely accepted that phagocytosis by macrophages is an important step in the handling of antigens, and that subsequent contact between macrophages and lymphocytes is necessary for antibody production. Schoenberg and co-workers [74] have claimed to demonstrate the presence of cytoplasmic bridges between macrophages and lymphocytes during antibody synthesis. There is, however, controversy over the way in which macrophages handle antigens. Fishman and co-workers [75] took macrophages from rat peritoneal exudate and incubated them with antigenic particles of bacteriophage. The macrophages were then removed, washed, and homogenized. The homogenate was added to lymphocytes from unimmunized rats and stimulated them to produce antibody. It was claimed that the immunogenic material which passed from the macrophages to the lymphocytes was of low molecular weight and was sensitive

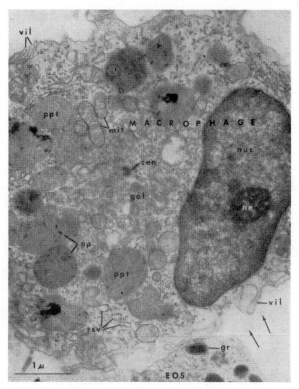

Fig. 33.—Electron micrograph of a macrophage. Phagocytosed masses of ferritin–antiferritin precipitate (pp, ppt) are seen in membranous sacs. Vil = villi, nuc = nucleus, ne = nucleolus, gol = Golgi apparatus, cen = centriole, mit = mito-chondria, rsv = rough-surfaced vesicles. Eosinophil (EOS) with granule (gr). (× 15,000.) *Reproduced from A. W. Ham (1965), 'Histology', 5th ed., by kind permission of Lippincott, Philadelphia. Preparation by H. Z. Movat.*

to ribonuclease. Fishman suggested that transfer of a special type of RNA was involved, and that this carried information about the antigen to the unimmunized lymphocytes. Askonas and Rhodes [76], however, found that the immunogenic material was in fact fragments of partly digested antigen bound to RNA. They called this material 'super-antigen'. The difference is important: it would not be particularly surprising to find that antigens can be rendered more antigenic by partial digestion in macrophages; but if it were established beyond doubt that lymphocytes can be

6

stimulated by antigen-free RNA derived from macrophages, the implications, both for molecular biology and for theories of antibody-production,
would be far-reaching. Fishman has subsequently been concerned to
show that antigen-free RNA can, in fact, carry the message which stimulates
the lymphocyte to produce specific antibody. In 1967 [77] he claimed to
have found two active fractions derived from sensitized macrophages.
One, a complex of RNA linked to fragments of antigen, appeared to be
responsible for the production of 7S antibodies. The other, apparently
pure RNA, was responsible for the 19S response. However, in 1968,
Unanue and Askonas [78], by transferring primed macrophages to
irradiated mice and later adding unstimulated lymphocytes, found that
macrophages were capable of holding antigen fragments in a relatively
stable pool, probably related to the cell membrane, for considerable
periods, and suggested that this might serve as a stimulus for lymphocytes
with which it comes in contact.

In summary, it is now clear that macrophages play an important role
in initiating antibody production. Whether they do so by processing the
antigen and presenting it to the lymphocytes in a more immunogenic form,
or whether they transfer information by means of antigen-free RNA, is
still ground for controversy, though the weight of evidence favours the
former alternative.

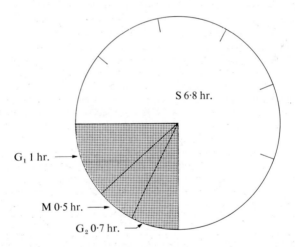

Fig. 34.—Cell cycle of lymphoblasts. This shows the approximate duration of
G$_1$, S, G$_2$ and M. (*After Sado and Makinodan* [80].)

4. CELLULAR PROLIFERATION AND ANTIBODY PRODUCTION

Having considered the nature of the cells which produce antibody, we
are now concerned with the question of how these cells arise in response
to an antigenic stimulus. In particular, do antibody-producing cells arise
by differentiation from precursor cells, or by cell-division, or by both
methods? A considerable amount of work on the cellular kinetics of the
antibody response *in vivo* and *in vitro* has been published in recent years.

It has important implications for theories of antibody production: unfortunately there is still a conflict of evidence in some vital areas.

In considering the question of cellular differentiation versus cellular division, an important limiting factor is the minimum duration of the cycle of cell-division in an individual cell. A mammalian cell passes through a number of stages during the process of growth and development. Howard and Pelč [79] first suggested that these could be represented as sectors of a clock-face through which the cell passes sequentially (*Fig.* 34). The phase during which DNA synthesis occurs has been termed 'S', the phase of mitosis 'M', and the two gaps in which no DNA is synthesized 'G1' and 'G2'.

Proteins and RNA are synthesized through G1, S, and G2. Sado and Makinodan [80] estimated the generation time of blast cells involved in the antibody response and concluded that it was about 9 hours. More recently Tannenberg and Malaviya [81] suggested a generation time of 13 hours for 19*S* plaque-forming cells in the log phase of both the primary and secondary responses in mice. It follows that any antibody-producing cell which has arisen in less than 9 hours after antigenic stimulation cannot have passed through more than one cycle (M to M).

a. Cellular Events during the Lag Phase

Makinodan and Albright [82], in a stimulating review, discussed cellular changes in all phases of the immune response. During the induction phase, antigen is localized in dendritic macrophages in the germinal follicles of lymph-nodes and in the white pulp of the spleen (*see* p. 127). At the same time, the germinal centres hypertrophy [83] and immature lymphoid cells (presumably the precursors of antibody-forming cells) migrate into the red pulp of the spleen. The relationship between macrophages and antibody-forming cells has been discussed previously (p. 140). Towards the end of the induction phase DNA synthesis begins. Dutton and Mishell [84] showed that at this stage (24–32 hours after the addition of antigen) spleen cells *in vitro* take up tritiated thymidine. A large dose of tritiated thymidine was added to the medium to kill dividing cells (the 'hot pulse' technique) and it was found that the production of plaque-forming cells was inhibited only if the pulse was given more than 24 hours after the administration of antigen. This suggests that, *in vitro*, the first 24 hours after antigen administration is taken up with the handling of antigen, and not with cellular division or DNA synthesis. Similar findings *in vivo* have been reported by Szenberg and Cunningham [85], who found that antibody-forming cells in mice immunized with sheep erythrocytes began to take up tritiated thymidine between 26 and 28 hours after antigenic stimulation.

b. Cellular Events during the Log Phase

During the logarithmic phase of antibody production there is a striking cellular proliferation. The germinal centres are the site of vigorous mitotic activity [83] and increasing numbers of plasma cells appear in the medulla of lymph-nodes [50, 51] and in the red pulp of the spleen [86].

During the primary response *in vivo* [87] and *in vitro* [84] the increasing rate of antibody production is paralleled by an increase in the number of antibody-forming cells, so that, for instance, when mice respond to sheep erythrocytes the rise in serum antibody is accompanied by a parallel rise in the number of plaque-forming cells in the spleen [87]. The same observations have been made for the secondary response [88]. It is therefore clear that the increased levels of antibody appearing in the blood after antigenic stimulation are due mainly to an increase in the number of antibody-producing cells. Most workers have accepted that the new antibody-forming cells arise as a result of mitosis, and that the doubling time of serum antibody represents the doubling time of the cells involved [89, 84]. Koros, Mazur, and Mowery [90] studied DNA synthesis in plaque-forming cells by taking spleen cells from mice immunized with sheep erythrocytes and incubating them with tritiated thymidine in vitro: their results suggested that the exponential increase in plaque-forming cells was due entirely to cellular proliferation, and that the rate of proliferation was proportional to the logarithm of antigen dose. Antigen appeared to shorten the G1 phase of the cycle, but did not affect the duration of S.

There have, however, been some dissident voices. Simonsen [91], who studied graft-versus-host reactions in mouse and chicken, and Bussard [92], studying peritoneal exudate cells in mice, concluded that lymphocytes had the potential ability to respond to more than one antigen, and that the primary response was not characterized by cellular proliferation. Tannenberg [93] also observed that if mice were immunized with sheep erythrocytes, their spleens contained cells producing 19S antibody which did not take up tritiated thymidine and had not therefore undergone mitosis. He has more recently [81] studied the generation time of 19S plaque-forming cells in mice and has claimed that, at a time when the doubling time for plaque-forming cells is 6 hours, their generation time is as long as 13 hours. This would suggest that a large proportion of the plaque-forming cells does not arise by mitosis. Tannenberg's earlier work has been criticized on technical grounds [90], and this is at present an area of lively controversy, where further experimental work will be needed to clarify the issue.

Up to now we have been considering the question of whether antibody-producing cells *arise* by cell division. We can now turn briefly to the question of whether antibody-producing cells can themselves divide. Although plasma cells are usually considered as end-cells incapable of further division, there is evidence that at least some antibody-producing cells are capable of further mitosis. Claflin and Smithies [94], studying spleen cells from mice responding to cow erythrocytes, found that a large number of plaque-forming cells was undergoing mitosis, and that each of the daughter cells was capable of producing antibody.

c. Cellular Events during the Plateau and Decline Phases

The burst of cellular proliferation which accompanies the exponential phase of antibody production slowly declines at the onset of the plateau phase. Jerne, Nordin, and Henry [87] showed that the rate of decrease in haemolysin titre was approximately the same as the rate of decrease in the number of plaque-forming cells in the spleen. During the plateau phase antibody-producing plasma cells which do not synthesize DNA appear in lymphoid tissue [95]. They have a half-life in tissues of less than 2 days [96]. Makinodan and Albright [82] conclude that the plateau phase and decline of antibody production are the result of suicidal differentiation of a series of plasma cells.

d. Cellular Basis of Memory

Immunological memory is a remarkably long-lasting phenomenon. It has been demonstrated after 20 years in humans [42]. To explain this tremendous time-scale it would be necessary to postulate either that antigen is retained within the animal throughout the whole period and produces a slowly declining stimulation of the immune apparatus, or that there are cells carrying memory which have an extremely long survival time in the body. Studies on the survival of antigen (reviewed *en passant*, by Uhr and Möller [97]) have shown that antigens are catabolized at varying rates, none of which is commensurate with the time scale of immunological memory. For the second possibility, evidence was provided by Gowans and Uhr [98], who showed that immunological memory could be transferred from an immunized rat to a syngeneic, irradiated recipient, by transferring small lymphocytes obtained from thoracic-duct drainage. Buckton, Court Brown, and Smith [99] showed that human circulating small lymphocytes have a mean life-span of 1574 days, with 95 per cent confidence limits that extended from 891 to 6743 days. The circulating small lymphocyte is therefore a cell with a life-span of the order required for immunological memory. Celada [100] introduced an elegant model for the study of memory cells. Mice were immunized with human serum albumin, and their spleen cells were injected into irradiated syngeneic hosts. The hosts were challenged at intervals with antigen, and the antibody titre was used to compute the survival of memory cells from the original immunization. He observed a biphasic decline in memory, corresponding with a short-lived cell population (half-life 15 days) and a long-lived population (half-life 100 days). The latter group correspond well with long-lived mouse lymphocytes. Celada also observed that the rate of decay of memory cells seemed to be independent of the number of times they were rechallenged with antigen, and suggested that a very small proportion of memory cells would transform under the influence of antigen into terminal plasma cells. Byers and Sercarz [101], using a different system for testing memory cells, found that they could in fact be exhausted by a very large dose of antigen. Bosman and Feldman [102] studied this problem directly, by injecting rats with tritiated thymidine during the primary response to keyhole limpet haemocyanin. Labelled cells were examined up to 50 days later, and the effect of a secondary challenge was observed. They concluded that the cells responsible for memory were 'mature, resting monoribosomal lymphocytes', and that antigenic restimulation converted them into polyribosomal lymphocytes and blast cells, which in turn gave rise to plasma cells, either by differentiation or by division.

e. Theoretical Implications of Cellular Studies

One of the great debates of immunology deals with the origin of the cells which produce antibodies. Do they arise by selection from committed precursors, destined since their origin to produce antibody of a single specificity, or do they arise from a pool of uncommitted totipotent cells, programmed to produce antibody by contact with a particular antigen? Theories supporting the first assumption are selectional: those accepting the second, instructional.

Theories of antibody production have recently been reviewed by Jerne [103], Haurowitz [104], and Smithies [106]. The two striking features of the immune response, which challenge any hypothesis, are (1) the extremely high degree of specificity of antibodies, which are capable of distinguishing between very closely related antigens (*see* p. 39), and (2) the very wide range of antibodies which can be produced by an individual animal.

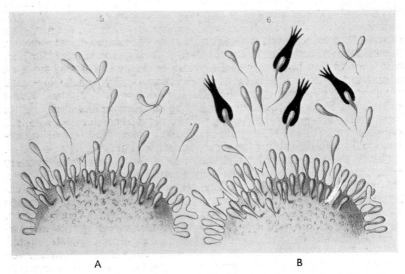

        A   B

Fig. 35.—**A**, Shows free antitoxins being liberated into the circulation. The cell also has bound antitoxins (and other receptors) on its surface. **B**, Shows free antitoxins and toxin/antitoxin complexes in the circulation. *Reproduced from P. Ehrlich, ' On Immunity with special reference to Cell Life', ' Proceedings of the Royal Society of London', vol. 66, 1899–1900, by kind permission of the Council of the Royal Society, London.*

The first convincing general theory of antibody production was devised by Ehrlich [107], who suggested that the organism produced cells bearing on their surface 'receptors' capable of reacting with particular antigens (*Fig.* 35). He proposed that the union of antigen and receptor stimulated the production by the cell of further receptors, some of which passed into the circulation as free antibodies. There are many features of this theory which are acceptable today. It is essentially a selective theory, since it assumes that antigen selects for interaction cells already capable of making a specific antibody.

When Landsteiner [108, 109] found that antibodies can be formed against synthetic haptens which are never found in nature, it became more difficult to visualize an appropriate selective theory. Why should an animal go to the extravagant length of holding available a highly specific antibody against an antigen which it would never encounter except at the hand of an inquisitive immunologist? Breinl and Haurowitz [110] put forward the first instructive theory of antibody production, suggesting that an antigen could interfere with the biosynthesis of gamma-globulin in such a way that the synthesized molecule contained a combining site complementary to the antigen. This theory was later taken up by Pauling [111], who suggested that the antigen acted as a 'template', and that the peptide chain of the antibody was folded to fit it.

The revitalization of selective theories began when Jerne [112] proposed his 'natural-selection theory of antibody formation'. This was modified by Burnet [113], who offered a 'clonal selection theory'. He suggested that individual cells of the lymphoid series were precommitted to produce a certain type of antibody. When a cell encountered the appropriate antigen it was stimulated to repeated cell-division, producing a clone of similar cells, all with the same antibody-producing ability. After a period in the doldrums, selective theories have become increasingly popular, and most recent experimental work is consistent with some kind of selective interpretation.

The purpose of this section is to examine the relevance of cellular studies to the debate. It will be useful first to dispose of some quantitative questions. (1) Can the wide diversity of antibody molecules be explained in terms of the known structural variability of the gamma-globulin molecule? In considering the number of possible antigens Haurowitz [104] concludes that '10^5–10^6 different immunoglobulins would be sufficient to combine specifically with all of the normal and synthetic haptens'. Jerne had previously suggested a figure of 10^6 as a reasonable estimate of the number of antigens to which an organism could be expected to respond. (2) Are there enough lymphocytes in the body to account for this diversity of antibodies, assuming that a lymphocyte can produce only one antibody? Jerne [103] takes 10^{12} as a reasonable figure for the number of lymphocytes in a man. Makinodan and Albright [82] suggest 6×10^8 as the number of lymphocytes in a mouse. These figures are sufficient to accommodate reasonable numbers of lymphocytes producing each of the antibodies of which the organism is capable.

A single plasma cell cannot be shown to produce more than one antibody. The crucial question now, from the theoretical point of view, is: What is the potential ability of the precursors of antibody-forming cells? Clearly, a selective theory would predict that they must themselves be unipotent, capable of developing into only a single type of antibody-producing cell, while an instructional theory would have them to be totipotent, capable, under the influence of antigen, of developing into any possible antibody-producing cell. There is very little experimental work on this point. Earlier work is reviewed by Shearer et al. [114], who studied the question by transplanting spleen-cell suspensions from unprimed donor mice into irradiated recipients. The host mice were challenged with sheep erythrocytes, and the development of cells producing three different types of antibody (19S haemolysins, 7S haemolysins, and haemagglutinins) was studied. The results suggested that each of the three types of antibody-producing cell was derived from a different type of precursor cell, and that the precursors of antibody-forming cells ('antigen-sensitive units') were themselves unipotent. This implies that the specificity of antibody-forming cells has developed before interaction with antigen.

The earliest precursors of antibody-forming cells are not antigen-sensitive. Papermaster [115] reviewed the question of when and how antigen-sensitive cells develop. The earliest precursor cells are found in the bone-marrow. For these to develop into antigen-sensitive cells, the thymus appears to be essential [115, 116, 117, 118]. Thymus lymphocytes, which are not themselves immunologically competent, appear to co-operate with bone-marrow precursor cells to produce antigen-sensitive units. Miller and his co-workers [116, 117, 118] have shown that the antibody-producing cells are descendants of the bone-marrow cells, and not of the thymocytes. The thymus cells take an indirect part, the details of which are still obscure. Miller suggests that they are themselves antigen-sensitive, but formal proof for the interaction of antigen and thymus cells is lacking. If further work confirms that antigen-sensitive cells are unipotent, we shall then have to ask whether thymocytes or the bone-marrow precursors of antibody-forming cells are unipotent. There is at present no experimental evidence on this point.

Evidence on the number of target cells available for a particular antigen suggests that one cell in 10^5 in the mouse spleen can respond to sheep erythrocytes. This figure is comparable with those obtained in other systems [103], and is quite compatible with the hypothesis that individual unipotent antigen-sensitive units exist for each antigen. The work of Dutton and Mishell [119] provides *in vitro* confirmation of the unipotency of antigen-sensitive units (*see* p. 143).

The evidence from cellular kinetics, which has been discussed earlier (p. 144), is less conclusive and less relevant. The central problem is whether antibody-producing cells arise by proliferation or by differentiation. This is indirectly connected with theories of antibody production: Burnet suggested that antigen would stimulate proliferation in a clone of sensitive cells, while an instructive mechanism would act on a cell after mitosis and lead it to produce antibody without undergoing cell division. Superficially, proliferation would seem to favour a selective mechanism, differentiation an instructive mechanism. However, a little thought will show that these are not necessary or absolute correlations, and that whichever cellular mechanism is eventually demonstrated, it would be possible to adapt either theory to fit the facts.

To sum up, cellular studies have shown that antibody-producing cells are committed to one antibody, and that their precursors, the antigen-sensitive cells, are probably unipotent. There is no experimental evidence on the degree of commitment of the precursors of antigen-sensitive cells. So far, all the evidence is compatible with selective theories. We are observing the death-agony of the Instructional Theory. Haurowitz, who gave it birth, disowned it in 1967 with the words: ' . . . the Selective Theory is now more attractive to me than it ever appeared before' [104].

If it can be confirmed that differentiation into unipotent cells takes place before interaction with antigen, then the Instructional Theory, already disowned by its progenitor, will be laid to rest.

If we accept that selective theories are now in the ascendant, the main problem of theoretical interest lies in the field of genetics. How can we account, in terms of genes, for the enormous number (10^6) of different immunoglobulin molecules which must be produced? This problem has been reviewed by Smithies [106] and is considered in more detail elsewhere in this book (*see* p. 113).

III. FACTORS WHICH INCREASE THE IMMUNE RESPONSE

Adjuvants

Some antigens, such as sheep erythrocytes, or the bacteriophage ϕX 174 will stimulate vigorous primary antibody production when given by a single intravenous or intradermal injection. Other weak antigens are ineffective when injected alone but can be made to stimulate antibody production if they are injected intradermally together with one of a number of non-specific stimulating agents or adjuvants. The one most widely used is Freund's complete adjuvant [120] which consists of a suspension of tubercle bacilli in an oil–detergent mixture. For the adjuvant to be effective, the antigen, in aqueous solution, must be thoroughly emulsified in the adjuvant. Freund's complete adjuvant increases delayed hypersensitivity, as well as antibody production. For some purposes it is convenient to use Freund's incomplete adjuvant, from which the tubercle bacilli are omitted. This stimulates antibody production, though generally less than the complete adjuvant, and produces only a transient, weak delayed hypersensitivity.

The action of Freund's complete adjuvant represents a combination of two effects: (1) The adjuvant effect of a water–detergent–oil emulsion of antigen and (2) the adjuvant effect of tubercle bacilli.

1. NON-ANTIGENIC ADJUVANTS

In Freund's incomplete adjuvant the antigen in solution is emulsified with a mineral oil (Bayol) and a detergent (Arlacel) and injected intradermally or subcutaneously. Paraffin oil or peanut oil can be used instead of Bayol, and lanolin will replace Arlacel. About 3 weeks after the injection of antigen in incomplete adjuvant granulomata form at the site of injection. The antigen can be identified in oily vesicles contained in macrophages (foam cells) [4]. The increased effectiveness of antigen under these conditions is presumably due to the delay in its absorption and elimination. Antigen is liberated in small amounts over a long period and thus produces the greatest possible stimulation of antibody production. Gall [121] has also suggested that adjuvant properties may be linked in some cases with surface-active molecules, which would help to unite antigens to the cell surface. Other non-antigenic agents are effective adjuvants. Diphtheria toxoid is a more effective antigen if absorbed on to mineral gels such as aluminium hydroxide, calcium, or aluminium phosphate or silicate. The effectiveness of antigens is also increased when they are absorbed on to silica particles [122] or cellulose [123], or mixed with acrylamide gel [124].

2. ANTIGENIC ADJUVANTS

The tubercle bacteria in Freund's complete adjuvant are, of course, strongly antigenic in their own right and may be effective as an adjuvant

7

in the absence of the oil–detergent emulsion. This was first demonstrated by Dienes and Schoenheit [125], who found that ovalbumin and horse serum, which are not normally antigenic in the guinea-pig, could be made to produce an immune reaction if they were injected into the lesions of a tuberculous animal. In this instance, the antigen produced delayed hypersensitivity rather than antibody. Killed tubercle bacilli greatly increase the effectiveness of many antigens, and White [4] showed that the adjuvant activity appeared to be associated with a peptidoglycolipid derived from the Wax D fraction. He suggested that its adjuvanticity might be associated with two features of the molecule: its surface-active properties and its strong affinity for gamma-globulin. Other bacteria (nocardia, corynebacteria, and pertussis) have been shown to act as adjuvants.

The histological changes observed after injection of an antigen in Freund's complete adjuvant are similar to those observed with incomplete adjuvant, but more marked [126]. The granulomata show large numbers of epithelioid cells and giant cells. Lymph-nodes adjacent to the injection show a similar granulomatous reaction, while the more remote ones show plasma-cell proliferation in the medulla.

Not all the activity of an adjuvant can be explained by its local effect, since it has been shown [127] that the immunogenicity of an antigen is increased if the adjuvant is given before the antigen, or into a different site. Some, at least, of the explanation of adjuvanticity may lie in the ability of adjuvants to stimulate phagocytosis by macrophages.

Immune Deviation

In cases where the administration of an antigen in Freund's complete adjuvant stimulates both antibody production and delayed hypersensitivity, it has been found that prior injection of the antigen alone may reduce delayed hypersensitivity, while leaving antibody production intact. This phenomenon has been referred to as 'immune deviation' and is reviewed by Asherson [128]. It is not yet clear whether this is a particular example of immunological paralysis (*see* p. 152).

IV. FACTORS WHICH DEPRESS THE IMMUNE RESPONSE

A. X-irradiation and Immunosuppressive Drugs

Irradiation of living tissues with X-rays produces striking damage to cells. The molecular basis of this effect has been reviewed by Hutchinson [129]; one of the main features is the disruption of strands of DNA. Since the immune response is dependent on protein synthesis, it is not surprising to find that it can be dramatically suppressed by X-irradiation. In general, the primary response and the secondary response seem to be equally radiosensitive [130, 131], while delayed hypersensitivity is considerably more resistant than antibody production [132, 133]. The time relationship between irradiation and administration of antigen is important. Taliaferro and Taliaferro [130] studied the formation of haemolysin in rabbits given 0·125 ml. of 1 per cent sheep red-cells per kg. intravenously. They found the greatest depression of antibody production when the antigen was given 24 hours after irradiation with 500 r. (*Fig.* 36). The length of the induction period was also increased. With longer intervals between the irradiation and immunization, haemolysin levels gradually returned to normal, though some reduction of antibody levels could be found when antigen was given as long as 4 weeks after irradiation. Irradiation given after immunization was less effective in inhibiting antibody production. Curiously it was found that irradiation 1–4 hours after the administration of antigen enhanced antibody production.

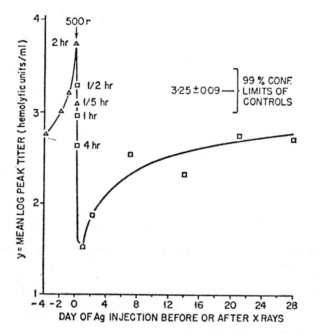

Fig. 36.—The effect of irradiation on antibody production in a group of rabbits injected with sheep erythrocytes at various times before and after irradiation with 500 r. *After W. H. Taliaferro and L. G. Taliaferro* [130]. *Reproduced from J. H. Humphrey and R. G. White (1964), 'Immunology for Students of Medicine', by kind permission of Blackwell Scientific Publications, Oxford.*

The effect of cytotoxic drugs on the immune response has recently been reviewed by Gabrielsen and Good [134]. Berenbaum [135] has discussed in detail the mechanism of immunosuppression. In general, their effects are similar to irradiation. They are most effective if administered 2 days before immunization. For a short period after immunization they may even enhance antibody production.

The immunosuppressive effects of irradiation and cytotoxic drugs should throw light on the mechanism of the immune response, but up to the present the light appears to be somewhat veiled. The handling of antigen by macrophages is relatively radioresistant [136] and Fitch et al. [137] found that antigen was taken up normally in the spleen and lymph-nodes of irradiated rats. The cells which are most clearly sensitive to irradiation and cytotoxic drugs are small lymphocytes, which would be expected to show the greatest radiosensitivity at a period when they are dividing rapidly. Dutton and Mishell [84] have shown that *in vitro* suspensions of spleen cells show a burst of mitotic activity 32–72 hours after the addition of antigen, and this is the stage at which they are most susceptible to destruction with high-activity tritiated thymidine (the 'hot-pulse' technique, *see* p. 143). There is, so far, no clarification from *in vitro* studies of the immunosuppressive effect of irradiation given before antigen. One possible interpretation is that the lymphocytes which react with antigen *in vivo* are formed by cell division 2 days before antigen is administered. If this hypothesis is supported by further work, it will provide support for a selective theory of antibody production.

B. Immunological Paralysis

Under certain circumstances a substance which would normally stimulate antibody production or delayed hypersensitivity may have the opposite effect and render an animal immunologically non-reactive. This phenomenon is usually specific, so that the non-reactivity is limited to the antigen itself or to closely related substances. This specific depression of immunological reactivity is known as 'immunological tolerance' or 'immunological paralysis'. It has recently been reviewed in detail by Dresser and Mitchison [73].

Immunological paralysis was first demonstrated in young animals, and it was thought that it depended on a specific and unique condition of the foetus. This aspect of tolerance is discussed in detail elsewhere (p. 332). However, a number of early observations had indicated that tolerance could also be induced in adult animals. Sulzberger [138] had shown that it was no longer possible to sensitize guinea-pigs to neoarsphenamine after they had been injected intravenously with the antigen. Chase [139] also showed that if guinea-pigs were fed repeated small doses of a chemical allergen, they became tolerant and could no longer be sensitized by skin applications. Felton [140] showed that while small doses (0·5 µg.) of pneumococcal polysaccharide caused antibody production in the mouse, larger doses (0·5–5·0 mg.) produced no antibody and rendered the animal specifically insensitive to the antigen for some months. He termed this 'immunological paralysis'. It is now recognized that the three phenomena of neonatal tolerance, the Sulzberger-Chase phenomenon, and Felton's paralysis are all related, and the terms 'immunological tolerance' and 'immunological paralysis' can be used interchangeably.

Mitchison [141] demonstrated clearly that for many antigens and for many animals increasing doses of antigen led, first, to a 'low-zone paralysis', in which the animal became specifically non-responsive to the antigen, without ever developing antibody. This was followed by a 'zone of immunization', in which the antigen provoked antibody production. Finally, higher doses of antigen led to the development of 'high-zone paralysis', when the animal was again specifically unresponsive. The concentration of antigen required to produce low-zone paralysis appears to be relatively constant for a wide range of antigens in a number of different animals. The dose of antigen required for immunization varies widely. Some (such as bovine serum albumin) are 'weak' antigens, requiring a high dose for immunization, while others, such as diphtheria toxoid, are 'strong' antigens and immunize in small doses. The dose of antigen required to produce high-zone paralysis is variable. For transplantation antigens it appears that weak antigens will produce paralysis at lower doses than strong antigens, but for purified protein antigens the dose required for paralysis is relatively constant and independent of the strength of the antigen. Dresser and Mitchison [73] suggest that high-zone and low-zone paralysis are similar phenomena.

Work which has already been mentioned (p. 140) shows that an antigen may immunize when it is administered in particulate form, and when in soluble form, paralyse. This may be because particulate antigens are processed by macrophages in an essential preliminary step to immunization, while soluble antigens, by gaining direct access to the lymphocytes, block their response.

Recovery from paralysis can be delayed by repeated injections of antigen. Pneumococcal polysaccharide, which is retained for an extremely long time in tissues, produces a correspondingly prolonged paralysis. In general, however, the duration of paralysis is not determined entirely by the catabolism of antigen, since, with many antigens, there is a gap of several months between disappearance of the antigen and the end of paralysis. The rate of recovery from paralysis is slower in adults than in young animals, and is further reduced by thymectomy and irradiation or antimitotic drugs [142]. The facts are best explained by assuming that immunological paralysis represents the destruction of immunologically competent cells by excessive amounts of antigen, and that recovery is due to the 'recruitment of a new population of reactive cells' [73].

The rate of recovery from paralysis and the rate of decay of antigen appear, then, to depend on different factors. We should expect that, in older animals and with short-lived antigens, antigen would disappear before appropriate immunocompetent cells reappear. The animal will therefore pass out of paralysis without producing antibody. This has been shown to be the case [73]. Alternatively, in young animals recovering rapidly from paralysis with long-lived antigens, we should expect that recovery of immunologically competent cells might take place before antigen was exhausted from the macrophages. In this case paralysis would be followed by spontaneous antibody production. This phenomenon has also been observed and is termed 'overshoot' [73].

CELLULAR BASIS OF PARALYSIS

At what stage does the paralysed immune mechanism fail? Macrophages from paralysed animals appear to ingest antigens normally [143], and antigen is trapped normally in the lymph-nodes and spleen [73]. The small lymphocytes from paralysed animals, however, appear to be defective. Lymph-node cells transferred from paralysed mice into syngeneic or irradiated recipients remain unresponsive [144, 145] to transplantation antigens. In animals paralysed with protein antigens it was impossible to demonstrate antibody after transfer of lymphocytes to irradiated hosts [146]. Studies with immunofluorescence [147] failed to demonstrate any antibody-producing cells in mice paralysed with bovine serum albumin. Dresser and Mitchison [73] discuss the theory that antigen immunizes when it reaches lymphocytes by way of macrophages and paralyses when it reaches them directly. This theory attractively fits most of the known facts about paralysis, though direct evidence for the paralysing effect of antigen on lymphocytes has not yet been produced. Whatever the means by which it is produced, the end-result of paralysis appears to be the death or irreversible inactivation of the lympoid cell. Dresser and Mitchison [73] point out that the specificity of paralysis, which leaves an animal free to respond to all other antigens, may imply that a single lymphocyte is capable of reacting only against a single antigen and therefore supports a selective theory of immunity.

An apparent exception to the specificity of immunological paralysis is the phenomenon described by Liacopoulos and Neveu [148], who found that massive doses of bovine gamma-globulin and other protein antigens produced a transient depression of the immune response to unrelated antigens. It seems likely, however, that this is a special form of antigenic competition (*see* p. 156).

C. Desensitization

The essence of immunological paralysis is that it is a specific unresponsiveness to an antigen which the animal has never previously encountered. It is possible to produce a similar state of immunological unresponsiveness in an animal which has already been immunized. This is known as 'desensitization'. It is, in general, much more difficult to desensitize an animal than to render it tolerant. There is, however, no reason to think that these are basically different phenomena. De Weck and Frey [149] have shown that guinea-pigs sensitized to dinitrochlorobenzene can be desensitized by the intravenous injection of large amounts of dinitrobenzene sulphonate. This effect was transient, lasting less than 5 days in most cases. However, with neoarsphenamine it was possible to sensitize guinea-pigs and then, by a combination of intravenous and intradermal injections, to produce a state of desensitization which lasted for more than 6 months.

Uhr [150] also showed that it was possible to desensitize guinea-pigs which had developed delayed hypersensitivity to ovalbumin or diphtheria toxoid by giving a large dose of the antigen intraperitoneally. This was, again, a short-lived desensitization: higher doses of antigen produced longer periods of unresponsiveness, but even with 60 mg. desensitization lasted only for a week. It is possible to produce prolonged desensitization of Mantoux-positive human subjects by repeated injections of tuberculin.

The term 'desensitization' is also used to describe a different phenomenon (*see* p. 246). Patients who develop immediate hypersensitivity to natural allergens and to drugs such as streptomycin can be 'desensitized' by repeated small injections, which result in the production of blocking antibodies.

D. Passively Administered Antibody

Shortly after antigenic stimulation, antibody production reaches a peak and then falls off. After restimulation there is a further peak: subsequent improvement is in the quality rather than the quantity of antibody produced. Cells explanted *in vitro* show no such limitation of quantity, and antibody production continues to increase far beyond the *in vivo* limitations [119]. There must exist control systems in the living animal which limit antibody synthesis and check the excessive proliferation of cells in response to an antigen. There are, in fact, two kinds of control. The first is crude and non-specific: a biological coarse adjustment. This is the regulation of gamma-globulin catabolism by the level of circulating gamma-globulin. This seems to affect IgG only and not IgA or IgM. If IgG is transfused intravenously into a normal animal, the rate of IgG catabolism is accelerated. Conversely, if an animal is depleted of gamma-globulin by plasmapheresis, the rate of gamma-globulin catabolism is decreased. Fahey and Robinson [151] showed that the portion of IgG responsible for increasing the rate of catabolism was the Fc fragment. This system is immunologically non-specific, and alterations in immunoglobulin synthesis occur without respect to its antibody activity.

The second control is a fine adjustment. The administration of specific antibody can, under certain circumstances, depress or inhibit antibody production in the recipient. This phenomenon is immunologically specific and has been recently reviewed by Uhr and Möller [97]. Uhr and Baumann [152] showed that the production of antibody to diphtheria toxoid could be suppressed by giving antibody up to 5 days after immunization. Fitch and Rowley [153] showed that passively administered antibody could inhibit antibody formation to sheep erythrocytes, and demonstrated that the primary response was affected to a greater extent than the secondary response. Subsequent work has shown that late, high-affinity antibody is more efficient at blocking the immune response than early antibody [154]. Delayed hypersensitivity is reduced little, or not at all, by passive antibody [97, 152].

The depression of antibody production by administered antibody has been shown to correlate with a diminution in the number of antibody-producing cells in the spleen [155]. There is some uncertainty about the comparative effects of 7S and 19S antibodies: Henry and Jerne [156] found that the number of cells in mouse spleen forming anti-sheep erythrocyte antibodies was reduced by passive administration of 7S antibodies but enhanced by 19S antibodies. They suggest that previous workers, who had found suppression by 19S antibodies, were using impure preparations.

The inhibition of 19S antibody-forming cells by 7S antibody may have an important role in limiting the 19S primary response [157]. Mishell and Dutton [158] showed that mouse spleen cells *in vitro*, when stimulated with sheep erythrocytes, produce more 19S antibody than *in vivo*. This excess antibody production could be blocked by adding immune serum to the culture medium. Some children with hypogamma-globulinaemia who are unable to produce IgG may produce IgM normally. They have been shown to develop IgM antibodies even in the secondary response, perhaps because of the absence of feedback inhibition from IgG [159, 160].

A recent dramatic application of the passive administration of high-affinity IgG antibody is the prophylactic injection of anti-D to prevent Rh-haemolytic disease of the newborn [161, 162]. Immunization of the mother by foetal erythrocytes leaking transplacentally at the time of delivery can be prevented by intravenous injection of suitable amounts of anti-D shortly after delivery. Controlled trials indicate that this method is likely to be of great value in the prevention of Rh-haemolytic disease.

E. Antigenic Competition

Michaelis [163, 164] first described the depression of the immune response to one antigen which may occur as a result of the injection of a second antigen. Recent experimental work has been reviewed by Adler [165], who studied the primary antibody response to ferritin in mice injected simultaneously with varying doses of bovine gamma-globulin (BGG). He showed that large doses of BGG (1·2 μg.N) depressed and abbreviated antibody production to ferritin, although smaller doses (0·016 μg.N) actually increased the level of ferritin antibodies. Competition could still be demonstrated if the BGG was given 12 weeks before the ferritin and was most effective if the animal had previously been sensitized to BGG, so that the competing injection evoked a secondary response.

The quantitative aspects of competition vary in different systems. Radovich and Talmage [166] studied antibody production to sheep red blood-cells (SRBC) in mice. As a competing antigen they used horse red blood-cells (HRBC) which show very little cross-reaction. They found that there was no diminution in the antibody production to SRBC when HRBC were given simultaneously. The greatest reduction of antibody production to SRBC occurred when HRBC were given 4 days previously (*Fig. 37*). They also studied the response to SRBC in irradiated mice which were reconstituted either with unimmunized spleen cells or with cells from animals immunized with HRBC, and showed that antibody production was lower when the cells were derived from animals pre-immunized with HRBC. Curiously, this effect of competition was more marked with a larger cell transfer (50×10^6) than with a smaller one (10×10^6).

The mechanism of antigenic competition is still obscure. It could represent competition for precursors of antibody-producing cells or a limitation on the rate of expansion of the lymphoid system. If all precursor cells are unipotent and precommitted, then clearly there can be no competition for them, since each antigen will select a different cell population. On the other hand, the work of Miller and his co-workers (p. 148) suggests that two cell types interact in the production of antibody-forming cells. If one of these cells (the thymocyte or the bone-marrow precursor cell) is precommitted, and the other multipotent, then competition might represent the exhaustion of the multipotent system.

There are two further hypotheses for the mechanism of competition. It might be that antigens compete for the antigen trapping system of macrophages and dendritic cells. If this were the case, however, it would be difficult to explain why an antigen given as a secondary stimulus should compete so much more effectively than a primary antigen. The results of Radovich and Talmage [166] on cell transfer would also be difficult to account for. A valuable test for this hypothesis would be to establish whether an antigen to which an animal has been made tolerant is still effective in antigenic competition, since there is some evidence [73] that antigen is trapped and handled normally in the tolerant animal. If tolerance were to abolish competition, this would suggest a site other than the antigen-trapping mechanism for the interaction of competing antigens.

Unfortunately, the evidence on this point is still conflicting. Weigle and High [167] found that antibody production in response to ovalbumin could be reduced in rabbits by simultaneous injection of bovine thyro-globulin, but that this antigenic competition was abolished in animals

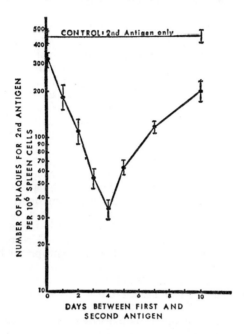

Fig. 37.—Antigenic competition. The antibody response to sheep erythrocytes (SRBC) in mice injected at various intervals previously with horse erythrocytes (HRBC). Antibody production is depressed most when the competing antigen (HRBC) is given before the standard antigen (SRBC). *Reproduced from J. Radovich and D. W. Talmage (1967), 'Science, N.Y.', vol. 158, pp. 512–514, Fig. 1, by kind permission of the Authors and of the American Association for the Advancement of Science. Copyright 1967 of the American Association for the Advancement of Science.*

rendered tolerant to bovine thyroglobulin. However, Schechter [168], using synthetic polypeptide antigens in rabbits, found that tolerance did not abolish competition. Further work will obviously be needed to show whether this difference is due to the use of synthetic instead of natural antigens.

A final possible explanation of the mechanism of competition is that the proliferating lymphocytes in the two simultaneous immune responses are in competition either for humoral factors necessary for their develop-ment or, simply, for space to develop within the reticulo-endothelial system. Radovich and Talmage favour the first of these hypotheses, but the experimental evidence is at present quite inadequate for a firm decision.

V. SUMMARY AND CONCLUSIONS

As a result of recent work on antibody production a general theory of the relationship between lymphocytes, antigens, and antibodies has emerged which provides a clear and valuable frame of reference. It is discussed by Mitchison [35, 169], Smithies [106], and formalized, with modifications, by Bretscher and Cohn [170]. Basically, it is suggested that antigen-sensitive cells bear on their surface receptor molecules capable of recognizing, and reacting with, the antigen against which they are committed to produce antibody. Now we already have a molecule capable of recognizing antigen and combining with it: this is the antibody itself. We can therefore visualize lymphocytes carrying at their surface bound molecules of that antibody which their genetic material enables them to produce. Interaction with antigen will act as a trigger (perhaps by distorting the antibody molecule) and will stimulate the cell to mitosis, or the production of further antibody, or both. There is a striking similarity between this theory and Ehrlich's original hypothesis of haptophores (*see* p. 146). There is direct evidence for the presence of antibody molecules at the surface of lymphocytes, which is summarized by Mitchison [35]. Antiserum directed against rabbit immunoglobulins (i.e., against antibodies) will produce blast-cell transformation in a number of rabbit lymphocytes. If the receptor on the cell surface is in fact antibody, and if combination with a whole antigen molecule is required in order to stimulate the cell, then it would be expected that an appropriate hapten would combine with and block the cell-bound antibody without stimulating further antibody production. Mitchison has shown [35] in elegant experiments that hapten can indeed block the secondary response, in accordance with the predictions of the receptor–antibody hypothesis.

This hypothesis also explains two further observations which have already been discussed. (1) The suppressive effect of passively administered antibody on antibody production (p. 154). If cell stimulation depends on the interaction of antigen with cell-bound antibody, passively administered antibody, by competing with cells for the available antigen, would be expected to depress the production of new antibody. Moreover late, high-affinity antibody would be expected to be more effective in this competition than early antibody. This has been observed (p. 156). (2) This hypothesis also neatly explains the increasing affinity of antibody produced later in the immune response (p. 136). Cells producing antibody of high affinity will obviously be more effective in competing for the available antigen than cells producing low-affinity antibody. In this way, during the immune response, a process of 'natural selection' will take place, in favour of those cells producing the most efficient antibody. Some quantitative aspects of this are considered by Smithies [106].

In summary, it now seems likely that antigen, on its first introduction into the lymphoid system, encounters lymphocytes which recognize it by virtue of specific antibody molecules which they carry on their surface. It seems most likely that these arise spontaneously and are selected by antigen. As immunization proceeds, those cells producing the most efficient antibody will proliferate. A second injection of antigen will provoke a secondary response, in which high-affinity antibody is produced rapidly and in large amounts.

REFERENCES

1. GLENNY, A. T., and SÜDMERSEN, H. J. (1921), 'Notes on the Production of Immunity to Diphtheria Toxin', *J. Hyg., Camb.*, **20**, 176.
2. GLENNY, A. T., and HOPKINS, B. E. (1922), 'Duration of Passive Immunity', *J. Hyg., Camb.*, **21**, 142.
3. WHITE, R. G. (1963), 'Functional Recognition of Immunologically Competent Cells by Means of the Fluorescent Antibody Technique', in *The Immunologically Competent Cell*, Ciba Foundation Study Group No. 16 (ed. WOLSTENHOLME, G., and KNIGHT, J.), p. 6. London: Churchill.
4. WHITE, R. G. (1968), 'Antigens and Adjuvants', *Proc. R. Soc. Med.*, **61**, 1.
5. ADA, G. L., PARISH, C. R., NOSSAL, G. J. V., and ABBOT, A. (1967), 'The Tissue Localization, Immunogenic, and Tolerance-inducing Properties of Antigens and Antigen-fragments', *Cold Spring Harb. Symp. quant. Biol.*, **32**, 381.
6. NOSSAL, G. J. V., ADA, G. L., and AUSTIN, C. M. (1965), 'Antigens in Immunity. IX, The Antigen Content of Single Antibody-forming Cells', *J. exp. Med.*, **121**, 945.
7. HALL, J. G., MORRIS, B., MORENO, G. D., and BESSIS, M. C. (1967), 'The Ultra-structure and Function of the Cells in Lymph following Antigenic Stimulation', *J. exp. Med.*, **125**, 91.
8. BOYDEN, S. V. (1966), 'Natural Antibodies and the Immune Response', *Adv. Immun.*, **5**, 1.
9. WIGZELL, H. (1967), 'Studies on the Regulation of Antibody Synthesis', *Cold Spring Harb. Symp. quant. Biol.*, **32**, 507.
10. STERZL, J. (1967), 'Factors determining the Differentiation Pathways of Immunocompetent Cells', *Cold Spring Harb. Symp. quant. Biol.*, **32**, 493.
11. MUSCHEL, L. H., GUSTAFSON, L., and ATAI, M. (1968), 'Effect of Anti-lymphocyte Serum on Natural Antibody', *Immunology*, **14**, 285.
12. KIM, Y. B., BRADLEY, S. G., and WATSON, D. W. (1968), 'Ontogeny of the Immune Response. V, Further Characterization of 19S γG- and 7S γG-immunoglobulins in the True Primary Immune Response in Germfree, Colostrum-deprived Piglets', *J. Immun.*, **101**, 224.
13. UHR, J. W., and FINKELSTEIN, M. S. (1967), 'The Kinetics of Antibody Formation', *Prog. Allergy*, **10**, 37.
14. NOSSAL, G. J. V., AUSTIN, C. M., and ADA, G. L. (1965), 'Antigens in Immunity. VII, Analysis of Immunological Memory', *Immunology*, **9**, 333.
15. WEI, M. M., and STAVITSKY, A. B. (1967), 'Molecular Forms of Rabbit Antibody Synthesized during the Primary Response to Human Albumin', *Immunology*, **12**, 431.
16. UHR, J. W., MARTIN, S., FINKELSTEIN, M. J., and BAUMANN, J. B. (1962), 'Antibody Formation. III, The Primary and Secondary Antibody Response to Bacteriophage φX 174 in Guinea Pigs', *J. exp. Med.*, **115**, 655.
17. JERNE, N. K. (1960), in *Mechanisms of Antibody Formation* (ed. HOLUB, M., and JAROSKOVA, L.). Prague: Czech Academy of Sciences.
18. SVEHAG, S. E., and MANDEL, B. (1964), 'The Formation and Properties of Polio-virus-neutralizing Antibody. I, 19S and 7S Antibody Formation: Differences in Kinetics and Antigen Dose Requirement for Induction', *J. exp. Med.*, **119**, 1.
19. BAKER, P. J., and LANDY, M. (1967), 'Brevity of the Inductive Phase in the Immune Response of Mice to Capsular Polysaccharide Antigens', *J. Immun.*, **99**, 687.
20. SERCARZ, E. E., and MODABBER, F. (1968), 'Antigen Binding to Cells: Determination by Enzymic Fluorogenic Group Hydrolysis', *Science, N.Y.*, **159**, 884.
21. LITT, M. (1967), 'Studies of the Latent Period. I, Primary Antibody in Guinea Pig Lymph Nodes 7½ Minutes after Introduction of Chicken Erythrocytes', *Cold Spring Harb. Symp. quant. Biol.*, **32**, 477.
22. WEIGLE, W. O. (1957), 'Elimination of I¹³¹ Labelled Homologous and Heterologous Serum Proteins from Blood of Various Species', *Proc. Soc. exp. Biol. Med.*, **94**, 306.

23. BENEDICT, A. A., BROWN, R. J., and AYENGAR, R. (1962), 'Physical Properties of Antibody to Bovine Serum Albumin as demonstrated by Hemagglutination', *J. exp. Med.*, **115**, 195.
24. DIXON, F. J., MAURER, P. H., WEIGLE, W. O., and DEICHMILLER, M. P. (1956), 'Rates of Antibody Synthesis during First, Second, and Hyperimmune Responses of Rabbits to Bovine Gamma Globulin', *J. exp. Med.*, **103**, 425.
25. NOSSAL, G. J. V., ADA, G. L. and AUSTIN, C. M. (1964), 'Antigens in Immunity. II, Immunogenic Properties of Flagella, "Polymerized Flagellin", and Flagellin in the Primary Response', *Aust. J. exp. Biol. med. Sci.*, **42**, 283.
26. TORRIGIANI, G., and ROITT, I. M. (1965), 'The Enhancement of 19S Antibody Production by Particulate Antigen', *J. exp. Med.*, **122**, 181.
27. TALIAFERRO, W. H., TALIAFERRO, L. G., and JAROSLOW, B. S. (1963), Argonne National Laboratory, Argonne. Unpublished data, quoted in [13].
28. DIXON, F. J., MAURER, P. H., and DEICHMILLER, M. P. (1954), 'Primary and Specific Anamnestic Antibody Responses of Rabbits to Heterologous Serum Protein Antigens', *J. Immun.*, **72**, 179.
29. DAVENPORT, F. M., HENNESSY, A. V., and FRANCIS, T., jun. (1953), 'Epidemiologic and Immunologic Significance of Age Distribution of Antibody to Antigenic Variants of Influenza Virus', *J. exp. Med.*, **98**, 641.
30. DAVENPORT, F. M., HENNESSY, A. V., and FRANCIS, T., jun. (1955), 'Persistent Antibody Orientation resulting from Primary Experience with Influenza Viruses. I, Type of Antibody Response after Vaccination', *Fedn Proc. Fedn Am. Socs exp. Biol.*, **14**, 460.
31. FRANCIS, T., jun. (1953), 'Influenza: The Newe Acquayantance', *Ann. intern. Med.*, **39**, 203.
32. FAZEKAS DE ST. GROTH, S., and WEBSTER, R. G. (1966), 'Disquisitions on Original Antigenic Sin. I, Evidence in Man', *J. exp. Med.*, **124**, 331.
33. FAZEKAS DE ST. GROTH, S., and WEBSTER, R. G. (1966), 'Disquisitions on Original Antigenic Sin. II, Proof in Lower Creatures', *J. exp. Med.*, **124**, 347.
34. LEVINE, B. B. (1967), 'Specificity of the Anamnestic Response to a Double Hapten Conjugate in Guinea Pigs primed with a Single Hapten', *J. Immun.*, **99**, 1173.
35. MITCHISON, N. A. (1967), 'Antigen Recognition responsible for the Induction *in vitro* of the Secondary Response', *Cold Spring Harb. Symp. quant. Biol.*, **32**, 431.
36. GLENNY, A. T., and BARR, M. (1932), 'The "Dilution Ratio" of Diphtheria Antitoxin as a Measure of Avidity', *J. Path. Bact.*, **35**, 91.
37. JERNE, N. K. (1951), 'A Study of Avidity based on Rabbit Skin Responses to Diphtheria Toxin-antitoxin Mixtures', *Acta path. microbiol. scand.*, Suppl. 87.
38. GREY, H. M. (1963), 'Phylogeny of the Immune Response. Studies on Some Physical Chemical and Serologic Characteristics of Antibody produced in the Turtle', *J. Immun.*, **91**, 819.
39. EISEN, H. N., and SISKIND, G. W. (1964), 'Variations in Affinities of Antibodies during the Immune Response', *Biochemistry*, **3**, 996.
40. FINKELSTEIN, M. S., and UHR, J. W. (1966), 'Antibody Formation. V, The Avidity of γM and γG Guinea Pig Antibodies to Bacteriophage ϕX 174', *J. Immun.*, **97**, 565.
41. TALIAFERRO, W. H., TALIAFERRO, L. G., and PIZZI, A. K. (1959), 'Avidity and Intercellular Transfer of Hemolysin', *J. infect. Dis.*, **105**, 197.
42. GOTTLIEB, S., McLAUGHLIN, F. X., LEVINE, L., LATHAM, W. C., and EDSALL, G. (1964), 'Long-term Immunity to Tetanus: A Statistical Evaluation and its Clinical Implications', *Am. J. publ. Hlth*, **54**, 961.
43. PFEIFFER, R., and MARX, F. (1898), 'Die Bildungsstätte der Choleraschutzstoffe', *Z. Hyg. InfektKrankh.*, **27**, 272.
44. HUEBSCHMANN, P. (1913), 'Das Verhalten der Plasmazellen in der Milz bei infectiösen Prozessen', *Verhandl. dt. path. Ges.*, **16**, 110.
45. RAMÓN Y CAJAL, S. (1896), *Manual de Anatomía patológica general*, 2nd ed. Madrid: Moya.
46. UNNA, P. G. (1881), 'Ueber Plasmazellen, insbesondere beim Lupus', *Mh. prakt. Derm.*, **12**, 296.
47. VON MARSCHALKO, T. (1895), 'Ueber die sogenannten Plasmazellen: Ein Beitrag zur Kenntniss der Herkunft der entzündlichen Infiltrationszellen', *Arch. Derm. Syph.*, **30**, 3, 241.

48. BING, J., and PLUM, P. (1937), 'Serum Proteins in Leucopenia', *Acta med. scand.*, **92**, 415.
49. FAGRAEUS, A. (1948), 'Antibody Production in Relation to the Development of Plasma Cells', *Acta med. scand.*, **130**, Suppl. 204, 1.
50. COONS, A. H., LEDUC, E. H., and CONOLLY, J. M. (1955), 'Studies on Antibody Production. I, A Method for the Histochemical Demonstration of Specific Antibody and its Application to a Study of the Hyperimmune Rabbit', *J. exp. Med.*, **102**, 49.
51. LEDUC, E. H., COONS, A. H., and CONNOLLY, J. M. (1955), 'Studies on Antibody Production. II, The Primary and Secondary Responses in the Popliteal Lymph Node of the Rabbit', *J. exp. Med.*, **102**, 61.
52. WHITE, R. G., COONS, A. H., and CONNOLLY, J. M. (1955), 'Studies on Antibody Production. III, The Alum Granuloma', *J. exp. Med.*, **102**, 73.
53. DE PETRIS, S., KARLSBAD, G., and PERNIS, B. (1963), 'Localization of Antibodies in Plasma Cells by Electron Microscopy', *J. exp. Med.*, **117**, 849.
54. HARRIS, T. N., HUMMELER, K., and HARRIS, S. (1966), 'Electron Microscopic Observations on Antibody-producing Lymph Node Cells', *J. exp. Med.*, **123**, 161.
55. VAN FURTH, R., SCHUIT, H. R. E., and HIJMANS, W. (1966), 'The Formation of Immunoglobulins by Human Tissues *in vitro*. I, The methods and their Specificity', *Immunology*, **11**, 1.
56. VAN FURTH, R. (1966), 'The Formation of Immunoglobulins by Human Tissues *in vitro*. II, Quantitative Studies', *Immunology*, **11**, 13.
57. VAN FURTH, R., SCHUIT, H. R. E., and HIJMANS, W. (1966), 'The Formation of Immunoglobulins by Human Tissues *in vitro*. III, Spleen, Lymph Nodes, Bone Marrow and Thymus', *Immunology*, **11**, 19.
58. VAN FURTH, R., SCHUIT, H. R. E., and HIJMANS, W. (1966), 'The Formation of Immunoglobulins by Human Tissues *in vitro*. IV, Circulating Lymphocytes in Normal and Pathological Conditions', *Immunology*, **11**, 29.
59. SELL, S., and ASOFSKY, R. (1968), 'Lymphocytes and Immunoglobulins', *Prog. Allergy*, **12**, 86.
60. PERNIS, B. (1967), 'Relationship between the Heterogeneity of Immunoglobulins and the Differentiation of Plasma Cells', *Cold Spring Harb. Symp. quant. Biol.*, **32**, 333.
61. COSTEA, N., YAKULIS, V. J., LIBNOCH, J. A., PILZ, C. G., and HELLER, P. (1967), 'Two Myeloma Globulins (IgG and IgA) in One Subject and One Cell Line', *Am. J. Med.*, **42**, 630.
62. NOSSAL, G. J. V., SZENBERG, A., ADA, G. L., and AUSTIN, C. M. (1964), 'Single Cell Studies on 19S Antibody Production', *J. exp. Med.*, **119**, 485.
63. ATTARDI, G., COHN, M., HORIBATA, K., and LENNOX, E. S. (1959), 'Symposium on the Biology of Cells modified by Viruses or Antigens. II, On the analysis of Antibody Synthesis at the Cellular Level', *Bact. Rev.*, **23**, 213.
64. ATTARDI, G., COHN, M., HORIBATA, K., and LENNOX, E. S. (1964), 'Antibody Formation by Rabbit Lymph Node Cells. I, Single Cell Responses to Several Antigens', *J. Immun.*, **92**, 335.
65. HIRAMOTO, R. N., and HAMLIN, M. (1965), 'Detection of Two Antibodies in Single Plasma Cells by the Paired Fluorescence Technique', *J. Immun.*, **95**, 214.
66. GREEN, I., VASSALLI, P., NUSSENZWEIG, V., and BENACERRAF, B. (1967), 'Specificity of the Antibodies produced by Single Cells following Immunization with Antigens bearing Two Types of Antigenic Determinants', *J. exp. Med.*, **125**, 511.
67. MÄKELÄ, O. (1967), 'The Specificity of Antibodies produced by Single Cells', *Cold Spring Harb. Symp. quant. Biol.*, **32**, 423.
68. NOSSAL, G. J. V., and MÄKELÄ, O. (1962), 'Autoradiographic Studies on the Immune Response. I, The Kinetics of Plasma Cell Proliferation', *J. exp. Med.*, **115**, 209.
69. GERSHON, H., BAUMINGER, S., SELA, M., and FELDMAN, M. (1968), 'Studies on the Competence of Single Cells to produce Antibodies of Two Specificities', *J. exp. Med.*, **128**, 223.
70. VAN FURTH, R., and COHN, Z. A. (1968), 'The Origin and Kinetics of Mononuclear Phagocytes', *J. exp. Med.*, **128**, 415.
71. FREI, P. C., BENACERRAF, B., and THORBECKE, G. J. (1965), 'Phagocytosis of the Antigen, a Crucial Step in the Induction of the Primary Response', *Proc. natn. Acad. Sci. U.S.A.*, **53**, 20.

72. DRESSER, D. W. (1962), 'Specific Inhibition of Antibody Production. II, Paralysis induced in Adult Mice by Small Quantities of Protein Antigen', *Immunology*, 5, 378.
73. DRESSER, D. W., and MITCHISON, N. A. (1968), 'The Mechanism of Immunological Paralysis', *Adv. Immun.*, 8, 129.
74. SCHOENBERG, M. D., NUMAW, V. R., MOORE, R. D., and WEISBERGER, A. S. (1964), 'Cytoplasmic Interaction between Macrophages and Lymphocytic Cells in Antibody Synthesis', *Science, N.Y.*, 143, 964.
75. FISHMAN, M., HAMMERSTROM, R. A., and BOND, V. P. (1963), '*In vitro* Transfer of Macrophage RNA to Lymph Node Cells', *Nature, Lond.*, 198, 549.
76. ASKONAS, B. A., and RHODES, J. M. (1965), 'Immunogenicity of Antigen-containing Ribonucleic Acid Preparations from Macrophages', *Nature, Lond.*, 205, 470.
77. FISHMAN, M., and ADLER, F. L. (1967), 'The Role of Macrophage-RNA in the Immune Response', *Cold Spring Harb. Symp. quant. Biol.*, 32, 343.
78. UNANUE, E. R., and ASKONAS, B. A. (1968), 'Persistence of Immunogenicity of Antigen after Uptake by Macrophages', *J. exp. Med.*, 127, 915.
79. HOWARD, A., and PELČ, S. R. (1953), 'Synthesis of DNA in Normal Irradiated Cells in Relation to Chromosome Breakage', *Heredity, Lond.*, 6, 261.
80. SADO, T., and MAKINODAN, T. (1964), 'The Cell Cycle of Blast Cells involved in Secondary Antibody Response', *J. Immun.*, 93, 696.
81. TANNENBERG, W. J. K., and MALAVIYA, A. N. (1968), 'The Life Cycle of Antibody-forming Cells. I, The Generation Time of 19S Hemolytic Plaque-forming Cells during the Primary and Secondary Responses', *J. exp. Med.*, 128, 895.
82. MAKINODAN, T., and ALBRIGHT, J. F. (1966), 'Proliferative and Differentiative Manifestations of Cellular Immune Potential', *Prog. Allergy*, 10, 1.
83. HANNA, M. G., jun. (1965), 'Germinal Centre Changes and Plasma Cell Reaction during the Primary Immune Response', *Int. Archs Allergy appl. Immun.*, 26, 230.
84. DUTTON, R. W., and MISHELL, R. I. (1967), 'Cellular Events in the Immune Response. The *in vitro* Response of Normal Spleen Cells to Erythrocyte Antigens', *Cold Spring Harb. Symp. quant. Biol.*, 32, 407.
85. SZENBERG, A., and CUNNINGHAM, A. J. (1968), 'DNA Synthesis in the Development of Antibody-forming Cells during the Early Stages of the Immune Response', *Nature, Lond.*, 217, 747.
86. THORBECKE, G. J., and BENACERRAF, B. (1962), 'The Reticulo-endothelial System and Immunological Phenomena', *Prog. Allergy*, 6, 559.
87. JERNE, N. K., NORDIN, A. A., and HENRY, C. (1963), 'The Agar Plaque Technique for recognizing Antibody-producing Cells', in *Cell Bound Antibodies* (ed. AMOS, B., and KOPROWSKI, H.). Philadelphia: Wistar Institute Press.
88. URSO, P., and MAKINODAN, T. (1963), 'The Roles of Cellular Division and Maturation in the Formation of Precipitating Antibody', *J. Immun.*, 90, 897.
89. ROWLEY, D. A., FITCH, F. W., MOSIER, D. E., SOLLIDAY, S., COPPLESON, L. W., and BROWN, B. W. (1968), 'The Rate of Division of Antibody-forming Cells during the Early Primary Immune Response', *J. exp. Med.*, 127, 983.
90. KOROS, A. M. C., MAZUR, J. M., and MOWERY, M. J. (1968), 'Radioautographic Studies of Plaque-forming Cells. I, Antigen-stimulated Proliferation of Plaque-forming Cells', *J. exp. Med.*, 128, 235.
91. SIMONSEN, M. (1967), 'The Clonal Selection Hypothesis evaluated by Grafted Cells reacting against their Hosts', *Cold Spring Harb. Symp. quant. Biol.*, 32, 517.
92. BUSSARD, A. E. (1967), 'Primary Antibody Response induced *in vitro* among Cells from Normal Animals', *Cold Spring Harb. Symp. quant. Biol.*, 32, 465.
93. TANNENBERG, W. J. K. (1967), 'Induction of 19S Antibody Synthesis without Stimulation of Cellular Proliferation', *Nature, Lond.*, 214, 293.
94. CLAFLIN, A. J., and SMITHIES, O. (1967), 'Antibody-producing Cells in Division', *Science, N.Y.*, 157, 1561.
95. MÄKELÄ, O., and NOSSAL, G. J. V. (1962), 'Autoradiographic Studies on the Immune Response. II, DNA Synthesis amongst Single Antibody-producing Cells', *J. exp. Med.*, 115, 231.
96. SCHOOLEY, J. C. (1961), 'Autoradiographic Observations of Plasma Cell Formation', *J. Immun.*, 86, 331.
97. UHR, J. W., and MÖLLER, G. (1968), 'Regulatory Effect of Antibody on the Immune Response', *Adv. Immun.*, 8, 81.

98. GOWANS, J. L., and UHR, J. W. (1966), 'The Carriage of Immunological Memory by Small Lymphocytes in the Rat', *J. exp. Med.*, **124**, 1017.
99. BUCKTON, K. E., COURT BROWN, W. M., and SMITH, P. G. (1967), 'Lymphocyte Survival in Men treated with X-rays for Ankylosing Spondylitis', *Nature, Lond.*, **214**, 470.
100. CELADA, F. (1967), 'Quantitative Studies of the Adoptive Immunological Memory in Mice. II, Linear Transmission of Cellular Memory', *J. exp. Med.*, **125**, 199.
101. BYERS, V. S., and SERCARZ, E. E. (1968), 'The X–Y–Z Scheme of Immunocyte Maturation. IV, The Exhaustion of Memory Cells', *J. exp. Med.*, **127**, 307.
102. BOSMAN, C., and FELDMAN, J. D. (1968), 'Cytology of Immunologic Memory. A Morphologic Study of Lymphoid Cells during the Anamnestic Response', *J. exp. Med.*, **128**, 293.
103. JERNE, N. K. (1967), 'Summary: Waiting for the End', *Cold Spring Harb. Symp. quant. Biol.*, **32**, 591.
104. HAUROWITZ, F. (1967), 'The Evolution of Selective and Instructive Theories of Antibody Formation', *Cold Spring Harb. Symp. quant. Biol.*, **32**, 559.
105. BURNET, F. M. (1967), 'The Impact of Ideas on Immunology', *Cold Spring Harb. Symp. quant. Biol.*, **32**, 1.
106. SMITHIES, O. (1968), 'Perspectives: Mutation and Selection in the Immune System', in *Regulation of the Antibody Response* (ed. CINADER, B.), p. 363. Springfield, Ill.: Thomas.
107. EHRLICH, P. (1900), 'On Immunity with Special Reference to Cell-life', *Proc. R. Soc.*, **66**, 424.
108. LANDSTEINER, K., and LAMPL, H. (1918), 'Ueber die Abhängigkeit der serologischen Spezifizität von der chemischen Struktur', *Biochem. Z.*, **86**, 343.
109. LANDSTEINER, K. (1947) *The Specificity of Serological Reactions.* Cambridge, Mass.: Harvard University Press.
110. BREINL, F., and HAUROWITZ, F. (1930), 'Chemische Untersuchung des Praezipitates aus Haemoglobin und Antihaemoglobin-Serum und Bemerkungen ueber die Natur der Antikoerper', *Z. phys. Chem.*, **192**, 45.
111. PAULING, L. (1940), 'A Theory of the Structure and Process of Formation of Antibodies', *J. Am. chem. Soc.*, **62**, 2643.
112. JERNE, N. K. (1955), 'The Natural-selection Theory of Antibody Formation', *Proc. natn. Acad. Sci. U.S.A.*, **41**, 849.
113. BURNET, F. M. (1959), *The Clonal Selection Theory of Acquired Immunity.* London: Cambridge University Press.
114. SHEARER, G. M., CUDKOWICZ, G., CONNEL, M. St. J., and PRIORE, R. L. (1968), 'Cellular Differentiation of the Immune System of Mice. I, Separate Splenic Antigen-sensitive Units for Different Types of Anti-sheep Antibody-forming Cells', *J. exp. Med.*, **128**, 437.
115. PAPERMASTER, B. W. (1967), 'The Clonal Differentiation of Antibody-producing Cells', *Cold Spring Harb. Symp. quant. Biol.*, **32**, 447.
116. MILLER, J. F. A. P., and MITCHELL, G. F. (1968), 'Cell to Cell Interaction in the Immune Response. I, Hemolysin-forming Cells in Neonatally Thymectomized Mice reconstituted with Thymus or Thoracic Duct Lymphocytes', *J. exp. Med.*, **128**, 801.
117. MITCHELL, G. F., and MILLER, J. F. A. P. (1968), 'Cell to Cell Interaction in the Immune Response. II, The Source of Hemolysin-forming Cells in Irradiated Mice given Bone Marrow and Thymus or Thoracic Duct Lymphocytes', *J. exp. Med.*, **128**, 821.
118. NOSSAL, G. J. V., CUNNINGHAM, A., MITCHELL, G. F., and MILLER, J. F. A. P. (1968), 'Cell to Cell Interaction in the Immune Response. III, Chromosomal Marker Analysis of Single Antibody-forming Cells in Reconstituted, Irradiated, or Thymectomized Mice', *J. exp. Med.*, **128**, 839.
119. DUTTON, R. W., and MISHELL, R. I. (1967), 'Cell Populations and Cell Proliferation in the *in vitro* Response of Normal Mouse Spleen to Heterologous Erythrocytes', *J. exp. Med.*, **126**, 443.
120. FREUND, J. (1947), 'Some Aspects of Active Immunization', *Am. Rev. Microbiol.*, **1**, 291.
121. GALL, D. (1966), 'The Adjuvant Activity of Aliphatic Nitrogenous Bases', *Immunology*, **11**, 369.

122. PERNIS, B., and PARONETTO, F. (1962), 'Adjuvant Effect of Silica (Tridymite) on Antibody Production', *Proc. Soc. exp. Biol. Med.*, **110**, 390.
123. OLOVNIKOV, A. M., and GURVICH, A. E. (1966), 'Immunization with Protein-cellulose Co-polymer (Immunosorbent)', *Nature, Lond.*, **209**, 417.
124. WEINTRAUB, M., and RAYMOND, S. (1963), 'Antiserums prepared with Acrylamide Gel used as Adjuvant', *Science, N.Y.*, **142**, 1677.
125. DIENES, L., and SCHOENHEIT, E. W. (1929), 'The Reproduction of Tuberculin Hypersensitiveness in Guinea Pigs with Various Protein Substances', *Am. Rev. Tuberc.*, **20**, 92.
126. ASKONAS, B. A., and WHITE, R. G. (1956), 'Sites of Antibody Production in the Guinea-pig. The Relation between *in vitro* Synthesis of Anti-ovalbumin and γ-Globulin and Distribution of Antibody-containing Plasma Cells', *Br. J. exp. Path.*, **37**, 61.
127. MURAMATSU, S. (1964), 'Shortening of the Period of Primary Immune Response by the Prior Injection of Freund's Adjuvant', *Nature, Lond.*, **201**, 1141.
128. ASHERSON, G. L. (1967), 'Antigen-mediated Depression of Delayed Hypersensitivity', *Br. med. Bull.*, **23**, 24.
129. HUTCHINSON, F. (1966), 'The Molecular Basis for Radiation Effects on Cells', *Cancer Res.*, **26**, 2045.
130. TALIAFERRO, W. H., and TALIAFERRO, L. G. (1954), 'Effect of X Rays on Hemolysin Formation following Various Immunization and Irradiation Procedures', *J. infect. Dis.*, **95**, 117.
131. MAKINODAN, T., KASTENBAUM, M. A., and PETERSON, W. J. (1962), 'Radio-sensitivity of Spleen Cells from Normal and Pre-immunized Mice and its Signifi-cance to Intact Animals', *J. Immun.*, **88**, 31.
132. SALVIN, S. B., and SMITH, R. F. (1959), 'Delayed Hypersensitivity in the Develop-ment of Circulating Antibody. The Effect of X-irradiation', *J. exp. Med.*, **109**, 325.
133. UHR, J. W., and SCHARFF, M. (1960), 'Delayed Hypersensitivity. V, The Effect of X-irradiation on the Development of Delayed Hypersensitivity and Antibody Formation', *J. exp. Med.*, **112**, 65.
134. GABRIELSEN, A. E., and GOOD, R. A. (1967), 'Chemical Suppression of Adaptive Immunity', *Adv. Immun.*, **6**, 91.
135. BERENBAUM, M. C. (1967), 'Immunosuppressive Agents and Allogeneic Trans-plantation', in 'Symposium on Tissue and Organ Transplantation', *Suppl. J. clin. Path.*, **20**, 417.
136. ELLIS, S. T., GOWANS, J. L., and HOWARD, J. C. (1967), 'Cellular Events during the Formation of Antibody', *Cold Spring Harb. Symp. quant. Biol.*, **32**, 395.
137. FITCH, F. W., BARKER, P., SOULES, K. H., and WISSLER, R. W. (1953), 'A Study of Antigen Localization and Degradation and the Histologic Reaction in the Spleen of Normal, X-irradiated, and Spleen-shielded Rats', *J. Lab. clin. Med.*, **42**, 598.
138. SULZBERGER, M. B. (1929), 'Hypersensitiveness to Arsphenamine in Guinea-pigs; Experiments in Prevention and in Desensitization', *Archs Derm. Syph.*, **20**, 669.
139. CHASE, M. W. (1959), 'Immunologic Tolerance', *A. Rev. Microbiol.*, **13**, 349.
140. FELTON, L. D. (1949), 'The Significance of Antigen in Animal Tissues', *J. Immun.*, **61**, 107.
141. MITCHISON, N. A. (1964), 'Induction of Immunological Paralysis in Two Zones of Dosage', *Proc. R. Soc.*, Series B, **161**, 275.
142. AISENBERG, A. C., and DAVIS, C. (1968), 'The Thymus and Recovery from Cyclophosphamide-induced Tolerance to Sheep Erythrocytes', *J. exp. Med.*, **128**, 35.
143. HARRIS, G. (1967), 'Macrophages from Tolerant Rabbits as Mediators of a Specific Immunological Response *in vitro*', *Immunology*, **12**, 159.
144. BILLINGHAM, R. E., BRENT, L., and MEDAWAR, P. B. (1956), 'Quantitative Studies in Tissue Transplantation Immunity. III, Actively Acquired Tolerance', *Phil. Trans. R. Soc.*, Series B, **239**, 357.
145. ARGYRIS, B. F. (1963), 'Adoptive Tolerance; Transfer of the Tolerant State', *J. Immun.*, **90**, 29.
146. FRIEDMAN, H. (1962), 'Transfer of Antibody Formation by Spleen Cells from Immunologically Unresponsive Mice', *J. Immun.*, **89**, 257.
147. SERCARZ, E. E., and COONS, A. H. (1963), 'The Absence of Antibody-producing Cells during Unresponsiveness to BSA in the Mouse', *J. Immun.*, **90**, 478.

148. LIACOPOULOS, P., and NEVEU, T. (1964), 'Non-specific Inhibition of the Immediate and Delayed Types of Hypersensitivity during Immune Paralysis of Adult Guinea-pigs', *Immunology*, 7, 26.
149. DE WECK, A. L., and FREY, J. R. (1966), *Immunotolerance to Simple Chemicals*, p. 71. New York: Elsevier.
150. UHR, J. W. (1958), 'Specific Desensitization of Guinea Pigs with Delayed Hypersensitivity to Protein Antigens', *Ann. N.Y. Acad. Sci.*, 73, 753.
151. FAHEY, J. L., and ROBINSON, A. G. (1963), 'Factors controlling Serum γ-Globulin Concentration', *J. exp. Med.*, 118, 845.
152. UHR, J. W., and BAUMANN, J. B. (1961), 'Antibody Formation. I, The Suppression of Antibody Formation by Passively Administered Antibody', *J. exp. Med.*, 113, 935.
153. FITCH, F. W., and ROWLEY, D. A. (1966), 'Feedback Mechanisms in the Regulation of Antibody Formation', in *Protides of the Biological Fluids* (ed. PEETERS, H.), p. 343. Proceedings of the Fourteenth Colloquium, Bruges. Amsterdam: Elsevier.
154. FINKELSTEIN, M. S., and UHR, J. W. (1964), 'Specific Inhibition of Antibody Formation by Passively Administered 19S and 7S Antibody', *Science, N.Y.*, 146, 67.
155. ROWLEY, D. A., and FITCH, F. W. (1964), 'Homeostasis of Antibody Formation in the Adult Rat', *J. exp. Med.*, 120, 987.
156. HENRY, C., and JERNE, N. K. (1968), 'Competition of 19S and 7S Antigen Receptors in the Regulation of the Primary Immune Response', *J. exp. Med.*, 128, 133.
157. MÖLLER, G., and WIGZELL, H. (1965), 'Antibody Synthesis at the Cellular Level. Antibody-induced Suppression of 19S and 7S Antibody Response', *J. exp. Med.*, 121, 969.
158. MISHELL, R. I., and DUTTON, R. W. (1967), 'Immunization of Dissociated Spleen Cell Cultures from Normal Mice', *J. exp. Med.*, 126, 423.
159. CHING, YI-CHUAN, DAVIS, S. D., and WEDGWOOD, R. J. (1966), 'Antibody Studies in Hypogammaglobulinemia', *J. clin. Invest.*, 45, 1593.
160. GLEICH, G. J., UHR, J. W., VAUGHAN, J. H., and SWEDLUND, H. A. (1966), 'Antibody Formation in Dysgammaglobulinemia', *J. clin. Invest.*, 45, 1334.
161. CLARKE, C. A. (1967), 'Prevention of Rh-haemolytic Disease', *Br. med. J.*, 4, 7.
162. FREDA, V. J., GORMAN, J. G., POLLACK, W., ROBERTSON, J. G., JENNINGS, E. R., and SULLIVAN, J. F. (1967), 'Prevention of Rh Iso-immunization', *J. Am. med. Ass.*, 199, 390.
163. MICHAELIS, L. (1902), 'Untersuchungen ueber Eiweisspraeziptine', *Dt. med. Wschr.*, 28, 733.
164. MICHAELIS, L. (1904), 'Weitere Untersuchungen ueber Eiweisspraezipitine', *Dt. med. Wschr.*, 30, 1240.
165. ADLER, F. L. (1964), 'Competition of Antigens', *Prog. Allergy*, 8, 41.
166. RADOVICH, J., and TALMAGE, D. W. (1967), 'Antigenic Competition: Cellular or Humoral', *Science, N.Y.*, 158, 512.
167. WEIGLE, W. O., and HIGH, G. J. (1967), 'The Effect of Antigenic Competition on Antibody Production to Heterologous Proteins, Termination of Immunologic Unresponsiveness and Induction of Autoimmunity', *J. Immun.*, 99, 392.
168. SCHECHTER, I. (1968), 'Antigenic Competition between Polypeptidyl Determinants in Normal and Tolerant Rabbits', *J. exp. Med.*, 127, 237.
169. MITCHISON, N. A. (1966), 'Recognition of Antigen by Cells', *Prog. Biophys. mol. Biol.*, 16, 3.
170. BRETSCHER, P. A., and COHN, M. (1968), 'Minimal Model for the Mechanism of Antibody Induction and Paralysis by Antigen', *Nature, Lond.*, 220, 444.
171. HUMPHREY, J. H., and WHITE, R. G. (1964), *Immunology for Students of Medicine*, 2nd ed., p. 133. Oxford: Blackwell Scientific.

CHAPTER 5

THE COMPLEMENT SYSTEM

By E. R. Gold and D. B. Peacock

I. Introduction
   Immune haemolysis

II. Components of complement
   A. C 1
   B. C 4
   C. C 2
   D. C 3, C 5, C 6, C 7, C 8, C 9

III. Mechanism of immune lysis

IV. Other biological functions of complement components
   A. Phagocytosis
   B. Hypersensitivity
   C. Properdin

V. Conglutinin

VI. Deficiencies of complement

I. Introduction

Complement is a substance, or strictly speaking a group of substances, present in the serum of man and animals, which combines with or is 'fixed' by many antigen–antibody complexes. We have noted elsewhere (Chapter 3) that all classes of immunoglobulins are not equally proficient in 'fixing' complement after their union with antigen; that often IgM is more effective in this respect than IgG (*see also* p. 174), and that IgA does not fix complement at all [1]. Complement was first recognized as a separate entity in blood by its capacity to lyse bacteria that had been 'sensitized' by homologous antibody. It is distinguished from specific antibody by its consistent presence in normal serum, by the level of its activity being unaffected by immunization, and by its inactivation on being heated to 55° C. for 30 minutes. Normal guinea-pig serum usually possesses a high level of lytic activity and is commonly used as a source of complement. The level in different species differs widely.

In 1901 Bordet and Gengou [2] introduced the principle of the complement fixation test and initiated thereby the first wave of interest in complement as a substance of fundamental importance in the immune mechanisms of the body. The second wave of interest followed Osborne's admirable review in 1937 [3], and the third wave is now in progress and stemmed from the development of suitable methods, chiefly ion-exchange chromatography, that permitted the isolation of undegraded protein with defined characteristics from mixtures of protein such as occur in serum. With this renewed interest has come the recognition that complement is probably involved in a number of immunological reactions not directly related to cytolysis.

Immune Haemolysis

Though the outcome of interaction between complement and bacterial cells and antibody may be death or lysis of the cells, perhaps the most striking and easily recognizable phenomenon associated with the fixation of complement is immune haemolysis. The release of haemoglobin from red blood-cells can be followed macroscopically and spectrophotometrically, and most of our knowledge of the way in which complement and antibody effect the lysis of cells has come from the study of this system.

Table XIX.—Optimal Proportions Titration of Haemolysin and Complement

Titre of Serum used to sensitize Cells	Titre of Complement									
	25	30	38	47	59	73	92	114	143	179
25	0	0	0	0	tr	1	3	3	4	4
50	0	0	0	0	0	tr	2	3	4	4
100	0	0	0	0	0	0	1	2	3	3
200	0	0	0	0	0	0	1	2	3	3
400	0	0	0	0	tr	1	2	3	3	4
800	0	tr	tr	tr	1	2	3	3	4	4
1600	1	1	1	2	3	3	4	4	4	4

0=100 per cent lysis. 2=50 per cent lysis. 4=No lysis.
At the 50 per cent end-point a 1 : 200 dilution of haemolysin represents the most sensitive system for the detection of free complement.

Examination of this system reveals that the amounts of antibody and complement required to produce lysis are to some extent inversely proportional to each other. However, a line drawn through points of equal haemolysis in *Table XIX* is typical of the results obtained in practice when different amounts of complement are used with red cells sensitized with varying concentrations of antibody (haemolysin). It will be seen that the situation is more complex than a straightforward inverse proportionality. Nevertheless, a point can be found where the least amount of complement suffices to cause a stated degree of lysis. Following this column down we can find the least amount of haemolysin which also suffices and this point represents the most sensitive combination of red cells and haemolysin for the detection of free complement. It is interesting that the older immunologists arrived at a very similar relationship between complement and haemolysin empirically by determining the least amount of haemolysin required to sensitize cells in the presence of an excess of complement (referred to as one minimum haemolytic dose) and then using five times this quantity (5 MHD) for maximum sensitization. The least amount of complement required to produce lysis of cells so sensitized is also referred to as one minimum haemolytic dose, or less confusingly perhaps as one haemolytic unit (1 HU).

For an analysis of the interaction between complement and antigen–antibody complexes and in the quantitative performance of the complement-fixation test, in which the haemolytic system is simply used as an indicator of free complement, it is necessary both to standardize the reagents in the above manner and to assess the degree of haemolysis, that

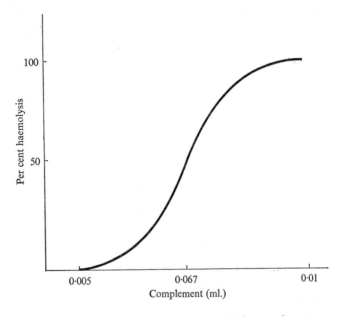

Fig. 38.—Lysis of sensitized red blood-cells by complement.

is obtained, accurately and reproducibly. If the degree of haemolysis induced is plotted against the amount of complement used a sigmoid curve is obtained (*Fig.* 38), indicating that we are dealing with a population of cells that are not all equally susceptible to the lytic action of complement. It means too that relatively large doses of complement are needed to effect the lysis of the last 5 per cent or so of cells and that 100 per cent lysis is not therefore the most sensitive or accurate method of determining the activity of complement. For this reason, as with most biological data, a

50 per cent end-point is taken where the dose–response relationship is undergoing the most rapid change. Since it is not possible under experimental conditions to choose exactly the dose of complement that would give a 50 per cent lysis, a method had to be devised with which a 50 per cent end-point can be calculated from any point or points on the curve of haemolysis.

The curve in *Fig.* 38 is described fairly accurately by von Krogh's equation,

$$x = K \left(\frac{y}{1-y} \right)^{1/n},$$

where x is the dose of complement, y, degree of haemolysis, and K and n are constants. K is equal to one 50 per cent haemolytic unit of complement since when $y = 0.5$ the function

$$\left(\frac{y}{1-y} \right)^{1/n} = 1.$$

Expressed logarithmically von Krogh's equation becomes

$$\log x = \log K + 1/n . \log \left(\frac{y}{1-y} \right),$$

and if $\log x$ is plotted against

$$\log \left(\frac{y}{1-y} \right),$$

a straight line is obtained with a slope of $1/n$. Under defined experimental conditions $1/n$ has a value of 0.2 [4]. If complement is to be estimated under these conditions the expression

$$K (1 \text{ HU}_{50}) = \frac{x}{\{y/(1-y)\}^{0.2}}$$

can be used to calculate 1 HU_{50} from any dose of complement that results in a degree of partial lysis. For reasonable accuracy values in the region of 20–80 per cent lysis should be taken.

II. COMPONENTS OF COMPLEMENT

The possibility that complement is not a single substance has already been hinted at on a number of occasions. The separation of complement activity into separate components is perhaps best approached in a semi-historical way so that the reader can appreciate how the concept arose and was developed.

Fresh serum can be separated readily into two fractions by dilution with distilled water at pH 5.2–5.4. The euglobulins are precipitated and can be redissolved in physiological saline. The pseudoglobulins remain in solution. Neither of these fractions is capable of lysing sensitized red blood-cells on its own, but mixed together the haemolytic property of the original whole serum is restored. In addition, both fractions are heat-labile (at 56° C. for 30 minutes).

Subsequently it was shown that complement activity could also be abolished by treating whole serum with yeast or with zymosan, a water-insoluble polysaccharide extract from yeast cell walls. Lytic activity can be restored to such a preparation by the addition of the euglobulin fraction or of heated serum. Since the first two fractions described were both heat-labile it follows that zymosan abolished the activity of a third component.

A fourth component, also heat-stable, can be demonstrated by treating whole serum with ammonia, hydrazine, or primary amines. After neutralization with acid this preparation can have its activity restored by the addition of heated serum, zymosan-treated serum, or the pseudoglobulin fraction. The four components so far characterized (C 1, C 2, C 3, and C 4) have been studied intensively in order to gain an insight into the mode of action of complement. For the quantitative estimation of each of these components reagents were prepared from the five preparations already described. Single preparations or combinations of them constituted the so-called R reagents [4] R1, R2, R3, and R4. Each of these reagents was designed to contain an excess of those components other than the one it was being used to detect. Thus R1 was used to detect C 1 since it contained an excess of C 2, C 3, and C 4, and in theory the amount of C 1 in a test solution could be found by diluting it out in the presence of constant amounts of R1 and sensitized cells.

Unfortunately, the R reagents have had to be used under widely varying conditions and in concentrations that approach dangerously close to anticomplementary or haemolytic levels, or both. It is not surprising then to learn that the results obtained in the same or different laboratories have shown a distressing lack of reproducibility. Osler [5] has pointed out some of the errors to which much of this earlier work led, partly due to the assumption that the component present in the lowest concentration necessarily determined the haemolytic activity of a preparation. Nevertheless, some of the conclusions based on the use of R reagents are still perfectly valid. Among these are the order in which the components of complement react with sensitized cells, i.e., C 1, C 4, C 2, C 3, and the importance of magnesium and calcium ions in particular stages of the reaction.

With the introduction of milder methods of protein separation it has become apparent that the situation with regard to C 3 is a good deal more complex than we had realized. It now seems that with the identification of six new components within the old 'C 3 complex' we have reached the position where the use of purified reagents will make it possible to avoid the inconsistencies which for so long bedevilled investigations into the mode of action of complement. It should also be possible to unravel the parts played by individual components in a number of reactions in which complement, in whole or in part, is involved. For the moment we will consider the components of complement separately in the order in which they are taken up in the process of immune haemolysis.

A. C 1

For the chromatographic separation of C 1 most workers used the euglobulin fraction of normal serum, to which was added the chelating agent, ethylenediamine-tetra-acetate (EDTA). In these circumstances three fractions, C 1q, C 1r, and C 1s, have been obtained which together display C 1 activity. It is suggested that the three subcomponents ordinarily form a macromolecular complex in serum and are held together by a calcium ion ligand [6]. The first step in complement fixation (or haemolysis) results in the adsorption of C 1 to the antigen–antibody complex with the generation of esterase activity. The activated component is referred to as C 1a. However, its substrate is not the red cell but the next two components in the reaction sequence, namely C 4 and C 2. The C 1 macromolecule sediments in the ultracentrifuge with the $19S$ globulins, but it is not an immunoglobulin. Its dissociation into three subcomponents by chelating agents was a purely fortuitous discovery that tended to confuse rather than clarify the picture at first, but that may nevertheless ultimately help in elucidating the nature and function of C 1.

The first step in the combination of complement with sensitized erythrocytes (EA) is set out in reaction I:—

$$\text{C 1} + \text{EA} \xrightarrow{\text{Ca}^{++} \; 4°\text{C.}} \text{EAC 1a.} \tag{I}$$

The reaction proceeds at 4° C., though much more rapidly at 30° C., and the resultant complex is stable for several weeks in a glucose–gelatin–veronal buffer [7]. This step also requires the presence of calcium ions in the reaction mixture. C 1 esterase (C 1a) can be eluted from the EAC 1a complex by EDTA and is associated with the C 1s subcomponent, but its enzymic activity is not simply due to dissociation of C 1 since C 1s can be similarly obtained from free C 1 in the form of a pro-esterase [6].

B. C 4

Under the action of C 1 esterase C 4 is bound to the EA complex. The presence of C 1a is necessary for the formation rather than maintenance of the union since the complex EAC 4 can exist separately. The second step in the fixation of complement is set out in reaction II:—

$$\text{C 4} + \text{EAC 1a} \xrightarrow{\quad 4°\text{C.} \quad} \text{EAC 1a, 4.} \tag{II}$$

This reaction will also proceed at 4° C., and the resulting complex is stable. Human C 4 has been characterized as a β_{1E}-globulin and again is not an immunoglobulin [8]. C 1 esterase will dissociate from the intermediate EAC 1a under a variety of conditions and is then capable of inactivating C 4 in solution. According to Lepow [6], the dissociation of C 1a is inhibited at reduced ionic strengths and this partly accounts for the increased haemolytic activity of complement under these circumstances.

C. C 2

In the next step, set out in reaction III, C 2 is added to the complex that has already been formed. Magnesium ions are required in order that the reaction may proceed. At 30–37° C. C 2 is activated by C 1 esterase and probably forms a union with a receptor site on C 4. This process is accompanied by the release of an inactive fragment, C 2i, which can be recognized in the fluid phase of the reaction mixture.

$$\text{C 2} + \text{EAC 1a, 4} \xrightarrow{\text{Mg}^{++} \; 30°\text{C.}} \text{EAC 1a, 4, 2a} + \text{2i.} \tag{III}$$

Though the EAC 1a, 4, 2a complex is fairly stable at 0° C. the decay rate of C 2a is considerably faster at activation temperatures and yields the complex EAC 1a, 4; to which C 2a can again be added by supplying more C 2 to the reaction mixture. C 2a is not fully stabilized until the next four components have been incorporated into the complex [7, 9].

At this stage, therefore, the situation is rather complex and the forward reaction depends on the temperature of the reaction mixture, on the number of sites (S) on an erythrocyte that are in the state EAC 1a, 4, on the concentration of C 2, and of the four components that follow it in sequence. Also, at this stage C 1a has finally fulfilled its function and the reaction can now proceed without its further intervention, even from the state EAC 4, 2a.

D. C 3, C 5, C 6, C 7, C 8, C 9

Theoretical considerations of the velocity of the reaction succeeding the formation of the complex EAC 1a, 4, 2a led to the suggestion that more than one extra component was involved [10]. Subsequently, three, four, five, and finally six distinct fractions replaced the old concept of a single component. Each of these fractions now enjoys the status of a separate complement component. Several groups of workers have been responsible for the difficult task of elucidating these problems; some of them have worked principally with human and others with guinea-pig complement. They have all employed different nomenclatures from time to time, and reagents have not always been compared in the different laboratories. General agreement appears to have been reached at a meeting in La Jolla, California [11], once it seemed fairly certain that the complement system in the two species was functionally the same and all the components taking part in immune haemolysis had been identified. The components are therefore now numbered from C 3 in the order in which they react; with the exception of C 4 which already had a place earlier in the sequence. Confusion can still arise because in the older literature C 3 was used to describe all the components reacting after C 2. The components have been reviewed and their nomenclatures compared on a number of occasions in recent years [6–8, 11, 12].

Human C 3 is a β_{1C}-globulin. It decays on heating or ageing to a β_{1A}-globulin which is haemolytically inactive. C 3 is also inactivated by dilute hydrazine or ammonia [8], which illustrates the difficulties the earlier immunologists were confronted with, since these are the reagents which were supposed to destroy only C 4. Though the decay of β_{1C} to β_{1A} can be observed *in vitro*, the process of immune haemolysis is apparently accompanied by a different conversion: from β_{1C} to a β_{1G}-globulin [8]. Evidence has been adduced suggesting that C 2a acts enzymatically to induce this change [*see* 8]. C 3 itself may have peptidase activity, normally masked by a serum inhibitor [13].

Human C 5 is a β_{1F}-globulin [8], and this component is heat-labile whether derived from human or guinea-pig serum [7]. This reaction step proceeds rapidly at 30–37° C., but very slowly at 4° C. [14], and according to Nelson [7] could be responsible for the known temperature dependence of the lytic stages that follow the formation of EAC 1a, 4, 2a.

C 6 and C 7 have been characterized more recently and correspond to Nelson's C 3e and C 3f of guinea-pig complement [7, 15]. It is only after the formation of EAC 1a, 4, 2a, 3, 5, 6, 7 that a really stable complex is formed that retains its reactivity with C 8 and C 9 after a period of several weeks if stored at 0° C.

The reaction of C 8 and C 9 with the previously formed complex is said not to deplete serum of these components [14, 16] and Nelson therefore proposed that they could be regarded as enzymes. The reaction of C 8 renders the red cell unduly fragile suggesting a partial disintegration of the cell surface; a process that is then completed by C 9 with the eventual formation of a damaged erythrocyte (E*) which spontaneously undergoes lysis.

The final stages of immune haemolysis are set out in reaction IV:—

$$\text{EAC 1a, 4, 2a, 3, 5, 6, 7} \xrightarrow{\text{C 8, C 9}} \text{E}^{\star}. \tag{IV}$$

It would appear that these nine components represent the complete complement complex with which are associated certain cofactors such as divalent cations, and inhibitors such as C 1 esterase inhibitor. That we have reached the final tally of complement components is suggested by the fact that purified reagents react in a manner consistent with their concentration and that those components that are depleted during the course of the reaction are depleted quantitatively [7]. Since the different components are present in serum and serum preparations in different concentrations a fixation reaction may use up the same number of *units* of each component but leave behind a different *percentage* of each. This has led to interpretative difficulties in the past, particularly with respect to the R reagents and to the properdin system. It should be recognized, too, that though we speak of 'purified reagents' we are normally only concerned with functional purity and not necessarily with chemical purity. In the absence of the latter it is necessary to be particularly careful about accepting evidence of the former.

III. Mechanism of Immune Lysis

While we have so far considered complement almost solely in terms of the lysis of sensitized red blood-cells, there remains a good deal to be said about the mechanism by which the components of complement effect lysis of these and other cells. We will therefore consider this aspect in more detail before moving on to consider some of the other functions of complement.

It should be recognized at the outset that reactions between antigens and antibodies involve ordinary physicochemical forces and have their characteristic rates of association and dissociation (*see* Chapter 6, 'Antigen–antibody Reactions'). The dynamic equilibrium between free antigen and free antibody and antigen–antibody complexes and the rate at which it is achieved might both be thought of as expressions of the 'avidity' of antibody for antigen, which might in turn affect the readiness with which complement is fixed. Nelson [7] has shown that rabbits inoculated with varying amounts of sheep red cells and administered over different inoculation schedules produced antibodies that were characteristically different in haemolytic efficiency. Such differences could partly be an expression of the firmness of union between antibody and antigenic site. Oddly enough Nelson equates highly avid antibody with low haemolytic efficiency, but explanations of such an apparent paradox have been sought and found. Talmage and his colleagues [17, 18] were the first to bring evidence to bear that low and high molecular weight antibodies behaved differently when lysing red blood-cells in conjunction with complement. They reported that the rate of haemolysis varied with the square of the 19S (IgM) antibody concentration, and with the fourth power of the 7S (IgG) antibody concentration. The inference to be drawn from these findings was that bi- and tetramolecular antibody complexes were required respectively in order to 'fix' complement and initiate lysis. Subsequently Humphrey and Dourmashkin [19] and still later Borsos and Rapp [1] held that one molecule of IgM and two or more molecules of IgG were necessary for haemolysis, or at least for the binding of C la to the cell surface. It is probably generally accepted now that two IgG molecules in close proximity to each other or attached to contiguous antigenic sites are necessary to initiate lysis. If we now return to the question of avid antibody and haemolytic efficiency we can see that antibody which does not bind too firmly but can flit from site to site may well be in a better position to form bimolecular complexes with other antibody molecules than firmly bound, highly avid antibody. Nelson goes on to point out that the situation is a good deal more critical than even this might suggest and that there is probably an optimal avidity of antibody that gives maximum haemolysis [7]. Experimentally the situation is also confused when whole serum is used because of the interplay between IgG and IgM molecules.

It is interesting to note in connexion with the requirement of two or more IgG molecules for fixation of complement that aggregated gammaglobulin is now known to adsorb complement without the intervention of antigen [20], and that at least one modern theory of immunological precipitation employs the notion that there is some kind of interaction between antibody molecules.

It is not clear at the moment, in the context of immune haemolysis in particular and of complement fixation in general, whether single IgM molecules are the functional equivalent of pairs of IgG molecules. If it were so, we are still faced with deciding how the two molecules of IgG are attached to antigenic sites on the cell surface: for example, each to two sites or each to one site. The adsorption of C 1 must be determined in some way by the form of attachment, and the charge configuration of the paired molecules must be mimicked by a single attached IgM molecule.

The impulse to generalize is always very strong, but are we at all justified in assuming that single bound molecules of IgM antibody and two or more of IgG are required for complement fixation? In the frequently used system, sheep erythrocyte, rabbit antibody, and guinea-pig complement, this could well be generally true. However, in contrast to this system, we have evidence that rabbit and mouse complements are more efficiently bound by IgG molecules than IgM [21, 22]. Until we know a great deal more about the fixation of complement to antigen–antibody complexes we would do well to reserve judgement on this score. It would be equally dangerous to infer, on the basis of *in vitro* experiments, that identical mechanism were at work *in vivo*, for it is rare under *in vitro* conditions for antibody and complement to be derived from the same species, let alone the same animal. In addition, where we speak of 'antibody' we often mean heat-inactivated serum, and similarly in the case of 'complement' we often mean uninactivated whole guinea-pig serum. Neither, of course, is functionally pure, and in the complement-fixation test proper we have at least one other such reagent. The functional activity of components of complement derived from different species could obviously be pertinent in this context. As one example of heterogeneity in this respect we can take the case of the fourth component. In the presence of guinea-pig C 4 one hundred times more human C 2 is needed to effect haemolysis than when the cells are coated with human C 4. Even guinea-pig C 2 is more active in the presence of human C 4 [23].

Because lysis of the red blood-cell is such an easily observable phenomenon it was both observed early and constantly used thereafter as a model for the examination of the lytic process. The fact remains that the non-nucleated red blood-cell is an unusual kind of mammalian cell, that *in vivo* immune haemolysis is a relatively rare occurrence, and that it is not the normal mechanism by which effete red cells are eliminated. It might be supposed on the contrary that the immune lysis of bacteria was an effective and common way for a host to rid itself of invading micro-organisms. Originally observed by Pfeiffer and Issaeff in 1894 [24] with cholera vibrios in the peritoneal cavity of immunized guinea-pigs, it is rather surprising to find that only a few genera among Gram-negative bacteria are susceptible to the lytic action of immune serum and complement. Among these genera are *Vibrio, Escherichia, Salmonella, Proteus, Haemophilus*, and *Brucella*. But by no means all species within a genus, nor all strains within a species, are equally susceptible. In particular, smooth strains of some species are notably more resistant than their rough counterparts.

The mechanism by which animal cells and bacteria are lysed by complement has not been worked out so far, and the two types of cell are very different in any case. In particular, bacterial cells have an outer cell wall that is not represented in animal cells; it gives rigidity to bacterial cells and determines their morphology. The composition of Gram-negative and Gram-positive cell walls differs considerably; that of the former contains much more lipid though the wall itself is only half the thickness of the latter. The high lipid content of the cell walls of Gram-negative bacteria finds a parallel in the cell membrane of animal cells. It is nevertheless not completely clear whether complement attacks the cell-wall structure of bacteria or the plasma membrane direct through the interstices of the cell wall. Muschel [25] points out that the action of antibody may be simply to concentrate complement at a particular site at the cell surface, and of complement fixation to activate enzymes of the complement complex or those of cellular origin, or both.

Muschel [25] also describes the effect of complement on spheroplasts of Gram-positive and Gram-negative bacteria. In a spheroplast the cell wall has been so degraded that it no longer supports the plasma membrane with its hypertonic contents so that the organism swells and loses its characteristic shape. Spheroplasts were prepared from the Gram-positive *Bacillus subtilis*. They could be lysed by both fresh and heated serum, and it was concluded that complement was not necessary in order to effect their lysis. Spheroplasts derived from Gram-negative organisms, on the contrary, were lysed only by fresh serum; this was so even when the spheroplasts were derived from strains resistant to immune lysis in the intact state. It was concluded, therefore, that there was a fundamental difference between the cell membranes of Gram-positive and Gram-negative organisms; that the cell walls and capsules of Gram-negative bacteria are responsible for the resistance that some of them show towards the action of complement; and that the greater thickness of the cell wall of Gram-positive bacteria is not the cause of their resistance to lysis, and that the high lipid content of the cell wall in Gram-negative bacteria is not a factor in susceptibility to lysis.

If the plasma membrane is the site of attack in immune lysis of bacteria, a parallel can be drawn between this reaction and passive haemolysis. In the latter case red cells are first coated with an unrelated antigen; antibody to this coating antigen is then allowed to react and is followed by the addition of complement. So-called 'passive' haemolysis results, but complement is less effective in this type of reaction than if it is allowed to adsorb to antibody attached directly to a red-cell antigen—presumably because it, or its active principles, have to act through a greater distance in order to affect the cell membrane.

It has long been held that in ordinary immune haemolysis complement binds primarily to the antibody and not directly to the red-cell surface. The mere fact that some classes of antibody fix complement whereas others do not cannot be taken as confirmation of this view. Until quite recently, however, there was no concrete evidence that complement acted enzymatically on the red cell, a circumstance that itself implies direct contact, even if only fleeting. Observations have now been made which strongly support the view that certain components of complement are bound directly to the red-cell surface as well as reacting with bound antibody [26, 27].

In the case of nucleated mammalian cells, and probably of red blood-cells as well, immune lysis is heralded by a loss of intracellular potassium and other micromolecular constituents, leading to osmotic changes that cause the swelling of cells. Deficiencies in the cell membrane sufficient to permit the escape of such ingredients are not large enough to allow haemoglobin to escape. Humphrey and Dourmashkin [19] describe lesions in lysed red cells and ascites tumour cells that they interpret as 'holes' 80 Å in diameter in the cell membrane; haemoglobin should have no difficulty in diffusing through holes of this size.

The final steps in the chain of events that results in the lysis of cells by complement remain unresolved. It is not even clear as yet whether C 8 and C 9 act directly on the cell membrane to produce lesions or whether this effect is produced by an intermediary substance. In this connexion it is reported that the cytolytic agent, lysolecithin, is formed as an end product of complement fixation [28, 29], but the quantitative aspects of this work have since been seriously questioned [8]. Even if its role were to be accepted, lysolecithin could still be derived from two sources: from a lipid component of complement itself, or from the cell membrane. Indeed, the lipid-rich cell wall of Gram-negative bacteria could be envisaged as a third possibility. However, if Muschel's work [25] is accepted then it is cell membranes rather than cell walls that determine sensitivity.

With the increasing availability of purified complement components the vagaries and uncertainties that beset the complement-fixation test and a number of other reactions in which complement plays a role should soon be a thing of the past. It is to a consideration of the part played by individual components of complement that we now turn.

IV. OTHER BIOLOGICAL FUNCTIONS OF COMPLEMENT COMPONENTS

A. Phagocytosis

Although the components of complement have been worked out using the system of immune haemolysis, it must be recognized that not all the components are necessarily involved in all the systems in which complement is implicated.

A case in point is immune phagocytosis where the availability of purified components has greatly clarified the role played by complement. It has been recognized for many years that complement may markedly enhance phagocytosis, that it is in this sense a heat-labile opsonin, but the exact manner in which it effects enhancement has not been known.

In a series of neat experiments Nelson [7] examined the phagocytosis of sheep red cells by guinea-pig leucocytes, also the same red cells but sensitized with antibody, and the intermediate erythrocyte–antibody–complement complexes ranging from EAC 1 through to EAC 1, 4, 2, 3, 5, 6. The complement components were derived from guinea-pig serum and a marked jump in phagocytic activity was noted first when the red cells were sensitized with antibody, and secondly when the intermediate EAC 1, 4, 2, 3 was tested. The addition of components C 5 and C 6 did not increase the degree of phagocytosis. Subsequently Ward [30] has claimed that an enzyme-split fragment of C 3 with a molecular weight of 6000 and derived from human and rabbit C 3 is a chemotactic factor. Nelson's work was done with washed intermediate complexes and only taken as far as the sixth component. Ward and his colleagues have studied the formation of chemotactic substances following the addition of antigen–antibody complexes to fresh human and guinea-pig serum [31]. In a note added in proof they state that this factor in human serum is the trimolecular complex, C 5, C 6, C 7. They also feel that the role of complement, and particularly of this trimolecular complex, in chemotaxis far outweighs the effect of a number of pharmacologically active agents such as bradykinin and kallidin (see Chapter 7) that alter vascular permeability.

B. Hypersensitivity

In hypersensitivity states tissue damage always ensues. We shall deal here only with immediate hypersensitivity and only with that part of it that might be associated with complement. Immediate hypersensitivity as a whole is dealt with separately in Chapter 7.

The cytotoxic action of complement in conjunction with antibody to cellular antigens is well documented, but this is not enough to explain the sequence of events that we describe as 'immediate hypersensitivity'. Nor, of course, is complement, free or fixed, responsible for all the manifestations of immediate hypersensitivity, and we know a number of substances that are pharmacologically active in this respect. Nevertheless, anaphylatoxin is by definition a property acquired by fresh guinea-pig and other sera on exposure to antigen–antibody aggregates; it induces anaphylactic shock in guinea-pigs. At one time this property was equated with the old C 3 complex, and until functionally pure components became available no advance on this position was possible. Even now some confusion still reigns, and while da Silva and Lepow [32] have produced most convincing evidence that anaphylatoxin is associated with the interaction of C 1 esterase with C 4, C 2, and C 3 in a system utilizing human components, they felt unable to refute entirely Jensen's claim [33] that in a guinea-pig system C 5 is also implicated.

One of the possibilities that might account for such discrepancies is that all the components of complement from man and guinea-pig have yet to be compared. In spite of this, a single numerical system has been adopted in this chapter for both sets of components in the interests of clarity, but it must be admitted that the functional and sequential identity of all the components has not been established at the moment. Furthermore, the two groups of workers have tackled the identification of anaphylatoxin in rather different ways. Da Silva and Lepow have used the novel approach of forming a complement complex directly on purified C 1 esterase, i.e., on the enzymatically active fragment of C 1. C 4, C 2, and C 3 are also purified reagents so that their system is functionally pure as far as can be determined and is also free of any antigen–antibody substrate. The reservations that remain to be made are again that functional purity is not necessarily chemical purity, and, as has been pointed out by numerous authors, function and sequence in one reaction, e.g., haemolysis, do not necessarily apply to every other reaction. In the same paper da Silva and Lepow also indicate that anaphylatoxin is a low molecular weight split product of C 3 that has been compared with and distinguished from the chemotactic factor derived from C 3 mentioned above [30]. It would therefore appear, over half a century after the idea was first promulgated, that we are approaching the point at which we can say with certainty that anaphylatoxin is a product of the complement system.

C. Properdin

The interest of properdin for the complement system is that, as originally conceived, properdin was a kind of universal antibody that reacted with zymosan, among other things, in the presence of magnesium ions to adsorb specifically the C 3 complex. This extreme view was partly due to the inherent difficulties associated with interpreting results obtained with the old 'R'-reagents, used for assessing levels of C 1, C 2, C 4, and the remaining components then lumped together under the heading of C 3. Later it was assumed that properdin represented a mixture of IgM antibodies, directed mostly against Gram-negative bacteria of the intestinal tract, and present in low titre in normal sera. More recently Lepow and his associates [34] have claimed to have purified properdin, and to have shown that it was not an immunoglobulin at all.

V. CONGLUTININ

All that it is necessary to say here is that conglutinin and immunoconglutinin both behave like antibodies with specificities principally directed towards the C 3 component, and perhaps to a lesser extent against C 4 [35]. The role of other components is still under investigation in this respect. It has been suggested that the determinant combining with conglutinin contains a mannotriose and the amino-sugar N-acetyl-D-glucosamine [36].

VI. DEFICIENCIES OF COMPLEMENT

Deficiencies of complement, usually described in terms of absence of haemolytic complement, have now been described on numerous occasions in a variety of species of animal and in man. The earliest observations were of lack of haemolytic complement, first in individual guinea-pigs and then in inbred strains. Early attempts to maintain complement-deficient strains ended in failure when infection wiped out the animal colonies. Subsequent observation of a human individual with a known defect of lytic complement did not bear out the suggestion that such individuals would necessarily be unduly susceptible to bacterial infections. The actual deficiency in this case was in the second component, but Gewürz et al. showed that the bactericidal activity of the patient's blood compared favourably with the sera of normal individuals when tested against a number of Gram-negative bacterial genera [37]. The authors felt that under the suboptimal conditions operating *in vivo* there was enough C 2 in this man's serum to protect him against recurrent bacterial infections. They go on to say that '... the addition of antibody and complement components served to exaggerate the extent of the deficiency of the subject'. This does not exclude the possibility that complement plays an important role in resisting infections, but it also indicates that too wide an interpretation should not be put on *in vitro* tests designed to detect optimal efficiency of reagents.

The interest in complement deficiency states stems directly from a desire to understand fully the biological role of complement and its components. In a number of cases this is beginning to be worked out. It is perfectly clear for instance that some functions of complement do not require all its components; capillary permeability and phagocytic factors have already been mentioned. In immune adherence preformed complexes of antigens and antibody, together with the decayed complement complex C 1a, 4, cause certain cells, chiefly of primate origin and including thrombocytes, to adhere to each other [*see* 7]. It is thought that this phenomenon may account for the thrombi and some of the other manifestations of the Schwartzman and Arthus reactions. Inbred strains of mice [38] and rabbits [39], with defined deficiencies in the fifth and sixth components, are currently under study. In the case of C 6-deficient rabbits it is suggested that allograft rejection may sometimes proceed as quickly as in normal animals, but their prolonged survival with some donor–host combinations suggested that an alternative mechanism of graft rejection involving complement is sometimes important.

It is of some interest that deficient animals will produce antibodies to the isologous components that are missing. Such antibodies constitute not only valuable reagents for further studies but also immunological proof of the absence of a component in the recipient.

Though not strictly germane to complement deficiencies, it is worth noting here that the hereditary condition of angioneurotic oedema has been associated with an absence of C 1-esterase inhibitor [40]. The C 1 esterase is also known to be associated with a capillary permeability factor; in the absence of normal serum inhibitor this mechanism may be overactive. Also the lysis of whole-blood clots probably involves complement. Platelets first adsorb IgM, followed by adsorption of at least the first four components of complement; enzymes associated with these components may participate in the activation of plasminogen with eventual lysis [41].

We might perhaps conclude by taking note of the fact that through the years following the discovery of complement and right up to modern times, it has occupied a curiously nebulous position with respect to *in vivo* reactivity. Only quite recently have we been able to assign rather general but quite definite roles to complement and its components—properties associated with phagocytosis and anaphylaxis, for instance. It is possible that a still wider role exists to be discovered in the field of cytotoxicity associated with the grafting of foreign tissues, as well as the lesions of auto-immune diseases.

REFERENCES

1. BORSOS, T., and RAPP, H. J. (1966), 'A New Complement Fixation Test: Enumeration of Antibodies at Cell Surfaces on a Molecular Basis', Complement Workshop, Abstracts, *Immunochemistry*, 3, 496.
2. BORDET, J., and GENGOU, O. (1901), 'Sur l'Existence de Substances sensibilisatrices dans la Plupart des Serums antimicrobiens', *Annls Inst. Pasteur, Paris*, 15, 289.
3. OSBORNE, T. W. B. (1937), in *Complement or Alexin*. London: Oxford University Press.
4. KABAT, E. A., and MAYER, M. M. (1961), *Experimental Immunochemistry*, 2nd ed. Springfield, Ill.: Thomas.
5. OSLER, A. G. (1961), 'Functions of the Complement System', *Adv. Immun.*, 1, 132.
6. LEPOW, I. H. (1965), 'Serum Complement and Properdin', in *Immunological Diseases* (ed. SAMTER, M.), p. 188. London: Churchill.
7. NELSON, R. A. (1965), 'The Role of Complement in Immune Phenomena', in *The Inflammatory Process* (ed. ZWEIFACH, B. W., GRANT, L., and McCLUSKEY, R. T.), p. 819. New York: Academic.
8. MÜLLER-EBERHARD, H. J. (1965), 'The Role of Antibody, Complement and other Humoral Factors in Host Resistance to Infections', in *Bacterial and Mycotic Infections of Man* (ed. DUBOS, R., and HIRSCH, J. G.), p. 181. London: Pitman.
9. NILSSON, U., and MÜLLER-EBERHARD, H. J. (1966), 'Requirement of C'3, C'5, C'6 and C'7 for the Formation of a Thermostable Intermediate Complex between Sheep Erythrocytes and Human Complement', Complement Workshop, Abstracts, *Immunochemistry*, 3, 500.
10. RAPP, H. J., SIMS, M. R., and BORSOS, T. (1959), 'Separation of Components of Guinea Pig Complement by Chromatography', *Proc. Soc. exp. Biol. Med.*, 100, 730.
11. MÜLLER-EBERHARD, H. J. (1966), 'Nomenclature of Complement', Complement Workshop, Abstracts, *Immunochemistry*, 3, 495.
12. KLEIN, P. (1965), discussion of 'Mechanism of Haemolysis', by MAYER, M. M., in *Complement* (ed. WOLSTENHOLME, G. E. W., and KNIGHT, JULIE), p. 36. Ciba Foundation Symposium. London: Churchill.
13. COOPER, N. R. (1967), 'Complement Associated Peptidase Activity of Guinea Pig Serum. II, Role of a Low Molecular Weight Enhancing Factor', *J. Immun.*, 98, 132.
14. LINSCOTT, W. D., and NISHIOKA, K. (1963), 'Components of Guinea Pig Complement. II, Separation of Serum Fraction Essential for Immune Haemolysis', *J. exp. Med.*, 118, 795.

15. INOUE, K., and NELSON, R. A. (1966), 'The Isolation and Characterization of a Ninth Component of Haemolytic Complement, C'3f', *J. Immun.*, **96**, 386.
16. NISHIOKA, K., and LINSCOTT, W. D. (1963), 'Components of Guinea Pig Complement. I, Separation of Serum Fraction Essential for Immune Haemolysis and Immune Adherence', *J. exp. Med.*, **118**, 767.
17. WEINRACH, R. S., and TALMAGE, D. W. (1958), 'The Role of Antibody in Immune Haemolysis', *J. infect. Dis.*, **102**, 74.
18. TALMAGE, D. W., FRETER, G. G., and TALIOFERRO, W. H. (1956), 'Two Antibodies of Related Specificity but Different Haemolytic Efficiency separated by Centrifugation', *J. infect. Dis.*, **98**, 300.
19. HUMPHREY, J. H., and DOURMASHKIN, R. R. (1965), 'Electron Microscope Studies of Immune Cell Lysis', in *Complement* (ed. WOLSTENHOLME, G. E. W., and KNIGHT, JULIE), p. 175. Ciba Foundation Symposium. London: Churchill.
20. ISHIZAKA, T., and ISHIZAKA, K. (1959), 'Biological Activities of Aggregated Gammaglobulin', *Proc. Soc. exp. Biol. Med.*, **101**, 845.
21. MOLLISON, P. L. (1965), 'The Role of Complement in Haemolytic Processes *in vivo*', in *Complement* (ed. WOLSTENHOLME, G. E. W., and KNIGHT, JULIE), p. 323. Ciba Foundation Symposium. London: Churchill.
22. WINN, H. J. (1965), 'Effects of Complement on Sensitised Nucleated Cells', in *Complement* (ed. WOLSTENHOLME, G. E. W., and KNIGHT, JULIE), p. 133. Ciba Foundation Symposium. London: Churchill.
23. TAMURA, N., and JENSEN, J. (1966), 'Purified Components of Guinea-pig Complement: Reaction of Erythrocytes with Antibody and the First Four Components', Complement Workshop, Abstracts, *Immunochemistry*, **3**, 504.
24. PFEIFFER, R., and ISSAEFF (1894), 'Über die spezifische Bedeutung der Choleraimmunität', *Z. Hyg. InfecktKrankh.*, **17**, 355.
25. MUSCHEL, L. H. (1965), 'Immune Bactericidal and Bacteriolytic Reactions', in *Complement* (ed. WOLSTENHOLME, G. E. W., and KNIGHT, JULIE), p. 155. Ciba Foundation Symposium. London: Churchill.
26. HARBOE, M. (1964), 'Interactions between [131]I Trace-labelled Cold Agglutinin, Complement and Red Cells', *Br. J. Haemat.*, **10**, 339.
27. GERLINGS-PETERSEN, B. T., and PONDMAN, K. W. (1964), 'Fonction de l'Anticorps et du Complément dans la Phagocytose', *Nouv. Rev. Franc. Hémat.*, **4**, 593.
28. FISCHER, H., and HAUPT, J. (1961), 'Das cytolysierende Prinzip von Serum Komplement', *Z. Naturf.*, **166**, 321.
29. FISCHER, H., ARGENTON, H., and FRITZCHE, W. (1961), 'Nichtimmunologische hämolytische Serum-Faktoren in der menschlichen Pathologie', *VII. Freiburger Symposium über Hämolyse und hämolytische Erkrankungen*. Berlin: Springer.
30. WARD, P. A. (1967), 'A Plasmin-split Fragment of C'3 as a New Chemotactic Factor', *J. exp. Med.*, **126**, 189.
31. WARD, P. A., COCHRANE, C. G., and MÜLLER-EBERHARD, H. J. (1966), 'Further Studies on the Chemotactic Factor of Complement and its Formation *in vitro*', *Immunology*, **11**, 141.
32. DA SILVA, W. D., and LEPOW, I. H. (1967), 'Complement as a Mediator of Inflammation. II, Biological Properties of Anaphylatoxin prepared with Purified Components of Human Complement', *J. exp. Med.*, **125**, 921.
33. JENSEN, J. (1966), 'Formation of Anaphylatoxin', Complement Workshop, Abstracts, *Immunochemistry*, **3**, 498.
34. PENSKY, J., HINZ, C. F., TODD, E. W., WEDGWOOD, R. J., BOYER, J. T., and LEPOW, I. H. (1968), 'Properties of Highly Purified Human Properdin', *J. Immun.*, **100**, 142.
35. LACHMANN, P. J. (1967), 'Conglutinin and Immunoconglutinins', *Adv. Immun.*, **7**, 479.
36. LEON, M. A., YOKOYARI, R., and ITOH, C. (1966), 'Chemical Specificity in the Conglutininin System and its Relation to Complement Structure', Complement Workshop, Abstracts, *Immunochemistry*, **3**, 499.
37. GEWÜRZ, H., PICKERING, R. J., MUSCHEL, L. H., MERGENHAGEN, S. E., and GOOD, R. A. (1966), 'Complement-dependent Biological Functions in Complement Deficiency in Man', *Lancet*, **2**, 356.
38. NILSSON, U. R., and MÜLLER-EBERHARD, H. J. (1967), 'Deficiency of the Fifth Component of Complement in Mice with an Inherited Complement Defect', *J. exp. Med.*, **125**, 1.

39. ROTHER, U., BALLANTYNE, D. L., jun., COHEN, C., and ROTHER, K. (1967), 'Allograft Rejection in C′6 Defective Rabbits', *J. exp. Med.*, **126**, 565.
40. DONALDSON, V. H., and EVANS, R. R. (1963), 'A Biochemical Abnormality in Hereditary Angioneurotic Oedema: Absence of Serum Inhibitor of C′1-esterase', *Am. J. Med.*, **35**, 37.
41. TAYLOR, F. B., and MÜLLER-EBERHARD, H. J. (1967), 'Factors influencing Lysis of Whole Blood Clots', *Nature, Lond.*, **216**, 1023.

CHAPTER 6

ANTIGEN ANTIBODY REACTIONS

By E. R. Gold and D. B. Peacock

I. Introduction

II. Mechanisms of reaction
   A. Forces involved
      1. Role of van der Waals's forces
      2. Role of electrostatic forces
      3. Hydration
      4. General considerations
   B. Thermodynamics and kinetics
      1. Introduction
      2. Application of thermodynamics
      3. Kinetics
      4. Detection and use of primary reactions

III. Secondary reactions
   A. Precipitation
      1. Equivalence zone
      2. Quantitative measurements
   B. Theories of precipitation
   C. Immunodiffusion and immuno-electrophoresis
   D. Agglutination
      1. Prozone phenomena
      2. Enzyme-treated red cells
      3. Antiglobulin test
   E. Passive agglutination
      Chemical supports
   F. Passive haemagglutination
      1. With unmodified red cells
      2. With modified red cells
         a. Chemical modification
         b. Chemical bonding
         c. General considerations
   G. Theories of agglutination

IV. Antigen–antibody reactions involving complement
   A. Complement-fixation test
   B. Complement-fixation inhibition test

I. Introduction

In preceding chapters we have discussed antigen, antibody, complement, and the events leading up to antibody production. In this and succeeding chapters we shall be dealing with the union between antigen and antibody and events that follow this union. A distinction into primary and secondary antigen–antibody reactions is in fact a convenient means of classification, providing that it is understood that under 'secondary reactions' are included all those reactions that consist of one or more steps beyond primary union. Complement fixation is an example of the complexity of events that may follow primary union, and at least nine separate reactions are involved, as we have already seen. The development of immediate hypersensitivity reactions is another example of a complex chain of events succeeding the initial reaction. Agglutination and precipitation are perhaps truly secondary reactions, though even they are complicated enough when considered at a fundamental level, as we shall see.

There are areas where even such a simple classification as this fails to separate events adequately. For instance, if an antibody reacts with an immunoglobulin that has already combined with homologous antigen, such a reaction might more properly be termed a 'second-stage primary reaction'. It is a situation that might obtain in certain auto-immune diseases.

II. Mechanisms of Reaction

A. Forces Involved

In the past immunologists have frequently stressed the high degree of specificity seen in immunological reactions. It is our opinion that this aspect has been overemphasized and that a similar specificity is exhibited in many biological processes at the molecular level.

However, our main concern now is what forces are active and how they are arranged in order that specificity may be achieved. In this respect we must count ourselves fortunate that the past two decades have seen the rapid development of physicochemical methods suitable for investigating these detailed biological problems. Physicochemical bonds may be regarded as either weak or strong according to the amount of energy that is involved in their formation. Pauling [1] gives a value of 10 kcal. per mole as forming a useful boundary line between bond strengths. Stronger bonds, such as the covalent bond, are not easily disrupted under physiological conditions and the ready reversibility of many biological reactions is due to the operation of weaker bonds. Those of particular importance in biology are listed in *Table XX* [2] and compared with the covalent bond.

Table XX.—Bonds of Importance in Biology [2]

Bond Types	Usual Bond Strengths (kcal.)
Van der Waals's bond	0·5
Ionic bond	5
Hydrogen bond	2–5
Reinforced ionic bond	10
Covalent bond	40–140

Perhaps the most general force of intermolecular attraction is van der Waals's force. It is the result of the motion of electrons in a molecule causing a momentary electric field that polarizes any other molecule in the neighbourhood. The instantaneous change in electric field in the first molecule induces an attractive force between the two which in practice is inversely proportional to the sixth power of the interatomic distance. Besides being weak, these forces are active over a very short range and are the first clear indication of the necessity for a close 'fit' between antigen and antibody.

The ionic bond, e.g., between sodium and chloride ions, is also a weak bond in media of high dielectric constant such as water or physiological saline. Coulomb forces of attraction also operate between charged (polar) groups and vary with the sixth power of the distance between them like van der Waals's force.

The third type of force is the hydrogen bond, with a significance possibly equal to that of van der Waals's force. The strength of the hydrogen bond depends on the atoms between which it forms a link. Oxygen and nitrogen are among the most electronegative of all atoms and form the strongest hydrogen bonds, of around 5 kcal. per mole. The hydrogen bond has strict stereochemical limitations; thus the atom attracted by a hydroxyl group, for instance, must come to lie in line with the axis of the hydroxyl group and within a fairly narrowly defined distance from the oxygen atom in order that a stable bond may be formed. Because of this hydrogen bonds have a greater influence on the steric configuration of polypeptide chains than, for instance, van der Waals's force.

The advantage of postulating that weak interatomic forces are involved in the union of antibody with antigen is that in order to explain the relative stability of the union we must accept (1) that several bonds are formed between each pair of molecules; (2) that the formation of several bonds in each case allows us to explain specificity on the basis of complementarity between antigen and antibody; and (3) that the relative ease with which antigen–antibody union can be disrupted by thermal agitation is consistent with this type of bond formation.

In previous chapters we have repeatedly stressed the importance of closeness of fit in antigen–antibody reactions. It now appears that this not only confers specificity on union, but looked at from the opposite point of view that it is necessary for the formation of stable complexes. It should, however, be recognized that the 'fit' need not necessarily be exact and, indeed, the theory of 'subcomplementarity' explicitly states this [3]. The evidence for such a viewpoint is that configurational changes have been observed in antibody after its union with antigen; presumably caused by mutual adaptation resulting from a less than perfect fit. 'Immunological denaturation' is also a well-recognized phenomenon in which structural alteration of the antibody molecule is the accepted explanation. An obvious parallel, too, lies in the flexibility of structure in the reaction between enzyme and substrate.

1. ROLE OF VAN DER WAALS'S FORCES

The importance of van der Waals's forces in the union of antibody with antigen lies in the spheres of both specificity and affinity. The strength of the attraction between two molecules will depend on how closely they can approach each other and over what surface area. Similarly, the specificity of the reaction will depend on the extent to which the complexity of the determinant pattern is mirrored in the antideterminant.

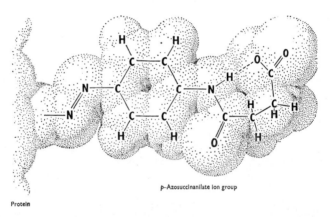

p-Azosuccinanilate ion group

Protein

Fig. 39.—The structure of the haptenic group of an azoprotein, ovalbumin-*p*-azosuccinanilate ion. *Figs*. 39, 40 *by kind permission of 'Endeavour'*.

By drawing the outermost electron orbits of the constituent atoms of a molecule a contour line representative of the van der Waals outline can be obtained (*Fig*. 39) [4]. Shown as a protuberance, there seem to be fairly good grounds for thinking that determinants fit into invaginations in the antibody molecule—a relationship shown in *Fig*. 40 [4], where apart from the van der Waals forces implied by the close fit, a hydrogen bond and an ionic bond also contribute to the reaction.

Such drawings are not entirely speculative and Pressman has investigated the binding energies involved in the combination of antibody with haptens under conditions where the goodness of fit is varied by introducing substituents into the structure of haptens [5].

With the introduction of any substituent that alters the van der Waals outline a lowering of binding energy may be recorded, but with the hapten *m*(*p*-hydroxybenzeneazo)-benzoate a disproportionately large reduction in the combining constant results when chlorine is substituted in either of the two positions adjacent to the carboxyl group (*Fig.* 41) [5], possibly because the carboxyl group is tilted out of the plane of the ring and hinders union. As might be expected the effect of increasing the size of a substituent group in a particular position is to increase the steric hindrance, and though the effect on the binding energy is often proportional to the size of

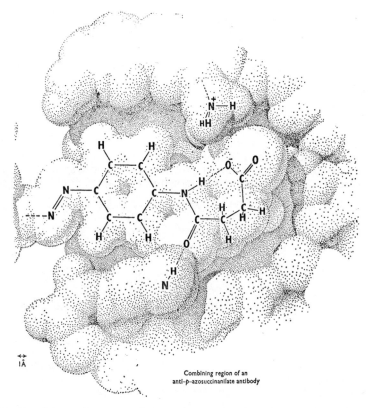

Combining region of an
anti-p-azosuccinanilate antibody

Fig. 40.—A haptenic group and a complementary region of its specific antibody.

the introduced group, in some cases, e.g., iodine for bromine, the larger group or atom actually increases the combining constant [6], presumably because other parts of the reacting surfaces are forced closer together in order to accommodate the larger group, leading to an increase in van der Waals's forces of attraction. Obviously this type of manipulation cannot be taken too far and Pressman has shown that antibody to a benzene-arsonate hapten fails to react at all with a hapten in which the arsonate group is separated from the benzene ring by a methyl group (*Fig.* 42) [5]. There is just one position where substituents can be introduced into the ring structure of haptens without altering their capacity to combine with homologous antibody, and this, of course, is where the diazo bond is formed in order to link hapten to carrier protein (*Fig.* 42).

In investigating problems of closeness of fit, the heterogeneity of the antibody response must always be borne in mind. In Chapter 2 we saw

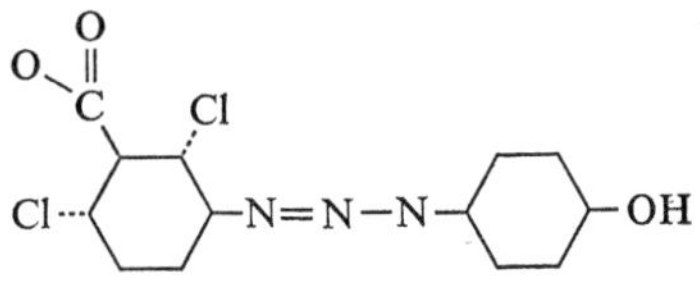

Fig. 41.—Effect of structural alterations on specificity. Substitution by chlorine in the positions indicated strongly affects the combining power between antiserum and hapten [*m*(*p*-hydroxybenzeneazo)-benzoate].

how immunologists have attempted to explain the various specificities detected by antisera by invoking the concept of partial antigens in some cases and different facets of a single sequence of sugars in others. Pressman has also considered the possibility that the orientation of a hapten with respect to the surface of a carrier protein may influence specificity [5]. In the case of a double benzene ring structure the hapten could be: (1) with

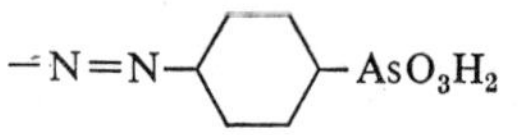

Hapten benzene-arsonate.

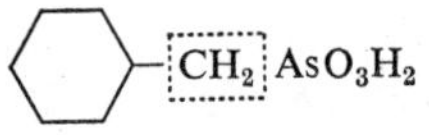

Antiserum to benzene-arsonate hapten gives no reaction with this hapten.

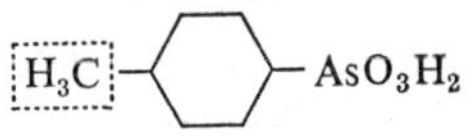

Substitution with a methyl group in the position occupied by the diazo in the conjugated hapten has no effect on the serological specificity of the benzene-arsonate hapten.

Fig. 42.—Effect of structural alterations on specificity.

the axis joining the rings vertical, in which case the antideterminant would have the form of a long invagination; (2) with the axis and the plane of the rings parallel to the surface, in which case the face of the ring structure would form the determinant; and (3) with the axis parallel and the plane of the rings vertical, in which case the antideterminant would have the form of a trench.

2. ROLE OF ELECTROSTATIC FORCES

Widely differing opinions have often been expressed about the influence of charged groups on antigen–antibody union. Boyd has taken the view [7] that experiments conducted by Singer [8] removed 'the role of Coulomb forces in holding antibody and antigen together . . . from the realms of pure hypothesis', and Hughes-Jones [9] that 'attempts to demonstrate the presence of any of these forces in antigen–antibody reactions have not been successful'. Pressman [6] has summed up the evidence in favour of the involvement of charged groups and we feel that the weight of evidence lies on his side; in spite of the fact that his earlier work and that of Singer quoted above could be criticized on the grounds that alterations in the pH of medium might have an effect on the antibody molecule as a whole, and thereby a secondary effect on the combining site. He describes the use of two haptens which differ only in that the nitrogen of one replaces the carbon of another and that the ammonium compound carries a positive charge (*Fig.* 43). Although the two haptens have virtually the same size and configuration, nevertheless their combining constants with antibody differed by a factor of ten.

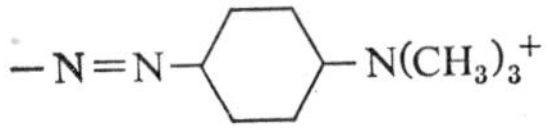

$$-N=N-\hexagon-N(CH_3)_3^+$$

p-azobenzene-trimethylammonium ion

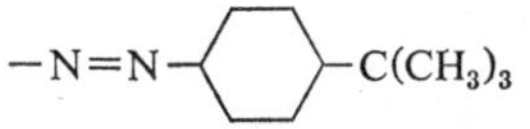

$$-N=N-\hexagon-C(CH_3)_3$$

p-azo-tertiary-butylbenzene

Fig. 43.—Similar haptens differing mainly in the charge they carry [6].

The argument is further strengthened, but perhaps not finally clinched even yet, by studies in which the combining sites of antibodies are protected during chemical treatment [6]. Protection is effected by combining antibody with its specific hapten during chemical treatment. After sufficient time has elapsed for the destruction of unprotected antibody, the hapten is eluted and the antibody shown to be still capable of reacting normally with homologous antigen. The theoretical implications of this work are already having practical applications. If one accepts that ionized groups are potentially important for antigen–antibody interaction then their action should be partly neutralized by ions in the surrounding medium. That this is so can be shown simply by carrying out the initial stages of a serological reaction in a medium of low ionic strength.

3. HYDRATION

In spite of what has been said previously not all antigenic determinants carry charged groups and not all antigen–antibody primary reactions are enhanced by lowering the ionic strength of the medium, for instance in the case of ABH and Lewis blood-group systems. Under these circumstances hydrogen bonds and van der Waals's forces must be operating and though they may not be interfered with by free ions they are still affected by the water molecules themselves. In the case of van der Waals's forces water has to be displaced from the interacting surfaces in order that they may come into sufficiently close proximity for these short-range forces to be effective. In the case of hydrogen bonds, water–solute bonds first have to be broken in order that solute–solute bonds may be formed.

Pressman indicates that the effect of hydration on combining power can be seen when the reactions of benzoate- and pyridine-derived haptens with antisera to the former are compared [5]. The combining power of the reaction would suggest that the nitrogen of pyridine is larger, not smaller, than the corresponding $=$CH— of benzene and Pressman attributes this to hydration of the nitrogen in aqueous solution.

4. GENERAL CONSIDERATIONS

It is now evident that specificity is achieved through the effect of several weak forces acting in concert and spread over a sufficiently large area so that the overall pattern of forces may present a unique arrangement. Though

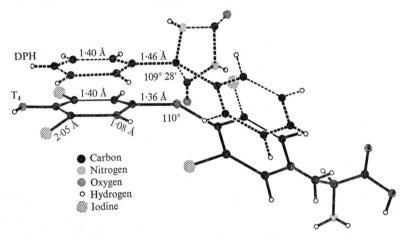

Fig. 44.—Three-dimensional representation of the proposed steric analogy between L-thyroxine (T_4) and 5,5-diphenylhydantoin (DPH). *By kind permission of the 'Journal of Clinical Investigation'* [11].

specificity is unique the mechanism by which it is achieved is not, and over twenty years ago Pauling was stressing the wide range of physiological, and indeed biological, reactions that exhibit a similar degree of specificity. A few examples will serve to illustrate the point.

A high degree of specificity is apparent in those drugs that act by blocking enzymes and can be classed as metabolite analogues. Albert has considered the action of such drugs in exactly the same terms that Pauling applied to serological reactions; first came considerations of steric configuration, then the assumption that van der Waals's and other weak forces operated between substrate and enzyme and that a drug substituted for the substrate [2]. In the field of enzymology itself the specificity and complementarity of active centres and substrates are seen over and over again. As an example we can take the operation of ionic and hydrogen bonds in the union of cholinesterase and its substrate.

Among the hormones we find that thyroxine can be displaced from thyroxine-binding alpha-globulin by all analogues of hydantoin which contain a particular diphenyl configuration [10]. In *Fig.* 44 is depicted the very close similarity of configuration in these seemingly rather different molecules. The same general conclusions regarding complementarity can be drawn from the difference in pressor activity between L- and D-adrenaline. The former is much more active and is said to make contact with the receptor at three points as against two points in the case of D-adrenaline.

Specific protein receptors with complementary configurations for pharmacologically active substances such as epinephrine, acetylcholine, and histamine are assumed by Bovet [11], and the same mechanisms are now being invoked to explain the sense of smell.

Looked at from another point of view, it might be asked: If so many biological reactions are specific by virtue of complementarity, what is the distinguishing feature of the immune response? The answer seems to lie only in the capacity of an antigen to call forth a response directed specifically towards itself. However, if one accepts that selection operates at some stage in antibody production, then the distinction reaches vanishing point, since in that case complementary sites for antigen would be supposed to exist in the host before stimulation, and changes leading to antibody production would be quantitative rather than qualitative.

In recent times biologists have been turning more and more to a consideration of events occurring at molecular and submolecular levels. As Szent-Györgi has put it, 'It is physics in the last instance which has to explain biological reactions' [12]. Achievements in these fields have already been striking. The concept of biochemical evolution preceding biological evolution, with laws similar to those postulated by Darwin, has been evolved; mutational events have been correlated with modifications of nucleic acid structure; diseases due to errors of inborn metabolism have been explained in biochemical terms; and pathological haemoglobins have been shown to produce 'molecular' diseases. Should it be possible some time in the future to rationalize biology completely, then the teleological explanations that are employed currently in order to explain immunological phenomena will no longer be necessary. Perhaps also cellular biophysics in the twenty-first century will be as complete as the magnificent edifice of quantum mechanics, as Setlow and Pollard [13] so enthusiastically foresee.

Studies of this sort have necessitated the use of experimental methods more akin to the physical sciences than to biology. At the same time the older qualitative methods have been replaced by newer quantitative ones, in some cases possessing the rigorous precision of those used in analytical chemistry. For further information on these subjects the reader is referred to textbooks of immunochemistry and experimental immunology [14, 15, 16].

B. Thermodynamics and Kinetics

1. INTRODUCTION

The physicochemical changes resulting from interaction between antibody and antigen can be interpreted kinetically and thermodynamically.

Studies of this kind have led to estimations being made of the bond strengths involved, and indirectly to a knowledge of the types of bonds formed.

It is beyond the scope of this book to deal with the fundamental aspects of these procedures, particularly with respect to thermodynamics, but the interested reader will find that a number of useful short accounts have been published recently [7, 1719]. For more detailed treatments textbooks of physical chemistry or more specialized books should be consulted.

For present purposes all that we need to do is to be able to recognize certain symbols and to understand something of what they mean. The first of these is the equilibrium constant (k), derived from the relationship between the concentrations of reactants and their product. Since antigen–antibody reactions are thought to be reversible bimolecular reactions we can consider them in these terms. A simple reversible reaction is represented by

$$A+B \rightleftharpoons C.$$

According to the law of mass action the speed at which a chemical reaction proceeds is proportional to the concentrations of the reacting substances, A and B, and their product C. The rate of the forward reaction is given by

$$v_1 = k_1[A].[B]$$

and of the reverse reaction by

$$v_2 = k_2[C],$$

where v_1 and v_2 are the rates of the forward and reverse reactions respectively and k_1 and k_2 are the respective specific rate constants. The state of equilibrium is expressed as

$$k_1.[A].[B] = v_1 = v_2 = k_2.[C]$$

or

$$\frac{[C]}{[A].[B]} = \frac{k_1}{k_2} = K.$$

K is the equilibrium constant of the reaction. It not only indicates how far to the right the reaction will proceed, i.e., defines how much of the product is formed, but from it may be derived information about the thermodynamics of the system.

The thermodynamic expression with which we are most concerned is the free energy (F) of a system. The Gibbs free energy, at constant pressure, is now usually denoted by G. It is related to total heat or enthalpy (H) and entropy (S) by the expression

$$G = H - TS,$$

where T is the absolute temperature. 'Free energy', 'enthalpy', and 'entropy' are all closely defined terms subject to strict limitations and it is not possible to explain their meaning exactly in a few sentences.

It is perhaps sufficient to remark that in the case of an antigen–antibody reaction, where two molecules combine, the change in free energy, ΔG, places a figure on the amount of energy by which the compound is more stable than the two isolated molecules. This quantity is sometimes called the 'affinity' of the reaction and is closely related to the strength of the bond formed between antibody and antigen. It is evident that this figure is most easily arrived at in the case of simple systems, e.g., univalent hapten and divalent antibody. The change in free energy at the standard concentration of 1 mole per litre is related to the equilibrium constant by the following expression

$$\Delta G^0 = -RT \log_e K$$

where R is the gas constant. In addition a value for ΔG^0 can be derived in the case of antigen–antibody reactions under conditions other than standard where the concentrations of reactants and products at equilibrium can be determined. Unfortunately, values are still often assigned to ΔG^0 when standard conditions do not apply.

2. APPLICATION OF THERMODYNAMICS

Thermodynamic data can, of course, be obtained by direct calorimetry and early attempts to obtain such data on antigen–antibody reactions employed this method. The results were rather variable and recent studies have mostly had the determination of K as their starting point, rather than of changes in enthalpy. As predicted by the proponents of template theories of antibody formation, the bond strengths involved in antibody–antigen interactions were low, and of the same order as those postulated between template and antibody.

Techniques have had to be adapted or devised for the determination of K. Some of them, e.g., equilibrium dialysis, are applicable only to systems using univalent haptens. In this case one of the reactants must be dialysable so that its concentration at equilibrium can be found. For protein antigens methods such as electrophoresis and ultracentrifugation have to be used to separate reactants, and in these cases the multivalence of the antigen has to be taken into account when determining the strength of single bonds.

Even so, unexpected results are not uncommon, and Epstein, Doty, and Boyd [20] have been forced to assume an unfavourable orientation of hapten on carrier protein in order to explain the larger energy changes observed when antibody combined with hapten compared with whole conjugate protein. On occasion, too, the union of antigen and antibody has been associated with negative values for entropy that would suggest an increase rather than decrease in the disorder of the system. It is possible that water molecules are released in the course of antigen–antibody union and that this does result in an increase in randomness of the system as a whole. Rather less likely is the explanation that union results in changes in tertiary structure of the antibody so as to allow a greater degree of freedom in the internal movements of the molecule.

In general the collection of thermodynamic data has confirmed the view that the fit between determinant and antideterminant is extremely close. For instance, the value for ΔG^0 in the reaction between lactose hapten and homologous antibody is $-5 \cdot 52$ kcal. per mole, but only $-1 \cdot 96$ kcal. per mole for cellobiose reacting with the same antibody, although the only difference between the two molecules is in the arrangement of atoms around carbon 4 of the terminal hexose. The alteration of van der Waals's outline by substitution has also been shown to affect the energy changes involved in union [21]. If iodine is introduced into a benzoate hapten in the ortho position to the antigenically strong carboxyl group, it reduces combining energy considerably more than if it is introduced in the meta position.

3. KINETICS

Apart from determining equilibrium constants, kinetics can also be used to study the union of antibody and antigen. Primary union between antigen and antibody can be very rapid, taking only a few milliseconds. Conventional chemical methods are unsuitable for studying such reactions in isolation since they are applicable only down to half-reaction times of 1 second. Also too slow are the more refined cathode-ray polarography [22] and 'stopped-flow' [23] techniques. In order to allow more precise measurements to be made, relaxation methods have been adapted to the study of hapten–antibody reactions.

Relaxation methods are based on the principle that reactants are first allowed to reach a state of equilibrium, which state is then disturbed rapidly and the establishment of a new equilibrium is registered. Equilibria can be disturbed in a number of ways, e.g., by changing the temperature, pressure, and electrical field strength. Eigen has used alterations of temperature [see 24] effected by the electrical discharge from a condenser, the establishment of new equilibria being registered spectrometrically.

Such methods can be used for determining association constants of antigen–antibody reactions. Theoretically the upper limiting value for the association constant in a diffusion-controlled reaction is a little over 10^9 per mole per second. Experimentally, a much lower figure of 2×10^7 has been obtained; it must, however, be taken into account that not all collisions in an antigen–antibody reaction will be fruitful so that diffusional separation can also occur. This may be the result of an unsuitable reciprocal orientation, and it must be remembered that an antideterminant probably occupies no more than 1 per cent of the surface area of an antibody molecule, so that every collision could not be expected to give rise to union.

Still lower association constants have been found in a system using human red-cell antigens [25]. In these experiments the authors took advantage of the fact that very high dilutions of the reactants could be used to slow down the reaction time, thereby avoiding the necessity for special methods of measurement. It was noticeable in this investigation that association and dissociation constants were heterogeneous due to heterogeneity of affinity—and not only with respect to different antisera, but also with respect to the antibodies of one antiserum. Nowadays, we would confidently expect to be able to relate some of these differences to the different classes of immunoglobulins.

4. DETECTION AND USE OF PRIMARY REACTIONS

· Some examples of methods which detect primary reactions have already been given in the section on kinetics. In principle any change in the physical or chemical properties of antigen or antibody, resulting from their union, can be used to signal that the reaction has taken place. However, we are not only interested in thermodynamic and kinetic data, but also in such things as the orientation and deformation of the molecules taking part; and whereas the older immunologists had to rely exclusively on secondary reactions such as agglutination, precipitation, and complement fixation, we are now able to detect primary union in a variety of ways.

Both physical and chemical methods can be used for detecting primary union provided that free and bound antigen can be neatly separated and that the antigen can be clearly distinguished from antibody. A number of methods is available for the separation of free and bound antigen; methods such as centrifugation, electrophoresis, filtration, and dialysis. The distinction between antigen and antibody is sometimes much harder to make and in immunochemistry use has often been made of purified polysaccharide antigens for this reason. We are fortunate, too, in that some antigens possess built-in markers in the form of characteristic colour or of readily identifiable elements, such as the heavy metals present in a variety of respiratory pigments. In rather similar vein enzymes and toxins can be used as biological markers, their neutralization signifying the attachment of antibody. It will be appreciated that a number of these methods can be used equally well for the detection of secondary reactions, but this in no way invalidates their use in primary reactions.

Since built-in markers are somewhat rare, artificial ones have been developed. They can be used to label either antigen or antibody, or both. Perhaps the most versatile form of marker is the radioactive isotope. It can be introduced in the form of radioactive iodine by the relatively simple procedure of iodination. Otherwise, for instance in the case of ^{35}S, a compound containing the isotope can be coupled to proteins by the recognized procedure of diazotization. Such labelling permits the ready estimation of free and bound antigen. For instance, in the immuno-assay of a hormone a standard amount of radioactive hormone is reacted with a standard antiserum. The ratio of free to bound antigen is then measured before and after the addition of the sample under test. Comparison with a calibration curve will indicate the concentration of hormone in the sample with considerable accuracy, amounts as little as $0.15 \mu g.$ per ml. being detected quite easily.

Another widely used method is the labelling of antibody with fluorescent dyes, so enabling antigen–antibody complexes to be seen with the aid of a light microscope. Ideally monochromatic light of the appropriate wavelength would be used to excite the dye and a barrier filter placed above the specimen would cut out wavelengths other than those arising from excitation of the dye. Unfortunately, such ideals are not attainable, but the method has achieved wide popularity because of its versatility. For instance, antigen can be detected in situ in tissue sections by labelled antibody, and vice versa. Antigen–antibody complexes can be detected by labelled anti-globulin, itself a most versatile application since one labelled antihuman serum will detect a whole range of reactions in which human immunoglobulin takes part. Similarly labelled antibody against complement can be used both to detect complement and, indirectly, to detect antigen–antibody complexes. Though it might be objected that we are dealing here with a number of secondary reactions, in each case we are ultimately dealing with the union between labelled antibody and its homologous antigen.

For further details of technique and practical applications of immunofluorescence the reader is referred to the monograph by Goldman [26].

A third type of substance used for labelling antigens and antibodies is ferritin, a protein obtainable from horse spleen and containing sufficient iron to render it electron-dense. Ferritin is also an antigen in its own right and has been used to detect antibody inside the endoplasmic reticulum of plasma cells.

Finally, a method already mentioned in connexion with the kinetics of antigen–antibody reactions is equilibrium dialysis [27]. The method requires the use of a dialysable hapten. Purified antibody solution is dialysed against the hapten. After a time a stage is reached at which the hapten is present in equal concentration on both sides of the membrane. Within the membrane the free hapten is also in equilibrium with hapten bound to antibody, and measurement of the concentration of hapten outside the membrane will tell us indirectly the relationship between free and bound hapten. The concentration of free hapten can be measured in a number of ways indicated above or by absorption-spectrometry.

III. Secondary Reactions

The words 'flocculation', 'agglutination', and 'precipitation' are often used indiscriminately in the literature of serology, so it is as well to begin by defining their meanings.

The derivation of 'flocculation' is the same as 'flake' and 'flock', and can therefore be properly defined as the formation of a loose aggregate. It is sometimes used in the sense of aggregates that fail to sediment, but more often, and correctly, as the formation of a loose, fluffy precipitate that is easily disturbed on shaking.

'Precipitation' means a 'throwing down', and has been used in this sense in chemistry to indicate a solid sediment formed in a liquid reaction mixture. It is used with the same meaning in serology to describe antigen–antibody aggregates that ultimately sediment under the force of gravity. 'Precipitation' is thus a general term that describes a certain type of visible reaction which follows the union of antigen and antibody; whereas 'flocculation' tells us something about the appearance of such a precipitate.

It might be thought that the distinction between agglutination and precipitation would be quite easy to draw, but it is in the area between frank agglutination of *cells* and precipitation of *soluble antigens* that the difficulties lie. There is an infinite gradation of size from cells, down through viruses to macro-molecules and beyond. We will speak of agglutination in connexion with the aggregation of mammalian, bacterial, and other cells, and of cells to which antigens have been artificially attached and of other non-cellular but insoluble supports, to which antigen has also been attached. The distinction between agglutination and precipitation may be more than a semantic and descriptive one. We shall, in fact, deal with the theories of precipitation and agglutination separately, because the detailed mechanisms leading to these phenomena may themselves differ in spite of the fact that interpretation in terms of electrostatic forces of attraction and repulsion are currently fashionable.

A. Precipitation

Because it is necessary only to mix two reagents together in order to observe them, precipitation and agglutination were the first serological reactions to be described. Both of them must be clearly distinguished from non-immunological (non-specific) aggregation even though they are ultimately physicochemical processes. The serological reaction is, of course, initiated by the immunologically specific union between antibody and its homologous antigen.

At first precipitin reactions were used in a purely qualitative way, but with time it came to be recognized that quantitative information was also available, and in 1926 Dean and Webb [28] described a method that allowed comparisons of potency to be made between different batches of antiserum. By their method constant amounts of antiserum were added to varying dilutions of antigen. The mixture showing most rapid precipitation under standard conditions was regarded as containing the reactant in optimal proportions. Within limits, sometimes quite wide, the same ratio of antigen to antibody at other antibody concentrations will still give most rapid precipitation. We can obtain, therefore, an optimal proportions ratio that is used to compare the potency of antitoxic sera *in vitro*. Differences in potency of 20 per cent or so can be recognized.

The Dean and Webb titration gives us a constant antibody optimal proportions ratio. Obviously, the titration can also be performed using a constant amount of antigen and varying the quantities of antiserum. This is the so-called 'Ramon' type of titration, and gives us a constant antigen optimal proportions ratio. It is widely used in estimating the antitoxic contents of horse antisera. Because of the different conditions in the two titrations, the values obtained for the ratios also differ—by up to 30 per cent in horse antitoxin–toxin titrations, though in other cases by much more. Such differences are more marked in some sera than in others. They result from the fact that at higher dilutions of antigen concentrations of serum above that required for optimal precipitation fail to accelerate and even slow down the rate of precipitation. The reason for this remains obscure, but is presumably connected with the relative concentrations of the various kinds of antibody that are normally produced in response to antigenic stimulation. It is of interest that in this respect rabbit and horse antisera classically behave so differently (*see below*).

1. EQUIVALENCE ZONE

In the precipitin reaction the zone of equivalence is that region where the relative proportions of antigen and antibody are such that neither remains free in solution. In practice it is taken to be the zone where no antigen, and little or no antibody, can be detected. Normally it overlaps the region of optimal proportions, but coincidence is not necessarily exact. Occasionally a little antigen is found in the zone too, and zone width varies considerably from system to system, probably depending on the choice of antigen and the method selected for immunization. Most of these qualifying remarks could be explained on the basis of reactions occurring between heterogeneous antigen and antibody populations.

On either side of equivalence lie the regions of antigen and antibody excess. Both these regions are characterized by incomplete precipitation. Antisera can be divided into two broad categories depending on their behaviour in these regions. Rabbit (R type) antisera form relatively insoluble complexes in both regions and particularly in the region of antibody excess. Horse (H type) antisera tend to have narrow zones of precipitation and to form soluble complexes in the region of antibody, as well as of antigen, excess. Furthermore, the speed of precipitation with R-type antisera tends to be uniform throughout the whole region of antibody excess so that with most such sera there is no single optimal proportions ratio in the presence of a constant amount of antigen. H sera, on the other hand, possess well-defined ratios with both constant antigen and constant antibody methods. Not all horse sera belong to the H type: antitoxic and antiprotein sera do, whereas antipolysaccharide sera do not. It is very well known that horse antisera to polysaccharide antigens are of high molecular weight (about 1 million), so it is tempting to speculate that the relative proportions of IgG to IgM antibodies determine whether an antiserum belongs to the H or R type.

The behaviour of antisera from other species of animals varies widely; for instance, it is difficult and sometimes impossible to get antiserum from guinea-pigs to precipitate or agglutinate, although it may actively neutralize.

2. QUANTITATIVE MEASUREMENTS

Macroscopic precipitation is usually preceded by a period in which there is a detectable opalescence. Quantitative estimates of the amount of precipitate can be made by examining the light-scattering properties of such mixtures in a nephelometer. Similar rather inexact estimates can be made by measuring the volume of a precipitate. Truly quantitative measurements can be effected chemically, for instance, by measuring the amount of antibody nitrogen in a precipitate [15]. Care has to be taken with washing precipitates which are normally formed in solutions containing extraneous protein that may be physically trapped, and in the case of protein antigens means have to be found of estimating the antigen nitrogen in the precipitate separately. It might be supposed, for instance, that in the zone of equivalence, or in antibody excess, all the antigen would be present in the precipitate, and while this is often so, the presence of a non-precipitating moiety of antibody in the antiserum would render the assumption quite invalid.

B. Theories of Precipitation

From the earliest days of immunology attempts have been made to explain the mechanism of precipitation and to extend these explanations to cover the whole field of antigen–antibody reactions. Omitting Ehrlich's purely speculative approach, Bordet was the first to propound a satisfactory theory [29] based on experimental evidence. He postulated a two-stage theory in which the first stage was specific union between antigen and antibody. The second stage, of precipitation, he considered was brought about non-specifically by the action of electrolytes and lipids.

In its time the theory was widely accepted. It was not until 1934 that Marrack produced the first serious contender in the form of the 'lattice' or 'framework' theory [30], which has stood the test of time and is still adequate to explain many of the observations associated with serological reactions. According to this hypothesis, precipitation is caused by the formation of a network of antigen and antibody molecules held together by specific interaction of their combining sites. Marrack also accepted the possibility that other forces could be involved in the formation of precipitates, at least under certain circumstances.

Goldberg examined the concept of the lattice theory mathematically [31] in a manner that was thought to explain many, if not all, of the quantitative aspects of the precipitin reaction. Starting from basic physicochemical principles and assuming that the most probable complexes are actually formed, he worked out the theoretical distribution of complexes of various size and composition, enabling predictions to be made about the quantitative course of the precipitin reaction. Goldberg made a number of other simplifications in order to reduce the problem to manageable proportions, for which he has been severely criticized. Chief among these, perhaps, are the assumptions of a homogeneity of combining sites and therefore of bonds between individual antigen and antibody molecules irrespective of the size of the aggregates formed, and of an absence of cyclical structures in the aggregates.

A lucid and more detailed account of the main lines of thought embodied in this examination, but without details of the mathematical treatment, is to be found elsewhere [18].

The theory predicts that in the region of heavy antigen excess complexes of the composition Ag_2Ab will be formed; with heavy antibody excess $AgAb_n$ complexes will be formed, where n is the valency of the antigen. Singer et al. have examined the behaviour of antigen–antibody complexes in the region of antigen excess by ultracentrifugation and electrophoresis [see 8]. Specific precipitates were dissolved in an excess of antigen and providing that the rate of re-equilibration was sufficiently slow a number of peaks, corresponding to fractions of different molecular weight, could be detected in the centrifugation pattern. In the region of heavy antigen excess the largest of these peaks is the uncombined antigen; next comes a peak equated with Ag_2Ab complexes, and this is followed in turn by smaller and smaller peaks containing less material but larger aggregates, e.g., of the composition Ag_3Ab_2. As the antigen concentration is decreased through moderate to slight excess so the faster sedimenting peaks increase in size at the expense of those containing smaller aggregates. Electrophoresis was also used to distinguish complexes of different size. The results were again consistent with the explanation that in the region of heavy antigen excess the main complex had the composition Ag_2Ab.

As indicated already, it is not enough to assume that specific union altogether accounts for the increasing size of aggregates and ultimately for precipitation. For instance, the ionic strength of the medium in which the reaction takes place has a profound effect on the outcome and this is just one of the reasons that suggest the possibility that forces other than those involved in primary union are important. The complexity of the situation is also indicated by the fact that the effects of alterations in ionic strength are by no means consistent. Thus raising the salt concentration in a reaction mixture to 1·79 M (12 × physiological) may more than halve the amount of antibody nitrogen precipitated when mammalian antisera are tested, but under the same conditions chicken sera may precipitate optimally [32].

The amount of precipitate formed also depends on the pH of reaction mixtures, but remains fairly constant in the range 6·6–8·5. Below pH 4·5 and above pH 9·5 precipitates do not usually form and formed precipitates can be dissolved. Singer has confirmed some of these observations and in addition has shown that the dissociation of antigen–antibody complexes is complete at pH 2·4, in the case of a bovine serum albumin/anti-BSA system at least [8].

It should be appreciated, of course, that under conditions far removed from physiological the molecules of antigen or antibody may themselves be so denatured that their combining sites are functionally destroyed in any case. It is with less extreme conditions that we are primarily concerned in order to shed more light on the secondary reaction of precipitation. It has to be admitted that we are still largely ignorant of the precise mechanism by which primary union leads on to precipitation, and that a true understanding is likely to come only when a great deal more is known about the nature of combining sites and the effect of primary union on the molecule as a whole. At the same time enough is known already for some kind of provisional picture to be drawn.

It is quite certain in the first place that a three-dimensional lattice arrangement is possible only when bivalent antibody and multivalent antigen are present together, unless the rather unusual case of multivalent antibody and bivalent antigen is accepted. At any rate these conditions constitute the minimum requirements and in their absence the formation of a lattice is a geometrical impossibility. Apart from what has already been said, the evidence that such structures actually exist comes from observations that suggest the formation of long chains when bivalent antigen was mixed with bivalent antibody [33], whereas a precipitate was formed when a small trivalent hapten was mixed with its homologous antibody [34]. Not all the evidence points in the same direction, however, and it has been reported that bivalent hapten and antibody can form precipitating polymers [35]. This could mean simply that long chains do precipitate, or that precipitating cyclical structures are formed, or that physicochemical forces other than those involved in primary union are instrumental in bringing about aggregation and loss of solubility. Even discounting the last piece of evidence, it would still be possible to take the view that it was the size of the antigen or hapten molecule that determined whether precipitation took place and not the number of determinants it carried. This aspect has been covered by investigations in which single determinants have been coupled to protein carriers such as albumin [36]; antisera to these artificially enlarged haptens fail to precipitate them. It has not proved possible as yet to obtain confirmation of these results with naturally occurring monovalent protein antigens, although such antigens undoubtedly occur; for instance, diphtheria toxin contains a single toxic group that is also antigenic. However, the molecule of toxin itself contains a variety of other antigenic determinants and possibly more than one of each specificity, but even if it carried only three determinants, each of a different specificity, a whole antiserum containing antibodies of all three specificities would be able to form a lattice with the toxin molecules. In rare cases antisera to diphtheria toxin have been found that neutralize but do not precipitate [37], and it is presumed that such antisera do not carry the full spectrum of antibody specificities for some reason of animal idiosyncrasy.

If lack of precipitation can be due to univalent hapten, then, taking a purely mechanistic view, it can equally well be due to univalent antibody. It has indeed been customary in the fairly recent past to refer to 'incomplete' antibodies that fail to precipitate or agglutinate as 'univalent'. In order to avoid unnecessary confusion it would be as well to point out immediately that incomplete antibody in this sense is not univalent. It is possible that truly univalent antibody could be produced during the course of certain diseases of the immunological system, but otherwise such molecules are only known as artefacts made by splitting immunoglobulins *in vitro* and allowing them to recombine to form antibodies of hybrid specificity. Such hybrid molecules are unable to form aggregates with one antigen. As far as it goes, then, the evidence of 'univalent' antibody supports the contention that precipitates arise because lattice-like structures are formed.

There are a number of conditions under which there can be failure to precipitate serologically and which should be accounted for in any theory of precipitation. So far we have considered monovalent antigen (or hapten) and antibody. Marrack [38] lists three other causes: (1) low affinity of antibody for antigen, (2) electrostatic repulsion, and (3) steric hindrance.

A lattice theory satisfactorily accounts for many aspects of the precipitin reaction, and in particular for the three zones that have become so well characterized (*Fig.* 45). Lack of precipitation in the zone of antibody excess is explained by postulating that all antigen sites are occupied by antibody and that in extreme cases all antigen sites are occupied by different antibody molecules; there is thus no mechanism by which a lattice can be built up. The relationship between antigen and antibody is reversed in the zone of antigen excess, and though the complexes formed have a different composition precipitation is again inhibited. What a lattice theory without modification fails to do is to explain why some potent antisera do not have a zone of inhibition in the region of antibody excess. In such cases one can postulate a rather high dissociation constant for the antigen–antibody reaction, permitting formed bonds to break and new bonds to be formed. The latter may be between one molecule of antigen and an antibody molecule already attached to another antigen molecule; in this way larger aggregates may be formed until eventually precipitation results. It is interesting to note, however, that Marrack invoked a lowered *affinity* of antibody for antigen to account for the failure of some cross-reacting systems to precipitate [38]. The fact that union does occur between heterologous antigen and antibody is proved by the fact that the homologous system can be inhibited, albeit usually by high concentrations of heterologous antigens. This does suggest all the same that a low affinity is associated with the lack of precipitation seen with

some heterologous, but reacting, systems. In terms of molecular interaction the meaning of 'lower affinity' is not quite clear, but in the context
of antigen–antibody reactions it could well be largely covered by 'higher
dissociation constant'. What is certain is that the heterogeneity of antibody
and antigen populations is so great that with the crude weapons at our
command we are only obtaining average or mean results and that it is not

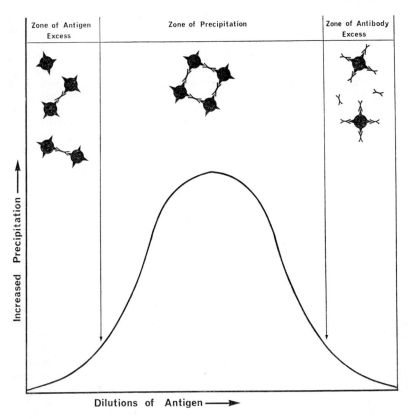

Fig. 45.—The possible consequences of varying the relative concentrations of
antigen and antibody on the formation of lattice-like structures. (*Drawn by
Dr. L. W. Greenham.*)

possible to generate rules governing the whole range of reactions by
observing those phenomena that occur at one extreme or another. In
other words, we are still in no position to explain all the anomalies seen in
the very complex situations where populations of antibodies react with
populations of antigenic sites.
    Even if we accept a simple lattice theory provisionally, there are still a
number of points that require clarifying. Under conditions of low ionic
strength that favour the union of antigen with antibody the formation of

aggregates is not necessarily equally favoured. Other observers have noted that altering the surface charge of antibody molecules by acetylation of the amino groups also reduces or abolishes the formation of a specific precipitate [39]. By increasing the net negative charge on antibody molecules in this way it is presumed that the net repulsive charge between them is increased, and since aggregates are largely made up of antibody molecules the growth of such aggregates is inhibited. Iodination, which reduces the net negative charge, has the reverse effect, as would be expected [6].

The formation of a precipitate can thus be viewed as a battle between the opposing forces, of association represented by the bonds formed between antigen and antibody on one side, and of disruption represented by the forces of repulsion acting mainly between antibody molecules on the other. Both these forces would be affected by the ionic strength of the medium.

Lastly, there is the question of inhibition of precipitation caused by steric hindrance. Described by a number of authors in connexion with a variety of systems and with both antibody and antigen, the fact remains that inhibition in all these cases can be put down to steric hindrance by other macromolecules forming complexes with either antigen or antibody. The subject does not really add to our understanding of the mechanism of precipitation. It may, nevertheless, be important in certain contexts to recognize that precipitation may fail if antisera, or, in some cases, antigens, are subjected to a variety of processes such as heating, ageing, photo-oxidation, and extraction with lipid solvents.

We are left with a rather unsatisfactory situation in which speculations about lattice formation are obviously inadequate at present to account for all the phenomena associated with serological precipitation. We know that the heterogeneity of antigen and antibody, particularly the latter, must introduce complications, and indeed that heterogeneity may extend to the presence of precipitating and non-precipitating antibodies in the same serum, a circumstance that is inferred from the descriptions of rare antisera that fail to precipitate at all. It could well depend on the relative proportions of such antibodies in an antiserum whether precipitation occurs at this or that concentration. Finally, the role of the medium in which the reaction is occurring must not be forgotten since, apart from any effect it may have on primary union, it may influence the course of precipitation through its effect on the net charge at the surface of immuno-globulins. It is the possibility that interaction between antibody molecules is finally responsible for precipitation that is currently engaging a good deal of attention.

C. Immunodiffusion and Immuno-electrophoresis

These two fairly recent developments of the precipitin reaction have provided us with a good deal of information about the precipitin reaction itself, but more particularly about the nature of the chief reactants. The main lesson affecting general serological principles to be gleaned from these techniques has been that both 'antigen' and 'antibody' are normally complex preparations consisting of a spectrum or population of molecules that in either case may differ quite widely within itself. As a result we now recognize that many antigenic preparations previously thought of as 'pure' antigens are, in fact, complex mixtures of antigens or their determinants.

The principle of immunodiffusion is that antigen and antibody are allowed to diffuse through a semi-solid medium such as agar gel. In single-diffusion techniques one of the reactants is incorporated in the gel and the other diffuses away from a reservoir. In double-diffusion techniques the reactants are allowed to diffuse towards each other from separate wells or troughs. In both cases bands of precipitation will appear where appropriate (optimal) concentrations of antigen and antibody are achieved. Precipitations such as these were described as long ago as 1905 by Bechhold [40], but in spite of new reports from time to time the technique of gel diffusion was used as a delicate tool for the study of precipitation only after its possibilities had been pointed out by Oudin in France [41], Ouchterlony in Sweden [42], and Elek in England [43]. With these

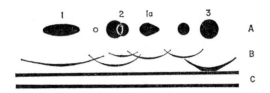

Fig. 46.—Diagrammatic illustration of the process of immuno-electrophoresis. A, Distribution of protein spots in gel following electrophoresis. I, Ia, Proteins of broad charge distribution; 2, Two different overlapping proteins; 3, Protein in high concentration against which there is little antibody. B, Areas of precipitates which form when diffusing antibody meets antigen. C, Trough containing 'polyvalent' antiserum. *Reproduced from R. R. A. Coombs and P. G. H. Gell (eds.) (1968), 'Clinical Aspects of Immunology', by kind permission of Blackwell Scientific Publications, Oxford.*

methods it proved possible to reveal hitherto quite unsuspected complexities in antigen and antibody preparations, but particularly in the former. For instance, antigens which had been highly purified chemically could subsequently be shown to be heterogeneous by immunological means. Thus, repeatedly recrystallized ovalbumin still contained con-albumin (serum albumin) as a contaminant.

A new dimension was added to the technique of immunodiffusion by Grabar and Williams [44] when they showed that one of the reactants could first of all be subjected to the action of an electric current in the gel before being allowed to diffuse through it. This is immuno-electrophoresis and it permits the separation of antigenic molecules in a mixture according to the net electric charge they carry as well as by the rate at which they diffuse. The principle of the technique is set out in *Fig.* 46 [45], and the large number of distinguishable antigens in a single preparation in *Fig.* 47 [46].

The high degree of serological resolution of which these methods are capable is largely due to the controlled rate of diffusion and the formation of narrow bands of precipitate. In the conventional precipitin reaction mechanical mixing and convection both play a part in bringing antigens and antibodies together as well as simple diffusion. A situation more analogous to immunodiffusion is set up in the interfacial technique when a preparation of antigen is carefully layered over an antiserum in a tube. As the reagents diffuse through each other all concentration ratios possible are theoretically achieved and precipitation occurs. The same sequence of events takes place in immunodiffusion, so that we can visualize the process as consisting, in the case of double diffusion, of two concentration

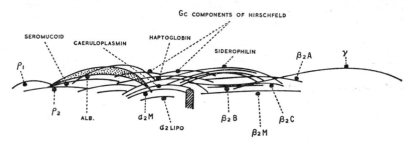

Fig. 47.—Diagram showing the principal precipitation arcs formed in an immuno-electrophoretic analysis of normal human serum. *Reproduced from J. F. Ackroyd (ed.) (1964), 'Immunological Methods', by kind permission of Blackwell Scientific Publications, Oxford.*

gradients formed between two wells cut into the gelled medium. As diffusion proceeds, a point is reached at which the concentrations of antigen and antibody are such that precipitation ensues. More antigen and antibody arriving from either side will simply add to the precipitate. The result is a sharp line of precipitate formed between two reservoirs, but such an explanation is really a gross oversimplification of the events; it does not, for instance, take into account the possibility of falling concentrations or exhaustion of reagents. It does, however, provide a sufficient basis on which the applications of the techniques can be discussed.

Perhaps the first thing to note is that the lines of precipitate may be clear and sharply defined with some sera and more diffuse with others. It will be remembered that H-type antisera have a relatively narrow zone of precipitation, whereas R-type antisera precipitate over a wide range of antigen–antibody ratios, principally because there is no inhibition zone of antibody excess. Antisera of the H type therefore give sharp lines of precipitation and those of R type give broad bands. The importance of balanced antigen–antibody systems also should not be overlooked. A balanced system contains antigen and antibody in appropriate concentrations and quantities of the reactants in wells placed at a suitable distance from each other. In unbalanced systems where antigen or antibody is in excess a formed precipitate may be dissolved. Under similar but less extreme conditions the line of precipitate may migrate over a period of time as a precipitate is dissolved in an excess of, say, antigen which moves on to meet higher concentrations of antibody when it is again precipitated. With R-type antisera the precipitates are less readily soluble and a migrating line often leaves a fuzzy trailing edge. This type of phenomenon can also sometimes be observed in the interfacial precipitin test carried out in a test-tube.

As indicated earlier, immunodiffusion and immuno-electrophoresis techniques are remarkably versatile. With a suitable arrangement of wells and troughs to act as reservoirs and a range of antigenic preparations and specific antisera, band patterns are formed that can convey a great deal of information about the relationships between different antigens and their determinants. With double-diffusion methods used in this way three kinds of band patterns can be recognized: the so-called reactions of 'identity', 'partial identity', and 'non-identity'. In *Fig.* 48 is illustrated a number of cases in which such reactions could be observed. In *Fig.* 48 a we see reactions of identity where two lines of precipitate meet in a smooth curve. A reaction of partial identity is shown in *Fig.* 48 c, where the spur extending the line formed between the homologous system indicates that some of the determinants on the homologous antigen molecule are not carried by the cross-reacting antigen. In *Fig.* 48 b we see a reaction of non-identity in which a multipotent antiserum detects two separate antigens in two preparations and the precipitation lines simply intersect since the two reacting systems are quite distinct.

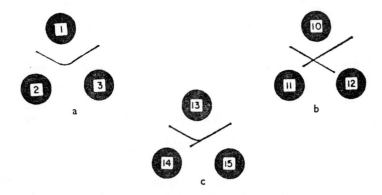

Fig. 48.—Simple gel-diffusion reactions. a. 1, Anti-A antiserum; 2, Antigen A: Preparation 1; 3, Antigen A: Preparation II. b. 10, Anti-(A+B) antiserum; 11, Antigen A; 12, Antigen B; c. 13, Anti-A antiserum; 14, Antigen A′; 15, Antigen A. *Reproduced from R. R. Coombs and P. G. H. Gell (eds.) (1968), 'Clinical Aspects of Immunology', by kind permission of Blackwell Scientific Publications, Oxford.*

Though the examples given above are quite clear-cut, it should not be assumed that the interpretation of band patterns is always simple. Even a single line between two cups may mean only that the resolving power of the system is inadequate; and a double line may indicate not two antigen–antibody systems but an unbalanced system. With multiple antigens and polyspecific antisera some systems may not form precipitates at all, depending on the relative concentrations and diffusion rates of the reactants. In other words, in complex mixtures it is not always possible for all systems to be in balance.

The wide variety of patterns that can be obtained and the interpretation to be placed on them is discussed in more detail elsewhere [45], and Ouchterlony has found it necessary to modify his original arrangement of identity, partial identity, and non-identity by dividing possible reactions into four groups [47]. But probably no system adequately embraces all the possibilities since we do not yet understand all the complexities of partial antigens, multiple determinants, and the vagaries of antibody production in response to such complex stimuli. What we can say is that with suitable reference antigens and antisera we can identify antigens and antibodies with a very fair degree of certainty even though they are present as mixtures. The importance of working with balanced systems must never be over-looked, although it may be difficult in some cases. As an aid to detection, measurement, and preservation, protein dyes have been widely used for staining the precipitates or the reagents before use in the test. The subject has been dealt with in some detail by Crowle [48].

The principles of immunodiffusion apply equally to immuno-electro-phoresis, but the methods differ in that the components of an antigen preparation are separated by subjecting them to electrophoresis before carrying out an immunodiffusion reaction. Individual antigens can be identified by this method by direct comparison with a reference antigen (*see Fig.* 49). Because separation is effected in two ways, immuno-electro-phoresis normally has a greater resolving power for antigen components than straightforward immunodiffusion. Sometimes this degree of resolution

Reference antigen

Test preparation

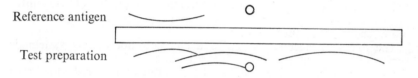

Fig. 49.—Identification of antigens by immuno-electrophoresis.

yields information that is not immediately useful, immunologically speaking. Thus, three kinds of ovalbumin can be detected electro-phoretically due to their different contents of phosphoryl groups, although they all have identical determinants. Similar observations have been made with globulins.

In immunodiffusion the position of bands of precipitate is a function of the relative concentration of the reagents, the optimal proportions ratio, and the respective diffusion rates. In immuno-electrophoresis the com-ponents of antigen are first separated in a direction at right-angles to their subsequent diffusion, and their respective rates of migration depend on the net charge of the individual molecules. At the alkaline pH's used, nearly all proteins carry a negative charge and would therefore be expected to move towards the anode. That this does not always happen is due to the phenomenon of electro-endosmosis. Agar, a commonly used gelling material, itself carries a negative charge and, since it cannot move towards the anode, pressure is exerted on the liquid of the gel to move in the opposite direction. The movement of charged particles in solution is thus a function of their own charge and the movement of liquid in the gel: they may migrate towards the anode, remain stationary, or even migrate towards the cathode. For this and other reasons agarose, a neutral polysaccharide constituent of agar, is sometimes preferred to agar. Electrophoresis and immunodiffusion can, of course, be carried out in a number of other media such as silica gel, gelatin, cellulose acetate, 'Cyanogum', and so on.

The usefulness of the techniques described in this section is evidenced by the immense wealth of literature that has grown up round the subjects in a short space of time. Between 1956 and 1960 1200 papers were published on the subject of immunodiffusion alone. Here we have been able to deal with only some of the main features of these reactions; for further details the reader is referred to books already quoted [15–17, 48], to the massive and authoritative review by Ouchterlony [49], and the monograph by Peetoom [50].

D. Agglutination

Agglutination in the immunological sense is aggregation of particles too large to be considered to be in solution. In practice this means cells of one sort or another, though exceptions can be found such as the agglutination of antigen-coated polystyrene latex particles.

For the detection of antibodies agglutination is a much more sensitive technique than precipitation, and whereas precipitin tests can detect as little as 2 μg. per ml of antibody, agglutination is 10–400 times as sensitive. In a few instances where the antigenic structure of a cell is highly repetitive as in the carbohydrate antigen of bacterial capsules, agglutination is no more sensitive than precipitation.

The following account is neither a complete nor even a systematic survey of agglutination but provides a basis on which the mechanism of the reaction can be discussed. If the agglutination of red blood-cells appears to receive more than its fair share of attention this is because the immense clinical importance of red-cell antigens has led to their intensive study, and thereby of the reactions associated with them. Many of the same phenomena have been observed with bacterial and other cells but have not been followed up with the same vigour; others probably occur but have not been looked for.

As with precipitation, the virtue and attraction of agglutination is that it can so readily be observed. The first description of red-cell agglutination is usually attributed to Landois [51] in 1875, though clumping of red cells in serum was actually observed some six years earlier by a German medical student [52], but published in an obscure journal that is not even mentioned in official lists of periodicals. Similarly, although the first description of bacterial agglutination is often ascribed to Gruber and Durham [53], in 1896, it seems certain that Charrin and Roger [54] observed it still earlier.

Agglutination, like precipitation, is a second-stage reaction that ordinarily follows primary union spontaneously. Once again like precipitation, the distinction between primary and secondary reactions is not an arbitrary one and the two parts of the reaction can be shown to occur optimally under markedly different physicochemical conditions.

First studied in detail in connexion with bacteria, the investigation of agglutination has followed rather a different course from that of precipitation. This was largely due to technical factors and stemmed partly from the fact that it is impossible to work with very heavy suspensions of bacteria because their very opacity renders it difficult to detect agglutination, and this predisposed to constant antigen titrations; and partly from the fact that the multiplicity of antigens on the cell surface was quickly recognized as a complicating factor in agglutination. For instance, the distinct specificities of somatic and flagellar antigens and their corresponding antibodies were clearly described by Smith and Reagh in 1903 [55]. At about the same time it was noted that the effect of heat on the same antigens and their antibodies also varied [56, 57]. The concept of heterogeneous antigens and antibodies was finally crystallized by Weil and Felix in their descriptions of flagellated and non-flagellated forms of *Proteus* bacteria [58, 59].

The essential role of electrolytes in precipitation has already been mentioned, but it was in connexion with agglutination that this role was first demonstrated by Bordet [60]. Specific agglutination can be shown to proceed in two stages by reacting bacteria with agglutinating antiserum in a salt-free medium. Usually no agglutination occurs, but the 'sensitization' of bacteria can be detected by the absence of antibody in the supernatant after centrifugation, and by the agglutination of resuspended cells after the addition of electrolytes. It was this kind of evidence that led Bordet to formulate his two-stage hypothesis for antigen–antibody reactions, which can be compared with the flocculation of colloidal suspensions of metals by salt; or the equally well-known phenomenon of the deposition of clay at a river mouth where muddy water mixes with the sea water.

Although electrolytes are essential if the reaction is to take place, agglutination (and precipitation) is inhibited or delayed by hypertonic concentrations of saline (0·2–0·5 M and above), resulting, for instance, in a reduced titre for isoagglutinins in the ABO blood-group system [61].

1. PROZONE PHENOMENA

The widespread use of the agglutination reaction for bacteriological diagnosis soon led to the discovery of prozone phenomena; that is to say that agglutination occurs in the presence of higher dilutions of antiserum but not in lower dilutions. Attention to detail led to the recognition that prozones were particularly noticeable when antisera had been stored for some time or had been heated. Shibley investigated the effect of heat on a high-titred antiserum to a dysentery bacillus that initially displayed no prozone [62]. Heating the serum induced three changes: at 60–70° C. a prozone was induced; at 76° C. the prozone was abolished and there was some reduction in the titre of the serum; and at 78° C. the capacity to agglutinate was abolished altogether. In 1931 Arkwright wrote that it seemed 'necessary to postulate two different kinds of agglutinins' and that 'these might be associated with serum proteins of different susceptibility to heat' [63], a conclusion which could prove perfectly acceptable even today.

The occurrence of prozone phenomena is not, of course, confined to heated sera. Prozones are found with particular frequency, for example, in sera that contain antibodies to the bacterium *Brucella abortus*. As in the case of precipitation, we have two possible explanations to account for inhibition in zones of antibody excess; either every available antigen site is occupied by an antibody molecule and larger aggregates cannot form, or we must postulate the existence of a separate kind of 'blocking' antibody molecule that is unable to agglutinate, and, as Arkwright foresaw, the effect of heat might be to alter the relative concentrations of 'blocking' and agglutinating antibodies in serum. The evidence for the existence of non-agglutinating antibodies is very strong. In 1944 Wiener [64] and Race [65] independently discovered such antibodies in unheated human sera directed towards Rh antigens. These so-called 'incomplete' antibodies are preferentially adsorbed to red cells and block the adsorption of and agglutination by 'complete' ('saline') antibodies. 'Saline' antibodies are so called because they agglutinate red blood-cells suspended in a saline medium whereas 'incomplete' antibodies agglutinate only when albumin or some other macromolecular substance such as serum, plasma, dextran, polyvinylpyrrolidone, gelatin, gum acacia, etc., is added to the medium. While the occurrence of incomplete or blocking antibodies may be an adequate explanation of some prozone phenomena at least, it does not of itself lead to a better understanding of the mechanism of agglutination. For this it would seem that a profitable approach would be to find out why some antibodies only agglutinate cells under special conditions and to define what these conditions are.

We have just noted the effect of a variety of macromolecules on incomplete antibody. In addition, blood-group serologists have devised two other methods for agglutinating red cells to which this kind of antibody has absorbed. The first of these is enzymatic digestion of the red blood-cell surface, and the second is the use of antiglobulin sera, both of them having some relevance to the problem of agglutinating mechanisms.

2. ENZYME-TREATED RED CELLS

A wide variety of proteolytic enzymes has been used for digesting the red-cell surface in order to render the cells susceptible to the agglutinating action of incomplete antibody. Such enzymes have been derived from animal, vegetable, and fungal sources and include trypsin, papain, ficin, bromelin, and protease G. The precise action of these enzymes on the red cell is still not known and doubt has been expressed as to whether it is proteolytic at all since most of them are known also to possess esterase activity, whereas a number of other proteolytic enzymes are ineffective in this respect. Nor is the activity of the effective enzymes identical. For instance, bromelin is the best of those mentioned above for the detection of antibody on the red cells of infants suffering from ABO haemolytic disease. Another pointer indicating that proteolytic activity may not be so important is that neuraminidase produces a similar serological effect, and that the activity of the enzyme is proportional to the amount of sialic acid released.

The technique of enzyme treatment can be combined with either of the other two methods, macromolecular medium or antiglobulin reagents, to enhance sensitivity [66], which perhaps suggests that the same mechanism is operating in each case. The discovery of incomplete antibodies associated with the Rh system initially led to the supposition that they were univalent. However, there is no doubt now that incomplete antibodies are at least divalent, and, indeed, incomplete anti-D sera are able to agglutinate certain kinds of cell carrying the D antigen. Before these facts were known the addition of macromolecular substances was thought to allow non-specific serum factors to effect agglutination. Once this idea had been discarded it was postulated that enzymes unmasked 'hidden' antigens, though this is not a very satisfactory explanation of enhancement by albumin, etc. More recently, attention has been turned towards physico-chemical factors common to all three methods, e.g., reduction of surface negative charge. Whether these latter-day explanations are correct or not, it is certain that it is at this level that answers to the problems associated with precipitation as well as agglutination must be sought.

Before going on to deal with theories of agglutination, however, we should first deal with the last of the three methods which enable incomplete antibodies to agglutinate.

3. ANTIGLOBULIN TEST

In antiglobulin tests incomplete antibody is first adsorbed to red cells and agglutination brought about by the action of antibody to the adsorbed immunoglobulin. The orthodox view of the mechanism involved was that the antiglobulin effected a bridge between immunoglobulins attached to different cells. Such a mechanistic viewpoint seems particularly reasonable when it is realized that in blood-group serology it was soon recognized that incomplete antibodies were predominantly IgG and complete were IgM. At the time it was supposed that the difference in molecular weight between the two classes was reflected in different lengths of molecule and whereas IgM molecules could span the distance between two red cells, IgG molecules could not.

In practice antiglobulin tests are described as 'direct' or 'indirect', although the serological principle is the same in both cases. In the direct test red cells that have been coated with antibody *in vivo* are used; in the indirect test antibody is adsorbed to the red cells *in vitro*.

The direct test is widely used in the diagnosis of haemolytic disease of the newborn caused by maternal antibodies to Rh and some other antigens finding their way into the foetal circulation. With ABO-haemolytic disease, however, the test is usually negative for reasons that are by no means clear. Possibly the red-cell antibody is orientated in such a way that antiglobulin is unable to attach to it. That antibody has actually been bound *in vivo* can be shown quite easily, either by eluting it and characterizing it separately, or by various modifications to the antiglobulin test itself. As we have mentioned before, the test can be used in conjunction with macromolecular media and enzyme treatment and the sensitivity of the test considerably enhanced thereby. It is of interest that enzyme treatment of cells already sensitized by antibody *in vivo* alters agglutinability because the antigenic sites themselves are in no way changed since they are protected in the same way as Nisonoff and Pressman protected antibody-combining sites while antibody molecules were being acetylated [39].

A wide variety of indirect antiglobulin tests has been devised. They are used not only for the detection of antibodies as such on the surface of red cells but also for the study of the antigenic structure of immunoglobulins. For diagnostic serology the sensitivity of a test is frequently of paramount importance. Many ingenious 'sandwich' and 'consumption' tests have been invented [45], with the ultimate objective of detecting antibody on the red-cell surface. Sometimes these methods are quite indirect in the true meaning of the word. For instance, in some cases antisera directed against components of complement are more successful than antiglobulin sera. Occasionally, several layers of antigen–antibody reactions have to be built up on the surface of a red cell before agglutination can be induced. In such cases it is not easy to understand from a mechanistic point of view why the first layer of antiglobulin was not adequate to bridge the gap between blood-cells. Antigens located in crypts in the cell membrane or determinants so orientated that antibody did not stick out from cell surface are among explanations offered to try to account for these phenomena.

Prozones have also been described in antiglobulin tests. They are rather characteristic of 'Raggs'. These are antiglobulins found in the serum of patients with rheumatoid arthritis, and they have been used as a natural source of antiglobulin reagent. 'Snaggs' are found in normal serum and characteristically are of much lower titre. Prozones have also been described in the case of rabbit antiglobulin sera. Inhibition by blocking antibody and saturation of antigenic sites have both been held to account for these zones of inhibition in the same way as they have been applied to bacterial agglutinins. The two mechanisms can be distinguished by carrying out a blocking test—the classic method used for the detection of incomplete antibodies, shown up by the fact that they can prevent agglutination by complete antibody added subsequently.

E. Passive Agglutination

Under this heading we shall consider a number of techniques that have as a common denominator the use of particulate supports to which antigen is attached before reaction with specific antibody is attempted. Passive agglutination, then, is the agglutination of particulate materials to which antigen has been attached, often by non-immunological means. Supports for this purpose can be cells, or they can be organic or inorganic particles. The virtue of the technique lies in its great sensitivity, upwards of 400 times as sensitive as corresponding precipitation techniques for the detection of antibody. Of course, it can legitimately be argued that passive agglutination is simply a modified precipitin reaction and as such it could more properly have been dealt with in that section. However, apart from its more obvious similarities to agglutination, in one important respect, to be discussed later, it is relevant to theories of agglutination. This is an aspect that has already been touched on lightly and is the orientation of an antigenic grouping at the surface of a particle. For these reasons we make no apology for introducing passive agglutination at this point.

It should be fairly obvious, too, that instead of antigens it should be possible to adsorb antibodies to the inert support and effect agglutination by adding antigen. In this event we refer to the reaction as 'reversed passive agglutination'. No significance attaches to this reaction other than that it is an alternative method to be used in appropriate circumstances. Also, in this section we shall refer from time to time to 'co-agglutination', a term used to describe a situation in which red cells are carried down or 'agglutinated' by *non-precipitating* complexes of antigen and antibody, even though the latter, mixed in different proportions or concentrations, are capable of precipitation. The mechanism of this reaction is not understood, and it differs in principle from passive agglutination in that neither antigen nor antibody is first adsorbed to the red cells [29]. Some reactions thought to be examples of passive agglutination may be partly or wholly co-agglutination.

In the preparation of particles for passive agglutination soluble antigens can be attached in three possible ways: by adsorption, by chemical bonding, and by immunological reaction. The most commonly used biological support is the mammalian red cell, but we shall deal first with attachment to organic and inorganic supports.

CHEMICAL SUPPORTS

A wide variety of chemical substances has been used for the adsorption of antigens, e.g., kaolin, barium stearate, charcoal, glass beads, china clay, carmine dye, and bismuth oxy-gallate particles, just to name some. We shall discuss shortly a few representative examples from among these and other materials.

Collodion particles were used as long ago as 1928 [67] but have not achieved wide popularity because of technical difficulties associated with the instability of suspensions and non-specific results. Once the antigen has been adsorbed to the particles, it is usual to wash them thoroughly before admixture with specific antibody in order to remove unadsorbed antigen which might interfere with the test by reacting with the antibody. It is of theoretical interest that a high degree of sensitivity is claimed for a test in which toxin, antitoxin, and collodion particles are simply mixed together. It is possible that the reaction is one of co-agglutination rather than passive agglutination.

Surface fixation has been used in connexion with serum albumin, bacterial, lipid, and red-cell antigens; it has also found application in routine blood group serology as a rough quantitative test for anti-A and anti-B. The test is based on the fixation of red cells and other antigenic substances, in the presence of antiserum, to the fibres of filter paper [68].

The *latex test* was devised by Singer and Plotz in 1956 [69]; the technique is now in widespread use and latex polystyrene particles coated with a variety of antigens and antibodies are readily available commercially. The spherical particles are 0·8–1·1 μ in diameter and provide an enormous surface area for adsorption, a single particle being able to absorb approximately 75,000 molecules of globulin. The mechanism of adsorption is not precisely known, but it is possible that the coated particle has more than one layer of antigen. Suggestions that the simultaneous adsorption of albumin and globulin is evidence of the presence of more than one kind of receptor site are therefore not necessarily true; the possibility that albumin could absorb to an intact protein coat of globulin and vice versa must also be entertained.

Although immunoglobulins remain attached to latex particles during washing, particles coated with thyroglobulin may fail to agglutinate in the presence of anti-thyroglobulin if they have been washed. It is possible that here again we are dealing with co-agglutination. Indeed, possibly co-agglutination should be suspected in a number of situations where sensitized particles are used without being washed.

9

Techniques and applications of the latex test have been reviewed by Singer [70] and by Goodman and Bozicevich [71].

The *bentonite test* employs sodium bentonite, a silicaceous earth that provides a very large surface area for adsorption. The test has the advantage that it can be used with polysaccharides and even with DNA, as well as protein antigens. In addition, the coated particles are often quite stable and can be stored for several months. Against it is its lack of sensitivity, at any rate compared with passive haemagglutination techniques.

As with other passive agglutination tests, non-specific agglutination has to be avoided by careful control of *p*H, salt concentration, and, most important, by the addition of stabilizing substances such as dilute normal rabbit serum or polyvinylpyrrollidone.

Bismuth tannate and *barium sulphate* have come into prominence as substrates rather more recently [72, 73]. The antigenicity of heavy chains of human immunoglobulins has been investigated using barium sulphate as a support [74]; its usefulness in reactions utilizing rabbit antihuman globulin has also been confirmed [74].

The barium-sulphate test has the considerable advantages of availability, cheapness, simplicity, and rapidity.

F. Passive Haemagglutination

1. WITH UNMODIFIED RED CELLS

As long ago as 1898, Nicolle [75] exploited the same principle, but instead of mammalian cells he used bacteria as supports.

As with chemical supports the exact mechanism by which antigens are attached is not known, but several interesting features are apparent. First, the method of extraction used for a particular antigen, from a bacterium say, is important. In other words, parts of the extracted molecule other than that governing serological specificity are important for adsorption. Then again adsorption is very greatly enhanced (one hundred to one thousandfold) by heating the antigen or treating it with alkali (probably the result of deacetylation). Finally, the same red cells can be sensitized, either consecutively or simultaneously, with the addition of eight or more different polysaccharides. Even if one polysaccharide is present at 250 times the concentration of the others it does not prevent adsorption of the latter. These facts, together and separately, have been taken to indicate, once again, that support surfaces possess several qualitatively different receptor sites for polysaccharides and other antigens. Once again it is also possible to envisage alternative explanations.

In the case of polysaccharides, auxiliary substances such as proteins or lipids are not necessary for adsorption to take place. On the other hand, only undegraded polysaccharides are adsorbed. It is assumed that they combine with lipoprotein, or possibly with phospholipid structures. Exceptionally, a polysaccharide is found that does not attach to red-cell surfaces.

The test has a number of practical applications and advantages. Its sensitivity can be exploited in a great many ways. In addition, antigens not normally located on the surface of cells can be studied by agglutination, as can surface antigens of cells that do not form stable suspensions.

Furthermore, we have seen that several antigens can be fixed simultaneously to the surface of red cells so that it is possible in one test to screen for a number of distinct specificities. The method also makes available highly sensitive techniques for the detection of incomplete or blocking antibodies. Finally, by the addition of complement, the whole test can be converted into a haemolytic reaction. On the whole, although considerable attention has to be paid to technical detail the test is simple to conduct and read. It has been reviewed by Neter [76] and by Goodman and Bozicevich [71].

2. WITH MODIFIED RED CELLS

a. Chemical Modification

We have seen that chemical treatment of bacterial antigens may alter their capacity to sensitize red cells. The red-cell surface may also be treated so that it adsorbs substances that otherwise it would fail to do.

Formalin-treated red cells not only adsorb polysaccharides [77] but proteins and haptens as well [78]. Tanning of red cells is also widely employed in order that protein antigens may be adsorbed and advantage taken of the sensitivity of passive haemagglutination. Applications of the test have been reviewed by Stavitsky [79] and techniques by Daniel and Stavitsky [80]. The use of pyruvic aldehyde as a tanning agent yields cells that retain a high degree of stability over considerable periods of time [81]. Formolization of red cells before or after tanning also produces stable, sensitive suspensions.

Simultaneous sensitization with several protein antigens is again possible with chemically modified red cells as was the case with polysaccharides and unmodified cells. The same inferences are to be drawn and reservations made.

Over the years a wide range of tanning agents has been employed, but on the whole attention has been mainly devoted to devising methods that produce stable suspensions reliably, rather than to their influence on the antigenicity of adsorbed materials. More recently advantage has been taken of the extreme simplicity of a technique associated with chromium-chloride treatment of cells [82]. In comparisons made with this and other methods it is becoming apparent that the tanning agent employed may have a very considerable influence on the specificities displayed by adsorbed antigens. The conclusion to be drawn from these data is that orientation of adsorbed protein on a cell support can play a major part in determining its serological behaviour. Such a viewpoint has a significant bearing when it comes to considering mechanisms of agglutination.

b. Chemical Bonding

Adsorption of antigenic material to modified or unmodified cells does not always result in a sufficiently firm union, so it is sometimes an advantage to be able to make use of stronger chemical bonds. A convenient method is to use the diazo linkage afforded by *bis*-diazobenzidine (BDB). The method suffers from the disadvantage that haemolysis may occur spontaneously before agglutination can be read. This can normally be prevented by treatment of the red cells with formalin before or after coupling. In order to avoid non-specific haemolysis the use of difluoro-dinitrobenzene as coupling reagent has been described [83].

c. General Considerations

In the case of chemical bonding a good deal is already known about the diazo link. In practice the concentration of the reagents has to be carefully controlled, since too little BDB may result in too little antigen being fixed to the cells, and too much may lead to non-specific agglutination from the formation of cell–BDB–cell complexes.

In the case of adsorption the mechanism of the process is still largely unknown, but sufficient evidence has been collected now to show that adsorption depends on both the chemical structure of antigens and on the nature of the red-cell surface. Exceptionally, proteins are adsorbed directly to the red-cell surface without the intervention of covalent bonds. On the other hand, bacterial and other polysaccharides are not invariably adsorbed. The relationship of structure of antigens to adsorption has been shown in the case of pneumococcal polysaccharides, SIII and SVI. The former is taken up untreated by human red cells, whereas the latter is adsorbed only after oxidation; presumably because some structure capable of reacting with a receptor on the red-cell surface is unmasked by this treatment. Similarly, the polysaccharide of *Klebsiella aerogenes* is adsorbed only after alkali reduction, a process that probably splits off an *O*-acetyl group; reacetylation reverses the picture.

There are numerous examples illustrating the importance of choosing the right support to demonstrate a particular reaction. For instance, a polysaccharide that does not adsorb to red cells may do so to bentonite. Also, although DNA is not fixed by tannin-treated red cells, it is by formolized cells and by bentonite. Richter and Cohen have emphasized that with the use of the same antigen–antibody system, BDB and tanned red-cell techniques can give widely different results, even quite contrary ones in the sense that one may fail to show agglutination while the other does [84].

It would appear from the foregoing that the reaction between antigen and antibody is strongly influenced by the nature of the surface to which the antigen is adsorbed. The same influence has been noted in the case of specific antibody attached to red cells acting as antigen in a globulin/anti-globulin reaction [85], indicating that in this context the nature of the attachment of antigen to support is unimportant; it can be immunological or not.

G. Theories of Agglutination

Basically, we must accept that some form of lattice is formed during agglutination. This is the simplest and most obvious explanation for the formation of stable aggregates, and until it is proved that antibody molecules do not link cells to each other it must be accepted that they do. At the same time it is obvious that this is not the whole explanation since, as we have been at pains to point out, in a number of instances where antibody can be shown to have been adsorbed, agglutination nevertheless does not follow.

It is for this reason that new attempts are being made to find explanations that cover all aspects of agglutination satisfactorily. Broadly speaking, three kinds of hypotheses have been put forward. The first of these maintains that the repulsive force between cells, due to the fact that they all carry the same charge, has to be overcome. The second holds that the most important feature responsible for holding cells in suspension is the layer of hydration that surrounds them. Removal or blockage of the hydrophilic groups on a cell therefore results in their agglutination. The third theory stresses the importance of the structure of the cell membrane; that antibodies can be bound but prevented from agglutinating cells through steric hindrance. It must be accepted that in many accounts no clear distinction is made between cell membranes and cell coats. Probably the outermost layer of cellular material is usually meant, but even here there can be a large measure of uncertainty since red cells can and do absorb macromolecular materials from the plasma in which they circulate. To a large extent the explanations offered, particularly in the first two of the above theories, fall within the realm of physical chemistry. It is not proposed, therefore, to give detailed accounts of them, but rather to examine them with a view to seeing how they fit in with the commoner serological observations that are not accounted for by a simple lattice hypothesis.

Pollack has proposed a comprehensive theory [86], embracing all aspects of red-cell agglutination associated with a reduction in the forces that normally hold them apart. The relevant parameters that have to be considered are the ionic strength (μ), pH, dielectric constant (D), and temperature. A number of these are also involved in the primary reaction of antigen–antibody union. It is sufficient to remind ourselves at this stage that a lowering of ionic strength increases the amount of antibody uptake and rate of binding; the optimum pH is about 6·7, and departures from this level in either direction decrease the amount of antibody bound; the effect of temperature is such that when it is raised the rate of association is raised, but so is the dissociation constant, so that, although equilibrium is reached more quickly, less antibody is in fact bound.

For a consideration of the secondary reaction, agglutination, Pollack starts with the long-held thesis that the interplay of two sets of forces determines whether charged particles, such as red cells or bacteria, remain in stable suspension. One set of forces probably includes van der Waals's forces and has been termed 'cohesive force' and 'interfacial tension'. The opposite force is stronger in stable suspensions and is the electrostatic repulsion between particles carrying the same charge. Red cells are negatively charged, probably due in large measure to the carboxyl groups of sialic acid residues at the surface. In the presence of electrolytes a red cell is surrounded by a diffuse layer of cations. Those nearest the red cell move with it so that a line of shear separates them from more distant ions. The zeta potential is the electric potential between these two layers and is a measure of the forces of repulsion between cells.

According to Pollack [86]:—

$$Z = \frac{-4\cdot137 \times 10^{-2}}{\sqrt{(D\mu)}} - \frac{3\cdot09 \times 10^{-1}}{D} \text{ volts,}$$

where sodium chloride is the electrolyte.

The zeta potential is directly proportional to the net surface charge on a cell, and inversely proportional to the dielectric constant and the ionic strength of the medium. The forces tending to keep cells in suspension apart will therefore be influenced by factors that affect the surface charge and by changes in the medium that alter the values of D and μ.

In the case of the former it is known that the adsorption of IgG and IgM antibodies to red cells can reduce the surface charge by up to 30 per cent; the 'blood-group enzymes' can similarly reduce the charge on human red cells from 20 to 53 per cent. Our present knowledge of the structure of immunoglobulins does not suggest that IgM molecules can stretch over much greater distances than IgG. On the basis of the present theory we would have to postulate only that IgM reduced the surface charge more effectively than IgG, which in view of the greater number of combining sites on IgM molecules is not unlikely. Confirmatory evidence of the importance of surface charge also comes from a comparison of the agglutinability of red cells of different species. Rabbit cells are regularly agglutinated by IgG antibodies in saline; human cells by IgM antibodies; and mouse and dog cells rarely even by IgM antibodies. The electrophoretic mobilities of these cells are 0·55, 1·31, 1·40, and 1·65 μ per second per volt per cm. respectively.

So far we have considered only the effect of physicochemical forces on agglutination, but it should be possible to narrow the gap between cells mechanically. Solomon has determined experimentally the effect of centrifugation on the agglutination of red cells by incomplete anti-Rh antibody [87]. He found that agglutination began at 4430 g and was complete at 17,750 g. Pollack calculated on theoretical grounds that spontaneous agglutination should take place at around 7340 g [88]. Allowing for the very considerable uncertainties inherent in the situation, this seems to be a remarkably close agreement between theory and practice.

So far, we have been concerned mainly with the effect of reduction of surface charge on the zeta potential. It is evident that the adsorption of antibody to the red cell and enzyme treatment may both decrease the distance to which the cells will approach each other in suspension. It remains to be seen what is the effect of alteration in the ionic strength and dielectric constant of the medium.

Since the zeta potential is inversely related to both these parameters, an increase in either should enhance agglutination. However, it will be remembered that increasing the ionic strength of a medium adversely affects the primary stage of the reaction. The result is that any increase in the concentration of sodium chloride above 0·17 M so decreases the amount of antibody bound that any increase of agglutination due to lowering the zeta potential is nullified.

The position with regard to alterations of dielectric constant is perhaps rather more clear-cut. Pollack et al. [86] have studied the effect of a number of polymers, Ficoll (a polysucrose), polyvinylpyrrollidone, and dextran (a glucose polymer), on the immunological agglutination of red cells. They were unable to find any evidence that the net surface charge was affected by these substances. Their effect on agglutination was, however, consistent with that on the dielectric constant and the zeta potential. They also found that by keeping Z constant through altering μ and D together they did not alter the agglutinability of a suspension. The picture presented thus far is perhaps deceptively simple.

For the moment at any rate it appears that in terms of zeta potential and intercellular distance Pollack has satisfactorily accounted for the inability of some antibodies to agglutinate and the effect of macromolecular substances on agglutination.

The fact that Hummel working independently has come to rather different conclusions [89] is, however, in some ways unimportant, since both workers agree that it is the intercellular distance that determines whether agglutination will take place in given circumstances. Hummel holds that the layer of hydration surrounding a cell, and which he conceives as a continuous transition from 'tightly bound' to 'freely mobile' water molecules, determines this intercellular distance. Both the action of linear colloids, such as polyvinylpyrrolidone, and of enzymes is regarded in terms of reduction in the layer of hydration. In contrast to Pollack he has found that correlation between absolute surface charge and agglutinability does not always exist. For instance, horse red cells carry a higher charge than cattle cells, but are nevertheless more readily agglutinated both immunologically and non-immunologically [90]. It has also been observed that treatment with enzymes, though leading to the same residual charge on red cells, may or may not result in spontaneous agglutination [91]. Brooks et al. [92] even disagree with the fundamental assumption of Pollack et al. [86] that the dielectric constant is inversely related to the potential energy barrier between charged particles.

Finally, it might be said that considerable importance should be attached to the formation of microvilli at the red-cell surface following the reaction between antibody and red-cell antigen. Such microvilli have been graphically demonstrated with the help of stereoscopic electron microscopy in the case of human red cells agglutinated by cold agglutinins [93]. The possibility that charge densities at the ends of microvilli could be sufficiently low to allow probes from one cell to approach within 5 Å of those from another cell has now been envisaged [94]. However this may be, it is evident that we shall have to abandon old ideas about enzyme treatment unveiling hidden determinants near the cell surface. Instead it would seem that we must embrace new notions of charge interactions between cells and cell probes, and of the effect of these interactions on intercellular distances and the formation of bonds between cells. It is possibly at this level, where microvilli approach each other, that the precise orientation of an antibody molecule at a cell surface, stressed by Uhlenbruck and Prokop [95], and indeed its location in relation to probe tip, could play an important part in determining whether a bond between two cells is formed.

IV. ANTIGEN–ANTIBODY REACTIONS INVOLVING COMPLEMENT

Antigen–antibody reactions in which complement takes part can be divided somewhat arbitrarily into three sections:—

1. Those in which the fixation of complement by antigen–antibody complexes is detected by an indicator system, haemolytic or conglutinating.

2. Those in which the action of antibody and complement at the site of a cellular antigen is revealed by lysis, conglutination, phagocytosis, or derangement of a number of physiological functions, such as mobility, to a minor or major extent.

3. Those in which the fixation of complement by an antigen–antibody complex is detected by the reaction with anti-complement antibody.

Biological processes are so immensely varied that almost every attempt at classification can be shown to be imperfect. In the example above, for instance, conglutination occurs as an indicator system in (1), reappears under (2), and overlaps with (3) since immunoconglutinin (*see later*) at least is antibody to certain components of complement. It is not possible, therefore, to adhere rigidly to the above classification in the description of a number of reactions involving complement that follows.

A. Complement-fixation Test

Whereas the conduct of agglutination and precipitation tests is relatively simple, that of the complement-fixation test is rather more complicated and usually gives the student of serology some difficulty. The

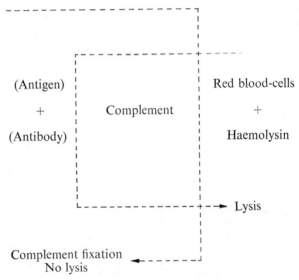

Fig. 50.—Diagram of a complement-fixation test. Either antigen or antibody must be present; the other reagent is then under test.

inherent confusion lies in the fact that five separate reagents are involved, some of them at critical concentrations, and the exact role that each has to play must be kept in the mind's eye all the time. The reaction should be considered in two parts, the test and indicator systems, both competing for complement. The reaction is illustrated in *Fig.* 50, where the test system shown on the left may be regarded as consisting of a known antigen and an unknown serum that may or may not contain antibodies to that antigen. Complement is added to this system and time allowed for union between antigen and antibody to occur and for complement to be adsorbed, i.e., for equilibrium to be established. If antibody was present complement will have been 'fixed'; if it was absent complement will have remained free. The indicator system, consisting of red cells already 'sensitized' with homologous antibody, is now added. The cells will remain intact in the absence of free complement, i.e., if antibody was present in the test system, and will lyse in the presence of free complement, i.e., if antibody was absent in the test system.

So far so good, but it is at this point that conceptual difficulties begin to arise, chiefly because we are unable to define complement, antigen, and antibody in absolute terms. It was pointed out in Chapter 5 that complement is most easily measured in terms of its ability to lyse sensitized red blood-cells. In the complement-fixation test, therefore, we have a situation in which the indicator system not only detects the presence of complement in the test proper but is also used to define the units in which

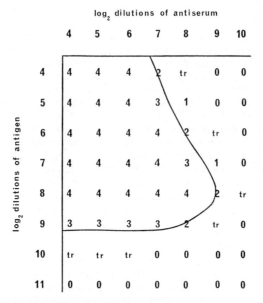

$\log_2$ dilutions of antiserum

	4	5	6	7	8	9	10
4	4	4	4	2	tr	0	0
5	4	4	4	3	1	0	0
6	4	4	4	4	2	tr	0
7	4	4	4	4	3	1	0
8	4	4	4	4	4	2	tr
9	3	3	3	3	2	tr	0
10	tr	tr	tr	0	0	0	0
11	0	0	0	0	0	0	0

($\log_2$ dilutions of antigen)

Fig. 51.—Block complement-fixation test, or test to determine optimal antigen dilutions. 0, 100 per cent lysis (no fixation); tr, 95 per cent lysis; 1, 75 per cent lysis; 2, 50 per cent lysis; 3, 25 per cent lysis; 4, 0 per cent lysis (full fixation).

complement is measured. The complexity does not end there, of course, since the amount of complement needed to lyse a given quantity of sensitized red cells (1 haemolytic unit) depends to some extent on the amount of antibody used to sensitize the red cells (*see* Chapter 5).

Also in Chapter 5 it was shown that a chequerboard titration would reveal the smallest quantity of antibody that could be used to sensitize red cells, consistent with maximum sensitivity.

Since haemolysis by complement is only a special case of complement fixation, exactly the same principle of chequerboard titration can be applied to a test system to find out what concentration of antigen is most effective in fixing complement in the presence of minimal amounts of antibody. A typical titration of this sort is set out in *Fig.* 51, and a moment's thought will show that the dilution of antigen providing the most sensitive indicator for the presence of antibody can be obtained from it. The resemblance of this titration to that shown in Chapter 5 for the titration of complement and sheep red-cell haemolysin is obvious; but here the sensitized red cells and complement have been added in measured doses to dilutions of test-system reagents. The line drawn through the points representing 50 per cent haemolysis makes it clear that at a dilution of 1 in 256 the antigen is capable of fixing as much or even more complement than at any higher concentration when in the presence of minimum quantities of antibody. This, then, is the dilution of antigen chosen to be used in all subsequent tests and if we make the (unwarrantable) assumption that the quality of antibody does not change from serum to serum, then this will remain the most sensitive test that can be devised for a particular system. This method of arriving at the dose of antigen to be used in the complement-fixation test is rather confusingly, but correctly, known as an optimal proportions titration.

Though the complement-fixation test has been described in terms of an unknown serum it is equally effective for the detection of antigen. The test is therefore extremely versatile and of wide applicability. Before the advent of such tests as passive agglutination, passive cutaneous anaphylaxis, and immune adherence it was often the most sensitive serological tool available. It is capable of detecting as little as 0·1 μg. of antibody nitrogen. As the Wassermann reaction the test has been universally accepted for the serological diagnosis of syphilis, and subsequently for a wide range of bacterial, mycotic, and viral infections in the fields of both diagnosis and epidemiological research, as well as a tool in the field of serological research itself. The best general account of the biological factors that affect the satisfactory performance of the complement-fixation test is that given by Fulton [96].

B. Complement-fixation Inhibition Test

It has already been noted in a variety of contexts that some antisera and/ or antibodies fix complement poorly or not at all. For example, chicken antisera, extremely useful though they are because of their high degree of specificity, suffer from the limitation that they fail to fix guinea-pig complement. An ingenious way of making use of the sensitivity of the complement-fixation test with such antisera has been devised [97]. This is the complement-fixation inhibition test, and it depends on the availability of another antiserum directed against the same antigen but capable of fixing complement. The test is conducted in three stages as opposed to the two of the haemolytic complement-fixation test. In the first stage chicken antiserum, say, is mixed with the antigen. In the second stage complement-fixing antibody and complement are added. If the antigen present has already reacted with the chicken antiserum it is no longer available to fix complement in the second stage. In the third stage sensitized red blood-cells are added. It will be noted that a positive reaction, i.e., one in which antibody is present in the chicken serum is indicated by lysis, the opposite of what happens in the direct complement-fixation reaction.

As might be expected, conditions in the second stage of the reaction are fairly critical; an excess of complement-fixing antibody may displace the antibody that has already reacted with antigen, thereby giving rise to a false negative reaction. The situation tends to be aggravated because complexes formed in the presence of complement are stabilized by its adsorption.

C. Conglutination

In the past conglutination has often been used to describe the enhancement of immunological aggregation due to a variety of causes. Nowadays it is most convenient to use it in its original sense [98, 99] of a component(s) of serum that strongly agglutinates complexes formed from antigen, antibody, and complement.

The modern view is that conglutination may be effected by two quite distinct mediators, called 'conglutinin' and 'immunoconglutinin'. Over the years the study of reactions involving these substances has been rather fitful; but more recently a continuing interest has been taken in the subject at the Cambridge School of Pathology and a number of illuminating monographs and review articles bears witness to the fact [100–104].

Conglutinin is a component of normal serum and as such has so far been found in the serum of ruminants only. It has a natural substrate in fixed complement, and presumably therefore takes part in a great many immune responses, though its role in defence against disease is still obscure. Chemically speaking, conglutinin is a euglobulin but with the high glycine content characteristic of many fibrous proteins. It has a molecular weight of 750,000 and the molecule is highly asymmetrical with an axial ratio of 1 : 10. The reaction between conglutinin and its substrates is strictly dependent on the presence of calcium ions, a fact which, together with its chemical composition, serves to distinguish it from antibody.

The conglutination reaction is most easily understood in terms of the direct reaction. Sheep red blood-cells sensitized with sub-agglutinating doses of homologous antibody, as in the complement-fixation test, are reacted with sub-lytic doses of complement. Such 'alexinated cells' are agglutinable by bovine serum which contains conglutinin. The source of complement is of some importance since conglutinating and haemolytic titres vary considerably in different species of animal. For instance, fresh horse serum is almost devoid of haemolytic complement activity, but serves very well as a source of conglutinating complement.

From what has just been said above it follows that the same components of complement are not equally involved in conglutination and haemolysis. Modern studies have revealed that conglutinin reacts with hidden determinants of the C 3 molecule [104]. To this extent the later-reacting components, from C 5 onwards, do not take part in the reaction. The nature of the determinant has been further defined in studies with the yeast cell-wall extract, zymosan, which also appears to be a substrate for conglutinin. In this case the reactive group appears to be a trimannose [105]; but since N-acetyl-D-glucosamine also inhibits the conglutination of alexinated cells it would seem that this amino-sugar must form part of the reactive group. It is assumed that C 3 exposes this specific grouping when it becomes attached to an antigen–antibody complex.

Immunoconglutinin, by contrast, is antibody produced in direct response to antigenic stimulation. It is not confined to any one species. By the relatively insensitive method of centrifugation and resuspension, usually used for the detection of conglutination, it is apparent that immunoconglutinin also reacts with hidden determinants of the C 3 molecule. More sensitive techniques indicate that sites on C 4 are also implicated [104]. Immunoconglutinins may develop as a result of stimulation with heterologous or autologous complement. Only autologous complement can form the stimulus under natural conditions, of course; heterostimulation is effected by immunizing animals with bacteria sensitized with antibody and alexinated with complement from some other species. It has been found in practice that such antibodies (immunoconglutinin) tend to be IgG, whereas those resulting from autostimulation are usually IgM. Such distinctions may be more apparent than real and could be due to the relative ease with which agglutination can be demonstrated with IgM antibody, or to different dosage levels of fixed complement under natural and experimental conditions. The analogy between immunoconglutinins and rheumatoid factor is very striking, both being autostimulated antibodies directed at components involved in the immune reactions themselves.

The biological significance of immunoconglutinins in particular is bound to be a matter for considerable speculation. As antibodies they are directed against a component, albeit altered, of the host's own tissues, and in this sense we have here an example of an auto-immune process (Chapter 12) that may be carrying out a physiological role. This is a concept that has been explored by Grabar [106] and may have wide implications in our understanding of the evolution and meaning of immunological processes. The possibility that auto-antibodies exercise a homeostatic control over the body has indeed been envisaged by many authors. In a rather limited sense, i.e., protection against infection, immunoconglutinins are the clearest, perhaps the only, example where such a role appears susceptible of proof in the near future. Some of the other possibilities of conglutinins and immunoconglutinins in the realms of protection against infection and amelioration of hypersensitivity states are discussed by Lachmann [104].

D. The Jerne Plaque Technique

In 1963 Jerne and Nordin [107] described an elegant technique for identifying and enumerating single antibody-forming cells which has proved to be highly adaptable and has since been widely used. A rabbit was inoculated with sheep erythrocytes and popliteal lymph-node cells were subsequently teased out in culture medium. The cells were then incubated in agar containing sheep erythrocytes for 1 hour, and at the end of this period complement was added. Those cells producing antibody to sheep erythrocytes were surrounded by a clear area of agar, in which the erythrocytes had haemolysed. Such cells are known as 'plaque-forming cells' (PFC).

The original technique revealed cells producing 19S antibody. Subsequent modifications have made it possible to demonstrate cells producing

$7S$ antibodies to erythrocytes. It is also possible to demonstrate cells producing antibodies to other antigens by using antigen-conjugated sheep erythrocytes in the detector system. The technical developments of this method are described by Dresser and Wortis [108].

V. CROSS-REACTIONS

No consideration of antigen–antibody reactions could be complete without some attention being given to the way in which specificity, or the lack of it, is expressed in serological reactions as a whole. It is by a study of cross-reactions that we can arrive at some assessment of the specificity of serological reactions in the context of biological materials as well as in immunochemistry. These two aspects are somewhat opposed, since in biology we are more concerned with the origin and function of materials, while in immunochemistry we are dealing with composition, configuration, and modes of function.

At first sight it would seem very simple to define a cross-reaction as a reaction in which an antibody produced in response to stimulation by one antigen reacts with another. (Exactly the same principles apply to cellular immunity. *See* Chapters 8 and 9.) Because one gets a cross-reaction between sheep red blood-cells and guinea-pig kidney, it is not necessary to abandon all ideas about specificity, since, as we know, the reaction between antigen and antibody is fundamentally one between determinant and antideterminant. Such a cross-reaction can therefore be entirely specific, and in this sense homologous. Indeed, Wiener and Wexler [109] go so far as to say that there is no such thing as a cross-reaction, and that all such reactions are simply the result of immunologically specific union.

Having said this much, we are now in a position to consider how cross-reactions might arise. There are four possibilities:—

1. The first of these has already been mentioned and concerns determinant structures that are found in antigenic material that comes from more than one source. Particularly where the biological source of the antigens appears very different, e.g., pneumococcal polysaccharide and human red-cell antigen, they are known as 'heterophile antigens'. Cross-reactions involving such antigens do not imply any heterogeneity of antideterminants; simply that configurationally identical determinants are to be found in diverse places.

2. Secondly, the more complex antigens, such as whole cells, contain a whole variety of antigens, some of which may be group- or species-specific and others strain-specific. Relevant examples in the fields of bacteriology and blood-group serology have been given in Chapter 2, ANTIGENS.

3. Thirdly, the antigenic stimulus may result in the production of a heterogeneous population of antibodies, each capable of reacting with its own specific determinant.

4. Fourthly, even a homogeneous population of antibody molecules may react with determinants that are similar to those that gave rise to their production in the first place. Indeed, this would be the rule rather than the exception: that determinants sufficiently the same, configurationally speaking, could always be found that would react with any given antibody.

It is more convenient to examine the above possibilities in terms of the strength of cross-reactions met with in the practice of serology. On this basis we can divide cross-reactions into four categories: (*a*) No cross-reactions observed; (*b*) Cross-reactions weaker than homologous; (*c*) Cross-reactions as strong or stronger than homologous; (*d*) Heterologous reactions only.

A. No Cross-reactions

This situation sheds no light on the problems we are considering and is adequately dealt with under (4) above (p. 225).

B. Cross-reactions Weaker than Homologous

This is, of course, the usual situation, otherwise specificity would have no meaning. All the possibilities envisaged above would give rise to this type of reaction, of which the first, dealing with heterophile antigens, was adequately covered in Chapter 2.

The second possibility dealing with the antigenic heterogeneity of cells also operates at molecular and submolecular levels. At the molecular level we need only take the example of immunoglobulins, which, apart from their antideterminant structures, carry Inv or Oz specificities on the light chains, and various Gm specificities on the heavy chains, as well as those specificities that serve to distinguish the different immunoglobulin classes from each other and divide light chains into two types.

At the submolecular level the complexities of antigenic relationships in the fields of blood-group serology and bacterial antigens have given rise to two explanations. The first postulates that different parts of a defined chemical structure, possibly overlapping sometimes, can act as the determinant, and that one or other of these determinants may be found in other related structures (*see Fig.* 52) [110]. The second postulates that different facets of the same three-dimensional structure act as determinants, so that the same sequence of sugars, for instance, could give rise to more than one specificity, apart from any configurational diversity such as that due to alpha- or beta-glycosidic links.

The third possibility envisages heterogeneity of combining sites due to inherent vagaries in the antibody-forming mechanisms of the host. All workers in fields of biology are familiar with the concept of a distribution about a mean. In the context of heterogeneity of antibody the 'mean' is represented by antibody with a specificity directed against the stimulating antigen; and deviations from the mean by antibodies with specificities directed against similar and therefore heterologous determinants. As Landsteiner put it, 'antibodies formed in response to one determinant group are, though related, not entirely identical' and 'vary to some extent around a main pattern' [111].

Finally, we can examine the situation where antibody is perfectly adapted to antigen, but is nevertheless able to react with determinants having slightly different configurations. No heterogeneity of antibody population is thereby implied, and in such circumstances one would expect that repeated absorptions with the heterologous antigen would ultimately abolish the homologous reaction as well as the heterologous one. However, even if the homologous reaction is only weakened we must still assume that some antibodies capable of reacting with more than one determinant were present in the original antiserum. In an example quoted by Landsteiner [111] an antiserum to the pentapeptide glycyl-glycyl-leucyl-glycyl-glycine is shown as reacting strongly with the homologous hapten, but also with ten other peptides containing glycine. Absorption with the pentapeptide of glycine abolished virtually all the

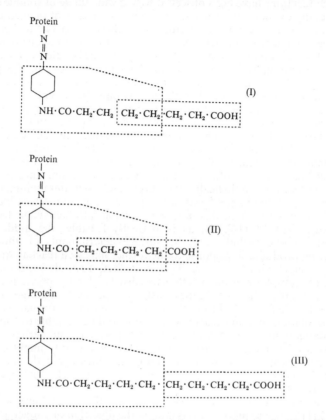

Fig. 52.—Cross-reactions between heterologous antigens. I, Homologous antigen; determinants (overlapping) outlined. II, Heterologous antigen; same determinants as in I. III, Heterologous antigen; same determinants as in I. *After Morgan* [110].

cross-reactions. Explanations that one poorly adapted antibody, capable of reacting with all the glycine-containing peptides, had been absorbed out may have been adequate at one time. We would perhaps be more likely to think in terms of antideterminants specific for the mono- or dipeptide of glycine, i.e., specific for a smaller area of hapten and therefore less discriminatory, rather than the vaguer concept of 'poorly adapted'.

Summarizing we can say that there are three mechanisms by which cross-reactions weaker than the homologous one can arise. These are due to: lack of absolute specificity, heterogeneity of antibody response, and heterogeneity of antigenic stimulus. It is perfectly possible, indeed, likely, that two or all three mechanisms are operative together in the same serological system.

C. Cross-reactions as Strong or Stronger than Homologous Reactions

Such reactions have been observed with a wide range of soluble antigens from complex molecules such as globulins to haptens of defined chemical structure. It is evident, in addition, that there is no bar to heterophile antigens giving rise to reactions as strong as the homologous one. Apart from this, reactions as strong as homologous ones could be visualized as arising occasionally by the same mechanisms as those in the previous category. More generally, however, and certainly in the case of stronger heterologous reactions, other explanations must be sought.

Modern theories of antibody production regard it as a multi-stage process in which one stage is the breakdown of the antigen molecule. With large molecules, such as immunoglobulins, 'hidden' determinants are exposed by digestion and they may form the specific inducers that determine the specificity of the immune response. The existence of such 'hidden' determinants is a simple matter of observation, since enzymatically digested, immunologically denatured, and even ammonium-sulphate-precipitated globulins can be shown to possess antigenic determinants that were not present, or at any rate not serologically active, in the native configuration [112–114]. If, as is perfectly feasible, the hidden determinants of one globulin are the surface determinants of another, an antiserum produced in response to the former may well react as strongly or more strongly with the latter. This is, in fact, a simple variation on the theme of multiple determinants that was discussed in the previous category.

Theoretically other possibilities exist. Acceptance that antigen performs some selective function during the process of antibody formation leads to the speculation that an occasional antigen would be unable to 'find' a cell that manufactures antibody of the correct specificity, but perhaps one that is only a fairly close approximation. Such an antibody might obviously react better with a 'heterologous' antigen. Once again this is a simple variation on a theme previously propounded, namely heterogeneity of antibody response.

An alternative possibility arises from the theory of 'subcomplementarity' [115], where more stress is laid on the digestion of antigen preceding antibody production. It is postulated that all antigenic determinants undergo some degree of structural alteration during this process. Antibody is produced that corresponds configurationally to the altered determinants, and when such antibody combines with the native determinant some degree of stress, and indeed configurational adaptation, is always involved. It is not impossible to visualize digestion of antigen proceeding to the point where a corresponding antibody is no longer able to conform to the structure of the native antigen, or would at least conform more readily to a heterologous antigen. This would not be an attractive hypothesis but for the evidence of immunological denaturation, i.e., of configurational change and therefore stress, resulting from the union of antigen and antibody.

D. Heterologous Reactions only

In the light of what has been said already it is obvious that if a host responds with the production of antibodies directed against hidden determinants, but not against surface determinants, then heterologous reactions without homologous ones will occur. The question is: Does the host ever respond in this way? It is not possible to answer such questions with certainty.

On the one hand, we have an accumulated body of evidence that the serum of normal human beings [112, 116] and of normal rabbits [117] contains antibodies to immunoglobulin fragments, i.e., hidden determinants. If this is true it is interesting to speculate whether a physiological mechanism for accelerating the disposal of denatured immunoglobulin is being described. As far as the present problem is concerned, such normal animals are immunologically tolerant towards surface determinants of their own immunoglobulins. Therefore in this sense the distinction between homologous and heterologous reactions does not arise. If they do produce antibodies against their own surface antigens then we immediately assume a pathological condition of the immune system, and indeed in such sera antibodies to both surface and hidden determinants occur together.

On the other hand, we have evidence such as that provided many years ago by Hooker and Boyd [118], when they prepared an antiserum against the hapten–protein conjugate, arsanildiazogelatin. This antiserum failed to precipitate the homologous antigen, but precipitated arsanildiazo-albumin instead. It is not easy to reconcile this finding with concepts of hidden determinants, since even the intact molecule (gelatin) is a poor antigen. A possible alternative would be some fault in transcription after specific induction or selection by antigen had occurred.

For the moment the only rational explanation of heterologous reactions stronger than the homologous ones that can be offered is that, by some idiosyncrasy of individual metabolism, no or little response is made to surface determinants, while the response to hidden determinants reaches higher levels. There is nothing inherently unlikely in such an idea since the response to a particular antigen or antigenic specificity is genetically determined, and immense variation in response is seen in any outbred population of animals.

It is clear from the foregoing discussion that, with the possible exception of the strongest heterologous reactions, no explanation other than the specificity of serological reactions needs to be invoked for cross-reactions. In other words, the immune response recognizes only physicochemical similarities, however diverse the biological source of materials. This being so, we can summarize by saying that cross-reactions can arise by three mechanisms:—

1. Because they carry a number of different determinants, in the native configuration and 'hidden', macromolecules stimulate the production of a population of antibodies. This is an antigen-induced heterogeneity of response.

2. Because the response to an antigenic stimulus is not uniform, individuals respond with a population of antibodies that vary about a 'mean'. This is a host-induced heterogeneity.

3. Because there is a limit to the resolving power or discriminating power of antibodies there must be some cross-reactions between antigens that present similar three-dimensional configurations. Discrimination may be affected by the size of the antideterminant, and this would constitute a host-induced heterogeneity of response.

Generally speaking, under natural conditions all three mechanisms will be operative. It is this complexity that has led biologists to consider cross-reactions as being in some way non-specific. From a biological point of view this may often be so when serological reactions are being used to

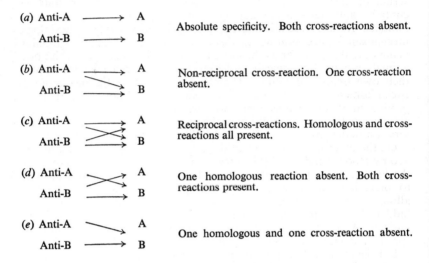

(a) Anti-A ⟶ A   Absolute specificity. Both cross-reactions absent.
     Anti-B ⟶ B

(b) Anti-A ⟶ A   Non-reciprocal cross-reaction. One cross-reaction
     Anti-B ⟶ B   absent.

(c) Anti-A ⟶ A   Reciprocal cross-reactions. Homologous and cross-
     Anti-B ⟶ B   reactions all present.

(d) Anti-A ⟶ A   One homologous reaction absent. Both cross-
     Anti-B ⟶ B   reactions present.

(e) Anti-A ⟶ A   One homologous and one cross-reaction absent.
     Anti-B ⟶ B

Fig. 53.—Reciprocal and non-reciprocal cross-reactions.

identify sources of material for instance. From the physicochemical point of view reactions are always 'specific'; and from the immunochemical point of view there are limitations to the resolving power of serological reactions.

In *Fig.* 53 are set out the various types of cross-reactions that could be encountered when two similar antigens are used to stimulate antibody production.

REFERENCES

1. PAULING, L. (1962), 'Molecular Structure and Intermolecular Forces', in *The Specificity of Serological Reactions* (rev. ed.), by LANDSTEINER, K., p. 275. New York: Dover.
2. ALBERT, A. (1965), *Selective Toxicity and Related Topics*, 4th ed. London: Methuen.
3. HARSHMAN, S., and NAJJAR, V. A. (1963), 'The Theory of Subcomplementarity as it pertains to the Mechanism of Antibody–antigen Reactions', *Immunodiagnosis of Helminthic Infections.* Monograph Series No. 22, *Am. J. Hyg.*
4. PAULING, L. (1948), 'Antibodies and Specific Biological Forces', *Endeavour*, 7, 43.
5. PRESSMAN, D. (1957), 'Molecular Complementariness in Antigen–antibody Systems', in *Molecular Structure and Biological Specificity* (ed. PAULING, L., and ITANO, H.). New York: American Institute of Biological Sciences.

6. PRESSMAN, D. (1963), 'The Chemical Nature of the Combining Site of Antibody Molecules', *Conceptual Advances in Immunology and Oncology. XVIth Annual Symposium on Fundamental Cancer Research, 1962, New York*. New York: Harper & Row.

7. BOYD, W. C. (1962), *Introduction to Immunochemical Specificity*. New York: Wiley.

8. SINGER, S. J. (1957), 'Physical-chemical Studies on the Nature of Antigen–antibody Reactions', *J. cell. comp. Physiol.*, **50**, Suppl. 1, 51.

9. HUGHES-JONES, N. C. (1963), 'Nature of the Reaction between Antigen and Antibody', *Br. med. Bull.*, **19**, 171.

10. OPPENHEIMER, J. H., and TAVERNETTI, R. R. (1962), 'Displacement of Thyroxine from Human Thyroxine-binding Globulin by Analogues of Hydantoin', *J. clin. Invest.*, **41**, 2213.

11. BOVET, D. (1959), 'Isosterism and Competitive Phenomena in Drugs; A Study of Structure-activity Relationships in Agents acting upon Automatic Effector Cells', *Science, N.Y.*, **129**, 1255.

12. SZENT-GYÖRGI, A. (1960), *Introduction to a Submolecular Biology*. New York: Academic.

13. SETLOW, R. B., and POLLARD, E. C. (1962), *Molecular Biophysics*. London: Pergamon.

14. KABAT, E. A., and MAYER, M. M. (1961), *Experimental Immunochemistry*, 2nd ed. Springfield, Ill.: Thomas.

15. KWAPINSKI, J. B. (1965), *Methods of Serological Research*. New York: Wiley.

16. WEIR, D. M., ed. (1967), *Handbook of Experimental Immunology*. Oxford: Blackwell Scientific Publications.

17. TALMAGE, D. W., and CANN, J. R. (1961), *The Chemistry of Immunity in Health and Disease*. Springfield, Ill.: Thomas.

18. HUGHES-JONES, N. C. (1963), 'Nature of the Reaction between Antigen and Antibody', *Br. med. Bull.*, **19**, 171.

19. PORTER, R. R., and PRESS, E. M. (1962), 'Immunochemistry', *A. Rev. Biochem.*, **31**, 625.

20. EPSTEIN, S. I., DOTY, P., and BOYD, W. C. (1956), 'Thermodynamic Study of Hapten-antibody Association', *J. Am. chem. Soc.*, **79**, 3380.

21. NISONOFF, A., and PRESSMAN, D. (1957), 'Closeness of Fit and Forces involved in the Reactions of Antibody Homologous to *p*-(*p'*-Azophenylazo)-benzoate Ion Group', *J. Am. chem. Soc.*, **79**, 1616.

22. SEHON, A. H. (1962), 'Antibody–antigen Reactions: Model Systems for the Specific Interaction of Biological Macromolecules', *Pure appl. Chem.*, **4**, 483.

23. STURTEVANT, J. M., WOFSY, L., and SINGER, S. J. (1961), 'Rate of a Hapten–antibody Reaction', *Science, N.Y.*, **134**, 1434.

24. EIGEN, M., and HAMMES, G. G. (1963), 'Elementary Steps in Enzyme Reactions (as studied by Relaxation Spectrometry)', *Adv. Enzymol.*, **25**, 1.

25. HUGHES-JONES, N. C., GARDNER, B., and TELFORD, R. (1963), 'Studies on the Reaction between the Blood Group Antibody Anti-D and Erythrocytes', *Biochem. J.*, **88**, 435.

26. GOLDMAN, M. (1968), *Fluorescent Antibody Methods*. New York: Academic.

27. EISEN, N. H. (1964), 'Equilibrium Dialysis for Measurements of Antibody–hapten Affinities', *Meth. med. Res.*, **10**, 106.

28. DEAN, H. R., and WEBB, R. A. (1926), 'The Influence of Optimal Proportions on Antigen and Antibody in the Serum Precipitation Reaction', *J. Path. Bact.*, **29**, 473.

29. BORDET, J. (1947), *Traité de l'Immunité dans les Maladies infectieuses*. Paris: Masson.

30. MARRACK, J. R. (1934), 'The Chemistry of Antigens and Antibodies', *Spec. Rep. Ser. med. Res. Coun.*, No. 194.

31. GOLDBERG, R. J. (1952), 'A Theory of Antigen–antibody Reactions. I, Theory of Reactions of Multivalent Antigen with Bivalent or Univalent Antibody', *J. Am. chem. Soc.*, **74**, 5715.

32. GOODMAN, M., RAMSEY, D. S., SIMPSON, W. L., and BRENNAN, M. J. (1957), 'The Use of Chicken Antiserum for the Rapid Determination of Plasma Protein Components. II, The Assay of Human Serum Orosomucoid', *J. Lab. clin. Med.*, **50**, 758.

33. EPSTEIN, S. I., and SINGER, S. J. (1958), 'Physical-chemical Studies of Soluble Antigen–antibody Complexes. IX, The Influence of pH on the Association of Divalent Hapten and Antibody', *J. Am. chem. Soc.*, **80**, 1274.

34. CAMPBELL, D. H., BLAKER, R. H., and PARDEE, A. B. (1948), 'The Purification and Properties of Antibody against p-Azophenylarsonic Acid and Molecular Weight Studies from Light Scattering Data', *J. Am. chem. Soc.*, **70**, 2496.

35. PRESSMAN, D. (1963), in the Discussion of a paper by MARRACK, J. R. [38].

36. SINGER, S. J., and PEPE, F. A. (1959), 'Physico-chemical Studies of Soluble Antigen–antibody Complexes. X, The Reaction of Univalent Protein Antigen with Antibody', *J. Am. chem. Soc.*, **81**, 3878.

37. POPE, C. G., and STEVENS, M. R. (1953), 'The Preparation of Non-flocculating Diphtheria Antitoxin by Absorption of Non-antitoxic Antibodies', *Br. J. exp. Path.*, **34**, 56.

38. MARRACK, J. R. (1963), 'The Nature of the Antigen–antibody Reaction', *Conceptual Advances in Immunology and Oncology. XVIth Annual Symposium on Fundamental Cancer Research, 1962, New York.* New York: Harper & Row.

39. NISONOFF, A., and PRESSMAN, D. (1959), 'Studies of the Combining Site of Anti-p-azobenzoate Antibody. Loss of Precipitating and Binding Capacities through Different Mechanisms of Acetylation', *J. Immun.*, **83**, 138.

40. BECHHOLD, E. (1905), 'Strukturbildung in Gallerten', *Z. phys. Chem.*, **52**, 185.

41. OUDIN, J. (1946), 'Méthode d'Analyse immunochimique par Précipitation spécifique en Milieu gélifié', *C. r. hebd. Séanc. Acad. Sci., Paris*, **222**, 115.

42. OUCHTERLONY, O. (1948), '*In vitro* Method for testing the Toxin-producing Capacity of Diphtheria Bacteria', *Acta path. microbiol. scand.*, **25**, 186.

43. ELEK, S. D. (1948), 'The Recognition of Toxicogenic Bacterial Strains *in vitro*', *Br. med. J.*, **1**, 493.

44. GRABAR, P., and WILLIAMS, C. A. (1953), 'Méthode permettant l'Étude conjugée des propriétés électrophorétiques et immunochimiques d'un Mélange de Protéines; Application au Serum sanguin', *Biochim. biophys. Acta*, **10**, 193.

45. COOMBS, R. R. A., and GELL, P. G. H. (1968), 'Diagnostic Methods in Serology and Immunopathology', in *Clinical Aspects of Immunology* (ed. GELL, P. G. H., and COOMBS, R. R. A.), 2nd ed. Oxford: Blackwell Scientific Publications.

46. GRABAR, P. (1964), 'Immunoelectrophoretic Analysis', in *Immunological Methods* (ed. ACKROYD, J. F.). Oxford: Blackwell Scientific Publications.

47. OUCHTERLONY, O. (1964), 'Gel-diffusion Techniques', in *Immunological Methods* (ed. ACKROYD, J. F.). Oxford: Blackwell Scientific Publications.

48. CROWLE, A. J. (1961), *Immunodiffusion*. New York: Academic.

49. OUCHTERLONY, O. (1962), 'Diffusion-in-gel Methods for Immunological Analysis, II', *Prog. Allergy*, **6**, 30.

50. PEETOOM, F. (1963), *The Agar Precipitation Technique and its Application as a Diagnostic and Analytical Method.* Edinburgh: Oliver & Boyd.

51. LANDOIS, L. (1875), *Die Transfusion des Blutes.* Leipzig: Vogel.

52. CREITE, A. (1869), 'Versuche über die Wirkung des Serumeiweisses nach Injektion in das Blut', *Z. rat. Med.*, 3rd series, **36**, 90.

53. GRUBER, M., and DURHAM, H. E. (1896), 'Theorie der activen und passiven Immunität gegen Cholera, Typhus und verwandte Krankheitsprocesse', *Münch. med. Wschr.*, **43**, 206.

54. CHARRIN, A., and ROGER, G. H. (1889), 'Note sur le Développement des Microbes pathogènes dans le Sérum des Animaux vaccinés', *C. r. Séanc. Soc. Biol.*, 9th series, 667.

55. SMITH, T., and REAGH, A. L. (1903), 'The Non-identity of Agglutinins acting upon the Flagella and upon the Body of Bacteria', *J. med. Res.*, **10**, 89.

56. EISENBERG, P., and VOLK, R. (1902), 'Untersuchungen über die Agglutination', *Z. Hyg. InfektKrankh.*, **40**, 155.

57. JOOS, A. (1901), 'Untersuchungen über den Mechanismus der Agglutination', *Z. Hyg. InfektKrankh.*, **36**, 422.

58. WEIL, E., and FELIX, A. (1917), 'Weitere Untersuchungen über das Wesen der Fleckfieberagglutination', *Wien klin. Wschr.*, **30**, 1509.

59. WEIL, E., and FELIX, A. (1920), 'Über den Doppeltypus der Rezeptoren in der Typhus-Paratyphus-Gruppe', *Z. ImmunForsch. exp. Ther. Orig.*, **29**, 24.

60. BORDET, J. (1899), 'Le Mécanisme de l'Agglutination', *Annls Inst. Pasteur, Paris*, **13**, 225.

61. YOKOYAMA, M., and FINLAYSON, J. S. (1961), 'The Effects of Salt Concentration, pH, and Certain Ions on the Agglutination of Human Erythrocytes by Isohaemagglutinins', *Transfusion, Philad.*, **1**, 175.
62. SHIBLEY, G. A. (1929), 'Studies in Agglutination. IV, The Agglutination Inhibition Zone', *J. exp. Med.*, **50**, 825.
63. ARKWRIGHT, J. A. (1931), *A System of Bacteriology in relation to Medicine*, vol. 6, chap. 12. Medical Research Council. London: H.M.S.O.
64. WIENER, A. S. (1944), 'A New Test (Blocking Test) for Rh Sensitization', *Proc. Soc. exp. Biol. Med.*, **56**, 173.
65. RACE, R. R. (1944), 'An "Incomplete" Antibody in Human Serum', *Nature, Lond.*, **153**, 771.
66. LODGE, T. W., ANDRESEN, J., and GOLD, E. R. (1965), 'Observations on Antibodies reacting with Adult and Cord Le(a-b-), with O_hLe(a-b-) Cells and a Soluble Antigen in Certain Salivas', *Vox Sang.*, **10**, 73.
67. JONES, F. S. (1928), 'Agglutination by Precipitin', *J. exp. Med.*, **48**, 183.
68. GURVICH, A. E. (1964), 'The Use of Antigens on an Insoluble Support', in *Immunological Methods* (ed. ACKROYD, J. F.). Oxford: Blackwell Scientific Publications.
69. SINGER, J. M., and PLOTZ, C. M. (1956), 'The Latex-fixation Test. I, Application to the Serologic Diagnosis of Rheumatoid Arthritis', *Am. J. Med.*, **21**, 888.
70. SINGER, J. M. (1961), 'The Latex-fixation Test in Rheumatic Diseases: A Review', *Am. J. Med.*, **31**, 766.
71. GOODMAN, H. C., and BOZICEVICH, J. (1964), 'Recently Developed Techniques for the Use of Inert Particles to detect Antigen–antibody Reactions', in *Immunological Methods* (ed. ACKROYD, J. F.). Oxford: Blackwell Scientific Publications.
72. PICK, E., and NELKEN, D. (1963), 'Passive Agglutination Tests. I, Bismuth Tannate Test', *Nature, Lond.*, **197**, 157.
73. GILBOA-GARBER, N., and NELKEN, D. (1963), 'Passive Agglutination Tests. II, Barium Sulfate Test', *Nature, Lond.*, **197**, 157.
74 GOLD, E. R. (1965), unpublished observations.
75. NICOLLE, C. (1898), 'Recherches sur la Substance agglutinée', *Annls Inst. Pasteur, Paris*, **12**, 151.
76. NETER, E. (1956), 'Bacterial Haemagglutination and Haemolysis', *Bact. Rev.*, **20**, 166.
77. WEINBACH, R. (1959), 'Die Verwendbarkeit formolbehandelter Erythrozyten als Antigenträger in der indirekten Haemagglutination, I and II', *Schweiz. Z. allg. Path. Bakt.*, **22**, 1 and 1043.
78. INGRAHAM, J. S. (1958), 'The Preparation and Use of Formalinised Erythrocytes with Attached Antigens or Haptens to Titrate Antibodies', *Proc. Soc. exp. Biol. Med.*, **99**, 452.
79. STAVITSKY, A. B. (1964), 'Haemagglutination and Haemagglutination Inhibition Reactions with Tannic Acid and *bis*-diazotised Benzidine–protein Conjugated Erythrocytes', in *Immunological Methods* (ed. ACKROYD, J. F.). Oxford: Blackwell Scientific Publications.
80. DANIEL, T. M., and STAVITSKY, A. B. (1964), 'Passive Haemagglutination in Study of Antigens and Antibodies', *Meth. med. Res.*, **10**, 152.
81. LING, N. R. (1961), 'The Attachment of Proteins to Aldehyde-tanned Cells', *Br. J. Haemat.*, **7**, 299.
82. GOLD, E. R., and FUDENBERG, H. H. (1967), 'Chromic Chloride: A Coupling Reagent for Passive Haemagglutination Reactions', *J. Immun.*, **99**, 859.
83. LING, N. R. (1961), 'The Coupling of Protein Antigens to Erythrocytes with Difluorodinitrobenzene', *Immunology*, **4**, 49.
84. RICHTER, M., and COHEN, J. (1965), 'Role of Non-specific Protein in the Sensitization of Red Blood Cells by Antigen', *Nature, Lond.*, **205**, 610.
85. GOLD, E. R. (1965), 'Studies on Human Antiglobulins', *Vox Sang.*, **10**, 731.
86. POLLACK, W., HAGER, H. J., RECKEL, R., TOREN, D. A., and SINGHER, H. O. (1965), 'A Study of the Forces involved in the Second Stage of Haemagglutination', *Transfusion, Philad.*, **5**, 158.
87. SOLOMON, J. M. (1964), 'Behaviour of Incomplete Antibodies in Quantitative Haemagglutination Reactions', *Transfusion, Philad.*, **4**, 101.
88. POLLACK, W. (1965), 'Some Physico-chemical Aspects of Haemagglutination', *Ann. N.Y. Acad. Sci.*, **127**, 892.

89. HUMMEL, K. (1964), 'Der Vorgang der Haemagglutination durch komplette und inkomplette Antikörper', *Dte GesundhWes.*, **20**, 321.
90. HUMMEL, K. (1955), *Die inkompletten Antikörper in der Immunbiologie*. Stuttgart: Fischer.
91. UHLENBRUCK, G., and KRUPE, M. (1965), 'Über ein merkwürdiges "Agglutinationsphänomen" enzymbehandelter Erythrozyten', *Ärztl. Lab.*, **11**, 114.
92. BROOKS, D. E., MILLAR, J. S., SEAMAN, G. V. F., and VASSAR, P. S. (1967), 'Some Physico-chemical Factors Relevant to Cellular Interactions', *J. cell. comp. Physiol.*, **69**, 155.
93. SALISBURY, A. J. CLARKE, J. A., and SHAND, W. S. (1968), 'Red Cell Surface Changes in Cell Agglutination', *Clin. exp. Immun.*, **3**, 313.
94. BANGHAM, A. D. (1964), 'The Adhesiveness of Leucocytes with Special Reference to Zeta Potential', *Ann. N.Y. Acad. Sci.*, **116**, 945.
95. UHLENBRUCK, G., and PROKOP, O. (1967), '"Inkomplette" Antikörper: ein Membranproblem', *Dt. med. Wschr.*, **92**, 940.
96. FULTON, F. (1958), 'The Measurement of Complement Fixation by Viruses', *Adv. Virus Res.*, **5**, 247.
97. RICE, C. E. (1948), 'The Inhibitory Effect of Certain Avian and Mammalian Antisera in Specific Complement Fixation Systems', *J. Immun.*, **59**, 365.
98. BORDET, J., and GAY, F. P. (1906), 'Sur les Relations des Sensibilactrices avec l'Aléxine', *Annls Inst. Pasteur, Paris*, **20**, 467.
99. BORDET, J., and STRENG, O. (1909), 'Les Phénomènes d'Adsorption et la Conglutinine du Sérum de Bœuf', *Zentbl. Bakt. ParasitKde*, Abt. I, Orig., **49**, 260.
100. COOMBS, R. R. A., COOMBS, A. M., and INGRAM, D. G. (1961), *The Serology of Conglutination and its Relation to Disease*. Oxford: Blackwell Scientific Publications.
101. COOMBS, R. R. A. (1964), 'Conglutinating Complement and its Use in Serological Tests', in *Immunological Methods* (ed. ACKROYD, J. F.). Oxford: Blackwell Scientific Publications.
102. LACHMANN, P. J. (1963), in *Clinical Aspects of Immunology* (ed. GELL, P. G. H., and COOMBS, R. R. A.). Oxford: Blackwell Scientific Publications.
103. LACHMANN, P. J., and COOMBS, R. R. A. (1965), 'Complement Conglutinin and Immunoconglutinins', in *Complement* (ed. WOLSTENHOLME, G. E. W., and KNIGHT, JULIE). Ciba Foundation Symposium. London: Churchill.
104. LACHMANN, P. J. (1967), 'Conglutinin and Immunoconglutinins', *Adv. Immun.*, **7**, 480.
105. LEON, M. A., YOKOBARI, R., and FROH, C. (1966), 'Chemical Specificity in the Conglutinin System and its Relation to Complement Structure', Complement Workshop Abstracts, *Immunochemistry*, **3**, 499.
106. GRABAR, P. (1963), in *Protides of the Biological Fluids* (ed. PEETERS, H.). Amsterdam: Elsevier.
107. JERNE, N. K., and NORDIN, A. A. (1963), 'Plaque Formation in Agar by Single Antibody-producing Cells', *Science, N.Y.*, **140**, 405.
108. DRESSER, D. W., and WORTIS, H. H. (1967), 'Localized Haemolysis in Gel', in *Handbook of Experimental Immunology* (ed. WEIR, D. M.). Oxford: Blackwell Scientific Publications.
109. WIENER, A. S., and WEXLER, I. B. (1952), 'The Mosaic Structure of Red Blood Cell Antigens', *Bact. Rev.*, **16**, 69.
110. MORGAN, W. T. J. (1937), 'A Conception of Immunological Specificity', *J. Hyg., Camb.*, **37**, 372.
111. LANDSTEINER, K. (1962), *The Specificity of Serological Reactions*, rev. ed. New York: Dover.
112. OSTERLAND, C. K., HARBOE, M., and KUNKEL, H. G. (1963), 'Anti-gamma Globulin Factors in Human Sera revealed by Enzymatic Splitting of Anti-Rh Antibodies', *Vox Sang.*, **8**, 133.
113. WILLIAMS, R. C., and KUNKEL, H. G. (1963), 'Antibodies to Rabbit-globulin after immunizing with Various Preparations of Autologous-globulin', *Proc. Soc. exp. Biol. Med.*, **112**, 554.
114. HAWKINS, J. D., and HAUROWITZ, F. (1961), 'The Recovery of Injected Antigens from Rat Spleens', *Biochem. J.*, **80**, 200.

115. HARSHMAN, S., ROBINSON, J. P., and NAJJAR, V. A. (1963), 'The Mechanism of Antibody–antigen Interaction and the Theory of Sub-complementarity between the Reactive Sites of Antibody and Antigen', *Ann. N.Y. Acad. Sci.*, **103**, 688.
116. EPSTEIN, W. V., and GROSS, D. (1964), 'Naturally Occurring Human Antibody reacting with Bence-Jones Proteins', *J. exp. Med.*, **120**, 733.
117. MANDY, W. J., and KORMEIER, L. C. (1966), 'Homoreactant: A Naturally Occurring Autoantibody in Rabbits', *Science, N.Y.*, **145**, 651.
118. HOOKER, S. B., and BOYD, W. C. (1933), 'The Antigenic Property of Gelatin-diazoarsanilic Acid', *J. Immun.*, **24**, 141.

CHAPTER 7

IMMEDIATE HYPERSENSITIVITY

By E. R. Gold and D. B. Peacock

I. Introduction

The immune hypersensitivities have proved over the years to be among the most, perhaps the most, confusing subdivisions of immunology for the student. This is partly because it is difficult to find grounds, teleologically, for the appearance of immune reactions that are often harmful to the host even to the point of causing death; and partly because it has been unclear whether hypersensitivity was the consequence of pathological changes in the immune system or not, and whether the increased resistance to infection noted in some hypersensitivity states is simply associated with or the direct result of it. Apart from this, there are two quite distinct kinds of hypersensitivity which arise through fundamentally different mechanisms. The so-called 'immediate hypersensitivities' are associated with circulating antibody; delayed hypersensitivity-type reactions are an expression of 'cell-mediated' or 'cellular' immunity. Delayed hypersensitivity will be dealt with separately in subsequent chapters, partly in order to reduce the confusion that results from dealing with two kinds of hypersensitivity together, but chiefly because the basic mechanisms are entirely different and this is therefore a logical division.

The immediate hypersensitivities can themselves be divided into two categories: (1) Those in which antigen reacts with antibody situated at the cell surface; and (2) those in which antigen reacts with precipitating antibody. Under the first category would fall such conditions as anaphylaxis, asthma, and hay fever; under the second, the Arthus reaction and serum sickness.

Clinically a third category, of drug sensitivity, might be said to exist. In conditions such as sedormid purpura the drug behaves as a determinant when attached to cell surfaces, with a consequent production of antibodies and cellular destruction. In this case circulating antibody reacts with antigen situated at the cell surface and the condition is more analogous to an auto-immune disease (Chapter 12) than to immune hypersensitivity. Of course, drugs may also combine with body proteins after administration and, acting as antigenic determinants, give rise to immediate hypersensitivities of either category (1) or (2). It is also true to say that clinical syndromes rarely fall neatly into a single category, and that mixtures of the above, with or without elements of delayed hypersensitivity, and other elements of humoral immunity are the rule rather than the exception. Nevertheless, it is often possible to recognize predominating features during the course of an immunological response, and it is helpful to make clear-cut distinctions between them. We shall therefore concern ourselves primarily with the classic experimental situations of anaphylaxis and Arthus reaction with occasional reference to clinical conditions in man.

II. ANAPHYLAXIS

The best-known, and in some ways the best-understood, hypersensitive response is anaphylaxis. It can be demonstrated by sensitizing an animal with suitably small single, or multiple, injections of antigen and subsequently challenging with a larger dose. In the guinea-pig 0·0001 ml. of horse serum may be sufficient to sensitize, and the animal may be responsive in 10–21 days. A characteristically striking response is obtained within a few minutes of challenge. In severe cases there is gross dyspnoea, due to an acute contraction of bronchiolar musculature, which may terminate in death by suffocation. At post-mortem the lungs are markedly distended and bloodless.

The discovery of anaphylaxis is generally attributed to Portier and Richet, in 1902 [1], but Bordet mentions [2] that as long ago as 1839 Magendie had observed a similar sequence of events in rabbits injected with ovalbumin, and that later Flexner had also done so following the injection of whole serum. However, the systematic study of anaphylaxis was certainly initiated by Portier, who also coined the expression 'phylaxis', meaning 'protection'.

The early immunologists were not unnaturally deeply concerned with the benefits deriving from the artificial induction of immunity to all manner of materials, but particularly toxins and poisons. During a scientific expedition at sea Richet, who had already observed anaphylaxis in dogs, attempted to immunize dogs against a poison extracted from sea anemones. A dose of 0·1 g. per kg. of body-weight was sufficient to kill the animals. His attempts at immunization with sublethal doses far from increasing resistance actually led to the death of dogs given doses of toxin that were completely innocuous for previously untreated dogs. The fact that the anemone extract was a poison was really incidental and merely provided a dramatic backcloth to the experiments. The distinction between toxic and hypersensitive reactions is often of some practical importance, however, as, for instance, in the Schick and Dick tests for susceptibility to diphtheria and scarlet fever respectively, where toxic reactions to the test material must be distinguished from hypersensitive ones. A similar situation exists with respect to phototoxic and photo-allergic reactions.

Although anaphylaxis has been widely studied for many years now, there are still extensive gaps in our understanding of these reactions and of the mechanisms through which shock is produced. Broadly speaking, it can be said that the initiating antigen–antibody reaction occurring at the surface of *target cells* leads to the release or activation of *biochemical mediators* that ultimately cause the contraction of smooth muscle in a susceptible *shock organ*, thereby inducing the typical picture of anaphylaxis in a particular animal species.

The experimental approach to the study of the mechanism underlying anaphylactic shock has been of three kinds, systemic, local, and *in vitro*, each method yielding information on different aspects of the same basic event. The study of systemic anaphylaxis has led to a wider understanding of the role played by 'primary target cells', i.e., where antigen–antibody reactions occur, of the biochemical mediators released from the target cells, and of the susceptible host organ, 'shock organ', to such mediators. Local cutaneous and passive cutaneous anaphylaxis reactions lend themselves particularly to quantitative studies of antigen–antibody interaction and have therefore illuminated the role played by antibody. *In vitro* techniques with isolated perfused organs or washed tissues have simplified the study of the pharmacological mediators.

One of the first things to be noticed about anaphylactic shock is that it pursues a very different course in different animal species. These differences are attributable to the organ principally affected in the species concerned. In the *guinea-pig* the shock organ is the lung, and more particularly the smooth muscle of the bronchioles. The immediate cause of contraction is of neuromuscular origin. If the animal dies after 5 minutes it is more likely to be due to oedema of the lung than to bronchiolar constriction. In the *rabbit* the most significant event is intermittent constriction of the branches of the pulmonary artery, and the animal dies in right-sided heart failure. Anaphylaxis in the rabbit is probably also associated with the deposition of antigen–antibody aggregates and platelet–leucocyte clumps in the lung capillaries. In a very general sense the lung is again the shock organ, but more particularly the musculature of the arterial walls, with platelets and leucocytes playing an undetermined role. In the *dog* a general dilatation of small blood-vessels is found. The organs most affected are kidney, spleen, and liver, with the liver occupying a central position in that its exclusion from the general circulation renders the animal insusceptible to shock. Otherwise a large volume of blood is 'lost' to the general circulation and the animal dies from 'haemorrhage' into its own vascular bed.

The mouse is of some interest in that it was first thought to be highly resistant to anaphylactic shock. However, the resistance varies from strain to strain, being genetically determined, and must be due to the failure of some strains to produce the appropriate kind of antibody since they can be sensitized passively with sera from other animals. The mechanism operating in non-fatal shock in the mouse seems to be one of general constriction of the vascular bed. In more severe cases this is followed by extreme dilatation of blood-vessels with a consequent fall in blood-pressure. At post-mortem the most striking features are congestion and haemorrhage of the stomach and intestines. These are therefore considered to be the shock organs.

It should be evident by now that anaphylaxis presents very different clinical pictures in different species of animal. In each case, however, the vascular musculature appears to be heavily involved, although the organ is not always the same. The question must arise, therefore, how is this distinction maintained? Is it perhaps that different biochemical (pharmacological) mediators are produced in response to the initial stimulation? We do not know the answers to these questions, but we can now go on to consider those substances that play an active part in inducing shocking mechanisms.

III. Biochemical Mediators

Only four biochemically active agents are known with certainty to mediate anaphylaxis. These are histamine, serotonin (5-hydroxytryptamine), bradykinin (a decapeptide), and slow-reacting substance-anaphylaxis (SRS-A). The interplay of these four factors, taken together with their local concentration, and the tissue susceptibility of the animal species concerned principally determines the various manifestations of anaphylactic shock that are seen.

As we have seen, the shock organ in the guinea-pig is the lung. Its importance receives confirmation from the fact that localization of antigen in this organ has been observed repeatedly. For instance, Dixon and Warren noted the uptake of labelled antigen by the lung in anaphylactic guinea-pigs [3], and the amount taken up has been found to be proportional to the intensity of shock [4]. The mediator is histamine, as evidenced by an associated increase in blood histamine in anaphylactic shock, in the level of histamine in the perfusate of sensitized, isolated organs, and by the protection against systemic anaphylaxis afforded by antihistamine drugs. Acute anaphylaxis in the guinea-pig is also associated with a marked degranulation of mast cells in the lung. Taken in conjunction with the known content of histamine loosely bound to heparin in these granules, this is an additional piece of corroborative, though circumstantial, evidence.

If a relatively large amount of antigen is given to the sensitized guinea-pig by the subcutaneous or intraperitoneal routes, instead of a small amount intravenously, respiratory distress is often absent, but death may still supervene after a period of hours. There is perhaps no convincing evidence that another of the mediators is responsible, but administration of SRS-A does cause some constriction of bronchiolar musculature [5].

The histamine content of guinea-pig lung varies considerably, from 5 to 25 μg., contrasted with the sensitivity of the bronchiolar smooth muscle, expressed as the minimum effective dose, of 0·4 μg. Histamine content is also closely correlated with mast cell population in the guinea-pig lung, and in anaphylactic shock a decrease in the histamine content of lung tissue is associated with a simultaneous drop in the number of mast cells and degranulation of the remainder [6]. The mast cell would then appear to be the prime target cell in guinea-pig lung, and if this is so we must suppose that the antigen–antibody reaction takes place at the cell surface. In this case the requirements of local concentration of pharmacological mediator and sensitive tissue are amply fulfilled. The sequence of events is none the less complicated, and Austen and Humphrey observe that 'the reaction of antigen with cell-fixed antibody releases an intracellular pro-enzyme that reacts with calcium to form a chymotrypsin-like enzyme; this in turn reacts with bound histamine, and releases it from the cell to produce the smooth-muscle contraction and vascular events that characterize acute shock' [7].

The very great similarity between the effects resulting from the administration of histamine to guinea-pigs and anaphylaxis in the same animal adds weight to the postulated role of mast cells in this immunological response. There are others, however, who hold that mast cells could be secondarily involved, following damage to other tissue cells by the antigen–antibody reaction, and, in addition, Benditt and Lagunoff conclude that 'histamine may only be a contributor to the phenomena of acute anaphylaxis even in guinea-pigs' [8]. Even so, the picture of systemic anaphylaxis is by no means as clear-cut in other animals, and, though mast cells and histamine can frequently be implicated, the action of antihistamines is not usually nearly as effective as it is in guinea-pigs.

Systemic anaphylaxis in the rabbit is associated with circulatory collapse and dilatation of the right heart, brought about by mechanical obstruction it is thought, as well as by the action of pharmacological mediators. The mechanical effect of the eosinophilic clumps found in the lung capillaries could well be enhanced by the release of histamine and serotonin from trapped platelets. The release of SRS-A *in vitro* and of plasma kinin (bradykinin) *in vivo* have also both been observed in the rabbit [*see* 7], so that all four recognized mediators may be acting together in this host. Neither antihistamines nor previous serotonin depletion protect the animal against anaphylactic shock.

Histamine, serotonin, and plasma kinin have all been implicated in the mouse at one time or another [7]. However, systemic anaphylaxis is not affected by antihistamines, while serotonin depletion has a marked effect. Nevertheless, the evidence is circumstantial at best, since neither method is specific in the sense that there are no side-effects.

With the dog, we return to a simpler picture with histamine apparently playing the predominant role, though the lung is no longer the shock organ. Circulatory collapse with congestion and stasis of the abdominal organs

are the principal findings and are associated with a high content of histamine in the liver (8–110 μg. per g.). Dog liver also contains considerable
amounts of serotonin, but it does not seem to be depleted during systemic
anaphylaxis. The levels of plasma kinin in the blood do not correlate well
with the degree of shock either.

Acute anaphylaxis in man is characterized by severe respiratory distress,
followed by circulatory collapse. Information on the pharmacological
mediators is fragmentary. Histamine and slow-reacting substance have
been released *in vitro* from the lung tissue of hypersensitive individuals by
exposure to the appropriate antigen. The human bronchiole appears to be
particularly susceptible to the action of SRS-A *in vitro* [9], but Austen
believes that 'extensive involvement of the *upper* respiratory region may be
an important species characteristic' in man [10].

Over the past few years a good deal of attention has been devoted to the
study of pharmacological mediators. In spite of this, relatively little is
known about their physiological activity; and this is all the more surprising
in the case of histamine which was found in animal tissues as long ago as
1910.

The pharmacological action of histamine (β-imidazolylethylamine) is
one of dilatation of capillaries, increase in permeability of venules,
contraction or dilatation of arterioles, depending on the species of animal,
and in general contraction of smooth muscle, though again with marked
species variation. As we have seen, histamine reproduces many of the
characteristic events in anaphylactic shock, notably the constriction of
bronchioles and the dilatation of the vascular bed. The latter, together with
increased vascular permeability, could account for the laryngeal oedema
associated with anaphylactic reactions in man. Histamine is found as such
in normal tissues, and in sensitized tissues before they are subjected to
shock. Presumably it exerts some control over smooth muscle, though how
such control is exercised is not understood at present. Mast cells can
release histamine without undergoing disruption, indeed probably without
degranulation as well, although the latter is often taken as indirect evidence
of release.

Serotonin has been found in platelets and chromaffinic cells; gut and
brain contain the largest amounts. Among its pharmacological actions is
stimulation of smooth muscle, though with a variable action on autonomic
ganglia depending on dose. Gangliosides have been implicated as receptors for serotonin [11].

Of the plasma kinins only the decapeptide, bradykinin, has a known
role as an active vasodilator and the capacity to increase vascular permeability and stimulate smooth muscle. Also known as kallidin-10, it occurs
in the body as a pseudoglobulin precursor from which it is released by
enzymatic action.

Slow-reacting substance was originally obtained from isolated lung
tissue by the action of the lecithinase A of cobra venom. It is probably an
unsaturated fatty acid and seems to occur in a precursor form since it has
not been detected in isolated sensitized tissues but does appear in the
perfusate after the tissue has been shocked. Slow-reacting substance
contracts guinea-pig ileum rather more slowly than does histamine; it also
acts on rabbit jejunum and human bronchiolar muscle, and some other

vertebrate muscle tissues, but on the whole it is remarkably selective in its stimulation.

The role played by any one of these mediators in anaphylactic shock is partly determined by the species of animal and partly by the kind of tissue or cell investigated. The importance of local concentration as well as sensitivity of tissues is underlined by the very variable concentrations found in different animals and their response to particular mediators. For instance, the histamine content of mast cells in dog tissue is 7–16 $\mu\mu$g., while that of rat mast cells is 10–40 $\mu\mu$g.; but these relative amounts in no way reflect the relative sensitivities of dog and rat to shock. Similarly, Austen and Humphrey [7] compare serotonin and histamine contents of the lungs in cat, dog, rat, guinea-pig, rabbit, and man and find a positive correlation only with serotonin in the rat. Possibly even more remarkable is the situation in the guinea-pig, where there are large numbers of mast cells in the ileum, an organ which is highly sensitive to the action of histamine, and yet the ileum is not the shock organ, nor is there evidence of histamine release at the site during systemic anaphylaxis.

So far we have listed four kinds of chemical mediators that are known to contribute to the general picture of anaphylactic shock. In very few instances, if any, can we be satisfied that a single one or any combination of these substances allows a complete explanation of all the phenomena we observe in an animal. The organs, tissues, and even cell types we have been considering are usually capable of releasing more than one of these mediators, and possibly other pharmacologically active substances as well. The participation of the latter in anaphylactic reactions has been suggested from time to time. Some of them, e.g., acetylcholine, are no longer regarded as mediators. The role of others, such as heparin which is frequently released with histamine from mast cells, is accepted by some authors [12] but not by others [7]. There certainly remain other mediators to be discovered and possibly the role of some known agents to be defined.

To sum up, we have the situation where anaphylaxis is often expressed in different ways in different animals. In some cases this may be due to the production of mediators in different concentrations, in other cases to the different susceptibility of those organs exposed to their action. It is remarkable, too, that extensive similarities at the molecular level can be found between tissues as different as unstriated molluscan muscle and striated vertebrate muscle [13]. At the other extreme in anaphylaxis we can see smooth muscle from different sites in the same animal reacting quite differently to the same stimulus, e.g., SRS-A produces contraction of the ileum but not of the bronchiole of the guinea-pig. It remains a task for the future to determine the molecular basis for such fine distinctions.

IV. PASSIVE CUTANEOUS ANAPHYLAXIS

Passive cutaneous anaphylaxis (PCA) is a local form of experimental immediate hypersensitivity. It provides a simplified model in which this type of reaction can be studied, and because of its great sensitivity in detecting antibody it has also been widely used in the examination of more basic problems of immunology. The test has been comprehensively reviewed by Ovary [14]. It has a counterpart in man: the Prausnitz-Küstner reaction.

The PCA is performed by injecting antiserum into the skin of an animal, usually the guinea-pig; after a few hours antigen is injected intravenously, and at the same time as or just after the injection of a dye such as Evans blue. During the time after injecting the antiserum, antibody becomes fixed to cells at the injection site, and when antigen is injected subsequently it reacts with the 'fixed' antibody to release pharmacologically active agents that increase vascular dilatation and permeability. The injected dye escapes from the blood-vessels at the site to stain the reaction site and render it more visible and measurable quantitatively. In man there is a characteristic weal and flare reaction at the injection site of antibody which is readily visible without the addition of dye.

It is evident that skin fixation depends on complementary sites being present on cells situated in skin and on reactive antibody, and the PCA reaction can take place only if both are present. One of the most confusing aspects of immediate hypersensitivity has been that, though passive transfer of hypersensitivity works perfectly conventionally within the species boundary, it is also possible to elicit hypersensitive reactions in heterologous species in the absence of such reactions in the donor animal, i.e., when the donor is not hypersensitive itself. Certain combinations are extremely sensitive in this respect, e.g., PCA reactions can be elicited in guinea-pig skin with as little as $0.003 \mu g.$ of antibody nitrogen of rabbit antibody. It is this kind of quantitative approach that has led to the recognition that reagins (antibodies causing hypersensitivity in the homologous species) are not necessarily involved when the species barrier is crossed.

In certain experimental situations it is sometimes convenient to change the way in which antigen and antibody are administered. In the particular situation where immunoglobulins are being studied antigenically the sensitivity of the PCA reaction can be used by taking advantage of the fact that the antigen (immunoglobulin) from a heterologous species will attach to guinea-pig skin. Anti-immunoglobulin is then injected intravenously after a suitable time interval. This is the so-called 'reverse passive cutaneous anaphylaxis' (RPCA) reaction. It has also been used to determine that the skin-fixing site on sensitizing antibody is on the Fc fragment of the molecule.

V. REAGINS

In man skin-sensitizing antibodies have been called 'reagins'. Because such antibodies are associated with immediate hypersensitivity-type reactions, we shall use 'reagins' as a generic term for all antibodies, in all species of animal, that give rise to hypersensitivity reactions in the homologous species.

The subject of reagins in man was informatively reviewed by Stanworth in 1963 [15], at which time he was constrained to say that 'reagin still represents a nebulous concept to many immunologists, some doubting the legitimacy of its classification as an antibody'. Happily there are few who still find themselves in this dilemma, since the work of Ovary, Benacerraf, and Bloch [16] and of White, Jenkins, and Wilkinson [17] identified

γ_1-immunoglobulin of guinea-pigs with the initiation of hypersensitivity reactions. In the field of human reagins the work of Bennich and Johansson and of Ishizaka and his colleagues culminated in the adoption of IgE as the name of a new class of immunoglobulin (*see* p. 117), which Ishizaka and his colleagues had shown was associated with reaginic activity in man [18].

With the characterization of anaphylactic-type antibodies in man and guinea-pig a great many puzzling features of immediate hypersensitivity reactions will fall into place, and a great many more avenues be opened to systematic investigation. Indeed, the importance of these advances in knowledge to this field of study cannot be overestimated. To mention just one example: in order to advance our understanding of the mechanisms of hypersensitivity an *in vitro* method of assaying human reagins was a paramount necessity [15], and eventually a rather complex but reasonably accurate method was devised [19]. Now, with the designation of immunoglobulin classes already applied to the immunoglobulins responsible for these reactions it is simply a matter of applying some quantitative precipitation technique using antisera to γ_1 and IgE respectively.

The properties of these two immunoglobulins are rather different, apart from any difference in antigenic structure that they may show, and it is obviously of interest to compare them and the kind of hypersensitivity responses for which they are responsible.

The immunoglobulin pattern in the guinea-pig is rather different from that in man and approaches much more closely that of the mouse (*see* Chapter 3). The immunoglobulin γ_1 has the same sedimentation coefficient ($7S$) but a higher electrophoretic mobility than γ_2. It is present in guinea-pig (and mouse) serum at a lower concentration than γ_2, but is nevertheless much more abundant than the IgE of human serum. Anaphylactic-type antibodies in the mouse and guinea-pig also require a relatively short time in which to fix to, or sensitize, tissues: for the PCA reaction this is 1 hour in the mouse and 3–5 hours in the guinea-pig. It should be remembered that these antibodies are species restricted, i.e., they do not sensitize tissues outside their own species. In parallel with the speed of sensitization the duration of the reaction is comparatively short: greatly reduced reactions are obtained at 24 hours in the mouse, and at 48 hours in the guinea-pig, following passive sensitization [20].

In contrast to the above pattern, human-type reaginic antibodies are found in the rat, rabbit, and dog, as well as in man, of course. They have not as yet been characterized as IgE, but in general their biological properties appear similar.

In the first place, the ordinary soluble antigens do not give rise to high titres of anaphylactic antibody, even with the help of adjuvants; PCA titres above 50 are only rarely seen [21]. In the rat peak titres are reached on the twelfth day after stimulation and antibody is not detectable after 30 days [22].

PCA reactions in the rat, obtained with rat antibody, attain their maximum 16–72 hours after sensitization, and may be elicited for a further 30 days. Other species in this group are probably comparable. The length of time over which reactions can be elicited after passive sensitization is an indication of the durability of this union.

The distinction between human- or IgE-type reagins and γ_1 antibodies can thus be made on biological grounds in that the former are usually present only in low titre, require a relatively long period for fixation to target cells, and effect a relatively long period of sensitization once fixed.

Our understanding of these distinctive roles was severely hampered in the past by the tacit assumption that since immediate hypersensitivity could be transferred passively by serum the same class of immunoglobulin initiated the hypersensitive response in both donor and recipient. This is indeed so with the transfer of isologous antibody, i.e., within a species; but between species the situation is different, and passive cutaneous anaphylaxis reactions can often be elicited, for instance in the guinea-pig, with γ_1 and IgG antibodies [23]. We are faced, therefore, with a paradoxical situation in which reactive sites for target cells within a species are found on immunoglobulins of a certain class, but when immunoglobulins from another species are used to induce sensitization, these neither belong to the same immunoglobulin class nor induce hypersensitivity in the donor. How, or why, they should carry specific sites of attachment for cell receptors in a heterologous species remains a mystery for the moment.

Structure of Reagins

Now that reaginic activity has been definitely associated with certain immunoglobulin classes with molecular weights of around 160,000, it should be assumed that they are built on the same general principles as other similar immunoglobulins until proved otherwise. We already know enough of their structure to render this hypothesis likely (*see* Chapter 3), and we can therefore postulate that each molecule contains two combining sites for antigen. There is, however, no direct evidence of this. What information we have that bears directly on this issue comes from PCA reactions employing heterologous systems.

As we have seen in earlier chapters, antibodies can be broken down and hybrid molecules reconstituted that carry combining sites of different specificities. These are truly univalent antibodies with respect to one specificity and can be used to sensitize tissues in the PCA reaction [14]. On the other hand, removal of the Fc fragment but leaving the combining sites intact destroys reaginic activity. It would seem, therefore, that fixation to tissues but not divalent antibody is necessary for sensitization. Monovalent hapten, on the other hand, is not adequate to produce a PCA reaction [14], so we must conclude that either both valencies of one antibody molecule or the formation of an antigen bridge between two molecules are needed to set off the release of pharmacological mediators under these conditions.

VI. BLOCKING ANTIBODIES

Hypersensitivity to a particular antigen can be abolished in laboratory animals by the rather simple expedient of passive sensitization to another antigen. Time has to be allowed for the transferred antibody to supplant reagin already fixed to tissue cells, and this time will vary according to the animal species and firmness of union. Heterologous and isologous immunoglobulin can be used.

There are a number of reasons why such methods should not be employed to treat patients with troublesome hypersensitivities such as hay fever, asthma, etc. First, there is the danger of introducing a new hypersensitivity; second, the limited duration of the protection afforded; third, the relative ineffectiveness of subsequent passive transfer, especially when heterologous serum was used, due to an accelerated secondary response by the patient against the injected serum; fourth, the dangers associated with the introduction of foreign protein into individuals who already show a propensity to develop hypersensitivity to foreign protein.

The only real alternative to such methods is practised quite widely and consists of the gradual desensitization of an individual with very small doses of antigen, in order to avoid untoward results, and then the build up of immunoglobulins of other classes with the repeated injection of antigen. Natural experience of the antigen will then be met with a humoral barrier of specific antibody. The chief drawback from an immunological point of view is that the active immunity induced is short-lived, and protective levels of antibody subside usually within a month or two. It is evident that passive immunity could be operated in this manner, too, but the same objections to the use of heterologous sera in such subjects apply here as above.

VII. ANAPHYLATOXIN

Over fifty years ago it was first noted that the addition of immune precipitates to serum led to the production of substances that would induce shock, so-called 'anaphylactoid' shock, in susceptible animals such as guinea-pigs. The term 'anaphylatoxin' was coined to describe this property of serum and as the years went by additional ways of inducing its formation were discovered. Early on it was found that the incubation of kaolin with normal serum had the same effect, and then that this property was shared by agar, inulin, talc, starch, and barium sulphate. Other polysaccharides added to the list in later years are dextran and zymosan.

It is not necessary to suppose that the pathway leading to the formation of anaphylatoxin is exactly the same in each of the above cases. However, Dias da Silva, Eisele, and Lepow conclude that complement is undoubtedly involved in the formation of anaphylatoxin [24], and that it is probably the product of interaction between C 1 esterase, C 4, C 2, and C 3. Cochrane and Müller-Eberhard believe that anaphylatoxin is not one substance but two, derived from the third and fifth components of complement respectively [25].

At all events, whatever its nature, the liberation of anaphylatoxin leads to the release of histamine with its usual accompaniment of mast-cell degranulation. It must be concluded that anaphylatoxin is an initiator, rather than a mediator, of anaphylactoid shock. As such, it plays a part more nearly analogous to reagin than to the pharmacological mediators.

Broder, Baumal, and Keystone [26] have devised methods of distinguishing between a number of those macromolecular substances, such as aggregated immunoglobulin, anti-immunoglobulin, soluble antigen–antibody complexes, Forssman, and other heterophile antibodies, as well as anaphylatoxin itself, that are known to induce shock. A number of these are also known to fix complement, but it is conceivable that others like the heterophile antibodies could react directly with antigens of the cell surfaces and so initiate shock by direct action, in the manner of reagins.

There are evidently many paths leading to the release of pharmacological mediators, just as there are many mediators that induce shock. As we shall see below, complement and anaphylatoxin are not implicated at all in the immediate hypersensitivities of the Arthus reaction and serum sickness. However, with the increasing availability of defined complement components, as well as of animal strains deficient in defined components, many of the obscurities associated with anaphylactoid shock could soon be clarified.

VIII. Arthus Reaction

As originally described, the Arthus reaction consists of tissue injury occurring at the site of antigen inoculation following repeated administrations of the same antigen [27]. Actually it is seen in its simplest form without a number of complicating factors as the passive Arthus reaction, when antibody is injected intravenously and antigen locally under the skin. The tissue injury is initiated by the formation of antigen–antibody complexes, with a subsequent alteration in vascular permeability followed by a characteristic infiltration of the inoculation site with polymorphonuclear leucocytes during the first 24 hours. This is then followed by a less dense infiltration of mononuclear cells—a reaction more in keeping with the delayed hypersensitivity type of reaction, which has led to the suggestion that the Arthus reaction is a mixture of immediate and delayed hypersensitivity responses.

What is certain is that, in the Arthus reaction, precipitating antibody, rather than reaginic-type antibody, is required. This distinguishes sharply the Arthus reaction from anaphylaxis.

IX. Serum Sickness

Chiefly noted in man in connexion with immune serum therapy, serum sickness has also been widely studied as an experimental disease in laboratory animals [28].

In the unsensitized patient serum sickness usually comes on 8–12 days after the injection of a large dose of heterologous (e.g., horse) serum. The manifestations may include a rise in temperature, itching, skin rashes, and joint pains. In the experimental situation it is fairly clear that we are dealing with a kind of systemic Arthus reaction in which pharmacological mediators are released as a result of combination of humoral antibody with antigen, with the formation of soluble antigen–antibody complexes in the region of slight antigen excess. Recent investigations suggest that only complexes with sedimentation constants greater than $19S$ undergo vascular localization [29]. Attachment to the endothelium of blood-vessels with associated release of pharmacological mediators from trapped platelets would seem to initiate the mechanism of tissue damage, a situation that is strikingly reminiscent of anaphylaxis in the rabbit. It is also reminiscent of the formation of anaphylatoxin, but Cochrane and Hawkins could find no evidence that complement was involved in the localization of complexes in the glomeruli of guinea-pigs [29].

The study of serum sickness in man has on the whole been less rewarding, since the situation is nearly always much more confused than in the experimental animal. In the first place, the injection of whole serum has usually been the starting-point, and with the multiplicity of antigens that that represents it is no wonder that investigators have found it impossible to identify the particular stimulus that leads to the hypersensitive response.

It is sometimes a source of confusion that an immediate hypersensitivity reaction does not occur until after a week has elapsed. The explanation is, of course, that time has to be allowed for antibody production to get under way. In some instances a second injection will induce a truly immediate reaction with preformed antibody; a circumstance that must not be confused with anaphylactic shock in an individual who is hypersensitive or 'allergic' to, for instance, horse dander.

X. Shwartzman Reaction

The characteristic lesion of the Shwartzman reaction (SR) is haemorrhagic necrosis of certain organs following two suitably placed and spaced injections of endotoxin. Among laboratory animals the rabbit is uniquely susceptible to the generalized form of the SR. The local SR is obtained if a rabbit is inoculated intradermally with a small dose of endotoxin and challenged 24 hours later with an intravenous dose of the same preparation. Petechial haemorrhages appear at the site of primary inoculation within a few hours of challenge, rapidly coalesce, and progress to complete necrosis within a further 24 hours. The interval of time between so-called preparative and provocative doses is fairly critical with outside limits of around 6 and 48 hours. The generalized SR is elicited if both doses are given intravenously; it is characterized macroscopically by bilateral, haemorrhagic, cortical necrosis of the kidneys. Histologically the two reactions present quite distinct features: cellular thrombi with enmeshed leucocytes and platelets are found in the small vessels of the dermis, while thrombi consisting almost entirely of fibrin occlude the glomerular capillaries.

On the face of it, immunological mechanisms would appear to have little to do with these reactions. There is evidently no time for antibody to attain significant levels before the acute reaction is virtually completed. We shall see, however, that antigen–antibody complexes can play a part in initiating the reactions, and, in the case of endotoxins derived from enterobacteria, it is difficult to exclude the possibility of pre-immunization in animals living under normal conditions. Apparently still more conclusive is the fact that preparative and provocative agents do not have to be antigenically related, or even antigens at all.

The preparative agent must nevertheless fulfil certain well-defined criteria. First of these is that it must be able, in the local SR, to cause a local accumulation of granulocytes. While endotoxin is capable of doing this, a number of other substances are just as effective: for instance, almost any antigen–antibody reaction, so that 'preparers' include tuberculin in the sensitized animal, and other antigens to which circulating antibody is present. The actual mechanism by which endotoxin prepares a site is difficult to define, and since endotoxin from the same organism need not necessarily be used for both inoculations, the non-specific element in these reactions is again underlined. However, our knowledge of the composition and antigenicity of endotoxins is fragmentary, so that lack of immunological specificity in this case could be more apparent than real.

The significance of leucocyte accumulations at prepared sites is that lysosomal acid hydrolases are released locally with resultant damage to the walls of small vessels. Later leucocyte–platelet–fibrin deposits are formed in these vessels under the influence of the provocative agent. Such deposits are characteristic of local but not general reactions. The importance of lysosomal enzymes is clearly seen from the fact that isolated leucocyte granules also behave as preparers, and that a number of inhibitors of proteolytic enzymes abort the local reaction. Similarly depletion of circulating polymorphonuclear leucocytes by X-irradiation or nitrogen mustard prevents local preparation. Inflammation produced by trauma or chemical irritants does not, however, prepare dermal sites for the SR, so factors other than local accumulation of granulocytes must also be involved.

With regard to the generalized SR the position is less well understood, and superficial resemblances to the local reaction SR do not bear detailed examination. Thus, although haemorrhagic necrosis occurs in both skin and kidney due to vascular occlusion, the thrombotic plugs in the latter consist almost entirely of fibrin; they also take several hours to develop after challenge compared with the 15–20 minutes required for the more cellular thrombi of the local SR. There is, in fact, no evidence of leucocytic accumulation in the kidney and reasons why this organ should be particularly affected must be looked for elsewhere. A possible clue to the way in which endotoxin acts as a provoking agent in the systemic reaction lies in the known capacity of blockading agents of the reticulo-endothelial system (RES), such as thorotrast, to perform the same function. Although, as mentioned elsewhere, endotoxins are known to enhance the antibody response by stimulating the RES, their initial effect is to depress the system, and, as we shall see later, malfunction of the RES is one of the factors leading to the appearance of Shwartzman reactions. It is possible, too, that a transient effect of this kind by the preparative dose is partly responsible for the critical levels of preparative and provocative doses, and of their temporal relationships. Only under special circumstances will a single dose of endotoxin suffice to provoke a reaction.

Classically, endotoxins of enterobacteria have been used for preparation and provocation in both local and general Shwartzman reactions. But the range of provocative agents in local reactions is very much wider than this. Substances as diverse as starch, agar, glycogen, kaolin, and antigen–antibody complexes also serve. There may, of course, be antibodies present in 'normal' serum to some agents, e.g., endotoxin, glycogen, but in other cases the possibility that they are acting as haptens, even to cross-reacting antibody, seems rather remote. The agents listed all have one property in common, however, and that is that they all promote intra-vascular clotting.

What, then, is the sequence of events following challenge which leads to the development of the SR? According to Hjort and Rapaport [30] it is as follows: first, fibrin or semiclotted fibrinogen must be formed intravascularly; second, this material must be deposited within small blood-vessels; and third, there must be failure of fibrinolysis.

In the local reaction accumulation of leucocytes in damaged vessels probably results in the liberation of acid mucopolysaccharides which precipitate the partly clotted fibrinogen. Induction of granulocytopenia thus inhibits both stages of the reaction. In the generalized reaction coagulation has to be more extensive, and possibly for this reason kaolin and starch are not effective as provocative agents, though antigen–antibody complexes are. In the local reaction occlusion of vessels leads to hypoxia of the tissues and lactic acid liberated by leucocytes cannot be removed [31]. This is probably sufficient to account for haemorrhagic necrosis. In the general reaction granulocytes are still necessary, probably again for liberating fibrinogen precipitants, even though there are no detectable local accumulations in affected organs. Deposition of fibrinoid material could be due to the combined action of the above and other factors, such as (1) depression of the RES, (2) diminished blood-flow, and (3) lack of fibrinolysis.

The effect of endotoxin and non-specific blockade on the RES is to diminish markedly the rate at which fibrin is cleared from the bloodstream. According to Lee and Stetson [31], this action of endotoxin combined with its ability to initiate a 'sustained low-grade intravascular coagulation' are the central events in the generalized SR. The remarkable susceptibility of the kidney is the direct result of retention of microthrombi in the glomeruli, apparently due to a filtration effect as indicated by the protection afforded a kidney by occlusion of its ureter [32].

The importance of diminished blood-flow is derived mainly from indirect evidence, including observations that vasodilators and sympathetic denervation of the renal artery protect the kidney. However, such actions might also be effective by altering glomerular filtration pressures [32].

The protective action of fibrinolysins has been mentioned previously, but it is of interest that pregnancy enhances the effect of endotoxin, probably because of a concomitant decrease in fibrinolytic activity in the serum.

Normally a subtle interplay of all the factors mentioned above is decisive in inducing a Shwartzman reaction, but if one of them is very potent it may suffice by itself. For instance, the condition can be mimicked by a single dose of thrombin injected into the renal artery; otherwise, if clotting is less severe, then one or more of the other factors are necessary.

It is strange that, although so much experimental work has been done since the local Shwartzman reaction was first described in 1937, its mechanism is still so imperfectly understood. Osler [33] has written that 'it is, at least in part, a tissue response mediated by an immune event in which the antigen has potent primary toxicity'. On the other hand, Wilson and Miles [12] hold that, just as non-specific non-immunological resistance exists, so the SR is an example of the converse, i.e., a nonspecific increase in sensitivity. The same view is taken by Hjort and Rapaport [30], who consider the local SR to be 'the product of a specific train of pathogenetic mechanisms set in motion by a variety of aetiologic factors', and by Chase [34], who states that 'it is not an antigen–antibody reaction'. Nevertheless antigen–antibody complexes do function in appropriate circumstances as preparative or provocative agents, and Stetson [35] remarks that it is possible to elicit 'both these phenomena' (i.e., local and generalized SR) with other antigens [i.e., other than endo-toxins] in suitably sensitized or immunized animals'.

As Hjort and Rapaport [30] point out, some of the confusion has arisen from the fact that endotoxin shock is not always distinguished from the Shwartzman reaction proper. The former probably requires the presence of antibody, since mice reared in a germ-free environment lack the suscep-tibility of normally reared animals to endotoxin. After exposure to enterobacterial infections they quickly become sensitive to its lethal effect. Conversely, the lack of dependence of the SR on antigen–antibody reaction is probably illustrated in the case of a patient with congenital 'agamma-globulinaemia' who died with generalized SR and cortical renal necrosis.

It must be admitted, though, that many similarities exist between endotoxic and anaphylactic shock, and that in the SR there is localization of macromolecules in the glomeruli, as is the case in a number of condi-tions where antigen–antibody complexes are formed in the circulation.

Because of its remarkable susceptibility, the rabbit has been almost exclusively used for the study of the generalized Shwartzman reaction. Other laboratory animals and man appear to be much more resistant, though they may be predisposed, e.g., by pregnancy, to overt reactions. In man, enterobacteriaemia is accompanied by endotoxin shock, but elements of the SR such as intravascular clotting may also be present, leading to a haemorrhagic diathesis secondary to thrombocytopenia and consumption of clotting factors. In addition, necrosis to a variable degree, chiefly of the kidneys and adrenals, may occur as well. However, the main and sometimes lethal effect is due to endotoxin shock.

Finally, perhaps we should conclude that Shwartzman reactions are not hypersensitive responses in the immunological sense, even though com-plexes of immunological origin are among the substances that initiate them; that the two kinds of Shwartzman reaction have superficial resem-blances in that their initiating mechanisms and gross lesions are very similar, but that their pathogenesis is rather different; and that they differ from the immune hypersensitivities in that immune reactions are incidental rather than central to Shwartzman reactions.

REFERENCES

1. PORTIER, P., and RICHET, C. (1902), 'De l'Action anaphylactique de certains Venins', *C.r. hebd. Séanc. Soc. Biol.*, **54**, 170.
2. BORDET, J. (1939), in *Traité de l'Immunité dans les Maladies infectieuses*. Paris: Masson.
3. DIXON, F. J., and WARREN, S. (1950), 'Antigen Tracer Studies and Histologic Observations in Anaphylactic Shock in the Guinea-pig', *Am. J. med. Sci.*, **219**, 414.
4. WEIGLE, O., COCHRANE, C. G., and DIXON, F. J. (1960), 'Anaphylactogenic Properties of Soluble Antigen–antibody Complexes in the Guinea-pig and Rabbit', *J. Immun.*, **85**, 469.
5. BERRY, P. A., COLLIER, H. O. J., and HOLGATE, J. A. (1963), 'Bronchostrictor Action *in vivo* of Slow-reacting Substance in Anaphylaxis (SRS-A) and its An-tagonism', *J. Physiol., Lond.*, **165**, 71P.
6. MOTA, I., and VUGMAN, I. (1956), 'Effect of Anaphylactic Shock and Compound 48/80 on the Mast Cells of the Guinea-pig Lung', *Nature, Lond.*, **177**, 427.

7. AUSTEN, K. F., and HUMPHREY, J. H. (1963), 'In vitro Studies on Anaphylaxis', Adv. Immun., 3, 1.
8. BENDITT, E. P., and LAGUNOFF, D. (1964), 'The Mast Cell: Its Structure and Function', Prog. Allergy, 8, 195.
9. BROCKLEHURST, W. E. (1962), 'Slow Reacting Substance and Related Compounds', Prog. Allergy, 6, 539.
10. AUSTEN, K. F. (1965), 'Anaphylaxis: Systemic, Local Cutaneous, and in vitro', in The Inflammatory Process (ed. ZWEIFACH, B. W., GRANT, L., and McCLUSKEY, R. T.), p. 587. New York: Academic.
11. WOOLEY, D. W., and GOMMI, B. W. (1965), 'Serotonin Receptors. VII, Activities of Various Pure Gangliosides as Receptors', Proc. natn. Acad. Sci. U.S.A., 53, 959.
12. WILSON, G. S., and MILES, A. A., eds. (1964), Topley and Wilson's Principles of Bacteriology and Immunity, 5th ed. London: Arnold.
13. HANSON, J., and LOWY, J. (1965), 'Molecular Basis of Contractility', Br. med. Bull., 21, 264.
14. OVARY, Z. (1965), 'PCA Reaction and its Elicitation by Specific Immunoglobulin Species and Fragments', Fedn Proc. Fedn Am. Socs exp. Biol., 24, 94.
15. STANWORTH, D. R. (1963), 'Reaginic Antibodies', Adv. Immun., 3, 181.
16. OVARY, Z., BENACERRAF, B., and BLOCH, K. J. (1963), 'Properties of Guinea-pig 7S Antibodies. II, Identification of Antibodies involved in Passive Cutaneous and Systemic Anaphylaxis', J. exp. Med., 117, 951.
17. WHITE, R. G., JENKINS, G. C., and WILKINSON, P. C. (1963), 'The Production of Skin-sensitizing Antibody in the Guinea-pig', Int. Archs Allergy appl. Immun., 22, 156.
18. ISHIZAKA, K., ISHIZAKA, T., and HORNBROOK, M. M. (1966), 'Physicochemical Properties of Reaginic Antibody. V, Correlation of Reaginic Activity with γE-globulin Antibody', J. Immun., 97, 840.
19. FITZPATRICK, M. E., CONNOLLY, R. C., LEA, D. J., O'SULLIVAN, S. A., AUGUSTIN, R., and MACAULAY, M. B. (1967), 'In vitro Detection of Human Reagins by Double Layer Leucocyte Agglutination: Method and Controlled Blind Study', Immunology, 12, 1.
20. BENACERRAF, B. (1968), 'Properties of Immunoglobulins which mediate the Release of Vasoactive Amines in Experimental Animals. Immunopharmacology', Int. pharmac. Meet., 11, 3.
21. MOTA, I. (1964), 'The Mechanism of Anaphylaxis. I, Production and Biological Properties of "Mast Cell Sensitizing" Antibody', Immunology, 7, 681.
22. BINAGHI, R. A., and BENACERRAF, B. (1964), 'The Production of Anaphylactic Antibody in the Rat', J. Immun., 92, 920.
23. OVARY, Z. (1968), 'The Mechanism of Passive Sensitization in PCA and RPCA in Guinea-pigs. Immunopharmacology', Int. pharmac. Meet., 11, 15.
24. DIAS DA SILVA, W., EISELE, J. W., and LEPOW, I. H. (1967), 'Complement as a Mediator in Inflammation. III, Purification of the Activity with Anaphylatoxin Properties generated by Interaction of the First Four Components of Complement and its Identification as a Cleavage Product of C'3', J. exp. Med., 126, 1027.
25. COCHRANE, C. G., and MÜLLER-EBERHARD, H. J. (1968), 'The Derivation of Two Distinct Anaphylatoxin Activities from the Third and Fifth Components of Complement', J. exp. Med., 127, 371.
26. BRODER, I., BAUMAL, R., and KEYSTONE, E. (1968), 'Studies into the Occurrence of Soluble Antigen–antibody Complexes in Disease. II, Criteria for distinguishing Soluble Complexes from other Macromolecular Histamine Releasers', Clin. exp. Immun., 3, 537.
27. COCHRANE, C. G. (1965), 'The Arthus Reaction', in The Inflammatory Process (ed. ZWEIFACH, B. W., GRANT, L., and McCLUSKEY, R. T.), p. 613. New York: Academic.
28. WEIGLE, W. O. (1961), 'Fate and Biological Action of Antigen–antibody Complexes', Adv. Immun., 1, 283.
29. COCHRANE, C. G., and HAWKINS, D. (1968), 'Studies on Circulating Immune Complexes. III, Factors governing the Ability of Circulating Complexes to Localize in Blood Vessels', J. exp. Med., 127, 137.
30. HJORT, P. F., and RAPAPORT, S. I. (1965), 'The Shwartzman Reaction: Pathogenetic Mechanisms and Clinical Manifestations', A. Rev. Med., 16, 135.

31. LEE, L., and STETSON, C. A (1965), 'The Local and Generalized Shwartzman Phenomena', in *The Inflammatory Process* (ed. ZWEIFACH, B. W., GRANT, L., and McCLUSKEY, R. T.), p. 791. New York: Academic.
32. COHEN, M. H., and LEE, L. (1964), 'Effect of Ureteral Blockade on Localisation of Circulating Fibrin Aggregates in the Kidney', *Fedn Proc. Fedn Am. Socs exp. Biol.*, **23**, 446.
33. OSLER, A. G. (1962), 'Skin Reactions of the Immediate and Delayed Types of Hypersensitivity: Some Aspects of their Mechanism', in *Immunodiagnosis of Helminthic Infections. Am. J. Hyg.*, Monograph Series No. 22.
34. CHASE, M. W. (1965), 'The Allergic State', in *Bacterial and Mycotic Infections of Man* (ed. DUBOS, R. J., and HIRSCH, J. G.), 4th ed, p. 293. Philadelphia: Lippincott.
35. STETSON, C. A. (1965), 'Endotoxins', in *Bacterial and Mycotic Infections of Man* (ed. DUBOS, R. J., and HIRSCH, J. G.), 4th ed., p. 304. Philadelphia: Lippincott.

CHAPTER 8

CELL-MEDIATED IMMUNITY: *IN VITRO* STUDIES

By T. E. Blecher

I. INTRODUCTION

THE term 'cell-mediated immunity' refers to that large group of specific immune reactions which can occur in the absence of demonstrable circulating antibodies. These immune states can be transferred to suitable neutral recipients by the transfer of cells alone, i.e., without plasma or serum, and in fact cannot be transferred by means of serum. Skin-delayed hypersensitivity is an important hallmark of this group of phenomena which includes immunity to certain micro-organisms and chemicals, allograft or tumour rejection (particularly 'first-set'), graft-versus-host reactions, and the animal experimental allergic diseases.

An obviously attractive way in which to try to gain insight into the mechanisms underlying these processes of cell-mediated immunity is to put the cells capable of transferring such states into culture tubes and to study their behaviour under controlled conditions particularly *vis-à-vis* their suspected complementary antigens, and it is with studies of this sort that the present chapter is concerned. Although in these studies the aim may have been primarily to study *in vitro* the reactions of the cells involved in immune reactions which are antibody-independent *in vivo*, evidence is accumulating of the production by such cells *in vitro* of gamma-globulins, soluble 'transfer factors', and possibly even humoral antibodies. However, experiments designed primarily to study the production of humoral antibodies by cells *in vitro* are dealt with elsewhere (Chapter 4).

What cells are capable of transferring reactions of cell-mediated immunity from one animal to another and thus might qualify for *in vitro* study as the carriers or agents of this immunity? Effective transfer of delayed hypersensitivity (DH) was first achieved in 1942 when Landsteiner and Chase used peritoneal exudate cells (of which two-thirds are monocytes/macrophages) to transfer DH to picryl chloride from sensitized to normal guinea-pigs [1]. Thereafter the transfer of tuberculin sensitivity was achieved using peritoneal exudate, lymph-node, spleen, or blood leucocytes. Lymph-node cells were found capable of transferring the capacity to reject tumours or allografts at an accelerated rate; thoracic duct cells (consisting of 98 per cent lymphocytes) transferred tuberculin hypersensitivity, the ability to reject a previously tolerated allograft, and could cause lethal graft-versus-host reactions. (*See review by* Bloom and Chase [2].) Experimental allergic diseases in animals can be transferred by the lymphoid cells of the sensitized animals but not by their serum, e.g., experimental allergic encephalomyelitis (EAE) in several species and experimental immune thyroiditis in the rat. (*See review by* Paterson [3].)

From these and many other studies it has become clear that cell populations rich in lymphocytes and/or macrophages are the most effective if not the only products by which cell-mediated immunity can be transferred, and it is these cells which have been intensively studied for immune reactivity *in vitro*.

Two approaches are possible in such *in vitro* studies: either the responses elicited in the transfer-competent cells by presenting them with specific antigen may be studied, or the effects of the transfer-competent cells upon specific target antigens in the form of living cells may be studied. In practice, three techniques have principally made it possible in certain situations to show a good correlation between *in vitro* cell reactivity with antigen and the presence of a state of cell-mediated immunity (without circulating antibodies) towards the same antigen in the donor of the cells tested. A strict correlation of this sort would strongly imply that the two reactions are both manifestations of one and the same immune reaction. Two of these techniques—the inhibition by antigen of macrophage migration and the stimulation of lymphocytes to transform into large 'blast cells' capable of mitosis—are examples of the first type of response; the converse situation is exploited in studies of the cytotoxic effects of lymphocyte/macrophage-rich cell suspensions on cells in tissue culture. These are now discussed in turn.

II. Macrophage Migration Inhibition

The principle of this technique is as follows. A compact cell population containing macrophages is cultured in suitable culture medium. After one or two days cells, principally macrophages, migrate outwards from the original explant over a fan-like area on the floor of the culture vessel. The pioneer study of Rich and Lewis, in 1928 [4], revealed that when the cells originated from an animal immunized against an antigen (in their experiments the tubercle bacillus) the addition of the antigen to the culture fluid specifically inhibited the outward migration of macrophages.

Rich and Lewis originally used plasma-clot explants of washed spleen cells or buffy-coat cells, and Aronson [5], three years later, bone-marrow and testicular explants, from tuberculous animals. Lung, liver, thymus, and other tissues have subsequently been found to yield suitable emigrating populations of macrophages which respond to antigen in similar fashion. In the individual animal the macrophages of various organs acquire this responsiveness at differing times after immunization [6].

Macrophage emigration from lymphoid tissue explants is preceded by that of polymorphonuclear leucocytes and lymphocyte-like small mononuclear cells, and succeeded after several days by fibroblast emigration. The macrophage migration is far the most sensitive to the presence of antigen [7]; inhibition of polymorph migration when it occurs appears to be non-specific. Cornea-, skin-, kidney-, and liver-cell migration are not significantly inhibited by specific antigen [*see* 8].

As a source of macrophages serous exudates offer certain advantages over tissue explants. Originally tuberculous pleural or peritoneal exudates were used, but these have been supplanted by the introduction of sterile peritoneal exudates induced by injections of glycogen, mineral oil, or other irritant substances. This allows the testing of cells from control unimmunized animals as well as from animals immunized to a variety of antigens other than the tubercle bacillus. George and Vaughan [9] described an improved quantitative technique: washed exudate cells were centrifuged in capillary tubes which were then cut at the cell-fluid interface. The cell-containing segment of capillary tube was then affixed to the lower cover-slip of a Mackaness chamber, antigen-containing culture medium added, and incubation at 37° C. begun. Within 24 to 48 hours macrophage emigration occurred fanwise from the open end of the capillary tube onto the floor of the chamber. Projection of the image of such cultures by transmitted light via a prism onto a sheet of paper or photographic plate allows measurement of the area of migration by planimetry, whether using plasma-clot or capillary-tube cultures.

A. Immunological Significance

In the present discussion the central question is: What is the relationship between *in vitro* macrophage migration inhibition (MMI) by antigen, and the state of immunity in the donor of the cells? In fact, from the start workers using this technique have observed remarkably good correlation between *in vitro* positivity and the presence in the cell donor of immune states of the type described as cell-mediated, and no correlation with the presence or absence of circulating antibodies. Rich and Lewis [4] showed that the migration of tuberculous, but not normal, guinea-pig macrophages was markedly inhibited by the addition of Old Tuberculin to the culture medium. However, hypersensitive guinea-pigs' serum did not confer this responsiveness onto normal macrophages. They concluded that '. . . allergy in tuberculosis results from a change in the individual fixed tissue and blood cells, which renders them more sensitive to the products of the tubercle bacillus. There are no humoral factors necessary for the production of the injurious local effects of allergy in tuberculosis'—a remarkable and early expression of the concept of purely cellular immunity which is in widespread acceptance today!

Aronson [10] further clarified the distinction between tuberculin sensitivity which is 'inherent in the cell' [5] and Arthus and anaphylactic sensitivity which are antibody-mediated reactions, at the same time confirming that MMI was related only to the former. Guinea-pigs showing marked Arthus and anaphylactic sensitivity to horse serum exhibited no MMI with this antigen even if they were also tuberculous and exhibited tuberculin-induced MMI. Using a similar antigen, Raffel [11] showed that the migration of bone-marrow macrophages of guinea-pigs showing Arthus sensitivity but no DH to ovalbumin was not inhibited by ovalbumin *in vitro*, whereas in animals with DH to this antigen migration was inhibited by ovalbumin. Many subsequent studies have confirmed these associations (*see reviews of the earlier work* [12, 8]) using these and other antigens, e.g., histoplasma, T4 bacteriophage, gamma-globulin, or picrylated guinea-pig skin [6].

Three other aspects of MMI reactivity further reinforce a close relationship between it and DH.

B. Failure of Transfer by Serum

David et al. [13], like many other workers, confirmed the classic observation [4] that serum did not confer reactivity onto normal macrophages, whether the serum was from animals manifesting DH and *in vitro* macrophage sensitivity to antigen or contained high titres of precipitating antibodies. Failure to transfer immunological reactivity to normal cells by serum accords well with the virtually universal failure to transfer states of cell-mediated immunity to the normal intact animal by means of serum mentioned earlier (*see review* [2]). It also strongly suggests that this particular reaction (MMI) which takes at least 24 hours for its manifestation is quite different from that which can be conferred onto macrophages within minutes by serum containing 'cytophilic antibody' (*see later*, p. 260).

C. Hapten versus Carrier-protein Specificity

Secondly, MMI reactions involving carrier-proteins and haptens have been found to show the identical pattern of specificity for the carrier-protein but not the hapten as Benacerraf and his colleagues [14] showed governs DH reactions *in vivo*, whereas humoral antibody-mediated reactions are specific only to the hapten. David, Lawrence, and Thomas [15] immunized guinea-pigs to four different proteins conjugated to 2,4-dinitrophenol by injecting the conjugates in complete Freund's adjuvant (CFA) into the foot pads, which induced DH as well as antibody formation. Migration of peritoneal exudate cells from these animals was specifically inhibited only by the immunizing conjugate and not by the hapten. The same animals' antibodies, on the other hand, reacted by passive cutaneous anaphylaxis and in gel diffusion equally well with either of two different dinitrophenyl–protein conjugates. Similarly Carpenter and Brandriss [7] immunized groups of guinea-pigs with one or other of five picrylated protein antigens in either complete or incomplete Freund's adjuvant (the latter does not produce DH). Only the macrophages of the CFA-immunized animals exhibited MMI and this only in response to the particular picrylated conjugate used for immunization, whereas the animals' antibodies reacted with any of a number of picrylated proteins.

D. MMI by Tissue Antigens

A third group of studies which further underline the close relationship between MMI *in vitro* and cell-mediated phenomena *in vivo* are those concerned with experimental allergic encephalomyelitis (EAE) and transplantation immunity. EAE is considered to be a primarily cell-mediated disease (*see* [3]) since, among other reasons, it is transferable by cells but not by serum taken from affected animals. David and Paterson [16] showed that the migration of peritoneal macrophages of animals suffering from EAE was inhibited by 'encephalitogenic antigen' (adult guinea-pig or rat brain plus spinal cord). Neonatal rat nervous tissue, which does not induce EAE, did not produce MMI. Again, their sera did not confer reactivity to control macrophages.

In their study of allograft sensitivity Al-Askari et al. [17] found that the migration of macrophages of sensitized mice (which had rejected skin-allografts) was inhibited when they were cultured together with macrophages from the skin-graft donor strain, or microsomal preparations of these cells [18]. Unsensitized macrophages of unrelated strains when cultured together showed no MMI in the 24-hour culture period used [17].

E. Cellular Mechanisms of MMI

Most of the more recent work on MMI has been concerned with attempting to discover the actual mechanisms involved. The results indicate that the visibly responsive cells, the macrophages, are in fact only non-specific indicator cells and that the actual bearers of the information for specific cellular reactivity are the minority population of lymphocytes present. Although immune serum does not transfer reactivity to normal peritoneal exudate cells, Paas et al. [19] found that the addition of 33 per cent, and David, Lawrence, and Thomas [20] that the addition of 5 per cent, or even on occasion 2·5 per cent of peritoneal exudate cells from tuberculin-sensitive guinea-pigs to normal peritoneal exudate cells resulted in *all* the cells of the mixed population showing inhibition of migration in the presence of tuberculin.

In 1963 Svejcar and Johanovsky [*cited in* 21] had found that the addition of antigen to sensitized and non-sensitized spleen explants cultured in the same vessel inhibited cell migration from both explants, and since then Bloom and Bennett [22] and others have established that a soluble migration-inhibiting factor (MIF) is produced. These workers [22] separated the macrophages from the lymphocytes of peritoneal exudates of tuberculin-hypersensitive guinea-pigs and found that the isolated macrophages when cultured showed no inhibition of migration by tuberculin. However, the addition of as little as 0·6 per cent of the separated sensitized lymphocytes (which do not themselves migrate) to *normal* peritoneal exudate cells resulted in the whole population of cells acquiring clear-cut responsiveness to tuberculin (i.e., MMI).

This was a significant advance in showing the macrophages to be merely passive indicator cells receiving instructions from the actual carriers of the immunologically specific 'know-how': the lymphocytes. Bloom and Bennett [22] were further able to show that if the lymphocytes of guinea-pigs having DH to tuberculin were incubated with tuberculin for 20 hours a soluble factor appeared in the supernatant fluid which imparted specific responsiveness (MMI) to normal peritoneal exudate cells. The factor did not result from the incubation of normal lymphocytes with tuberculin, or of the sensitized lymphocytes without tuberculin or with a different antigen, e.g., coccidioidin. Moreover, incubation with the appropriate antigens of the lymphocytes of animals having high titres of circulating antibodies but no DH to the purified protein derivative (PPD) of tuberculin, bovine serum albumin, or ovalbumin respectively did not result in the production of MIF. The factor was non-dialysable and its appearance was prevented by mitomycin C. They have subsequently shown [23] that MIF first appears in the supernatants after 6 hours of incubation with antigen, which would suggest its new synthesis rather than the release of preformed material. Very similar results have been obtained by David [24] using guinea-pig lymph-node instead of lymphocytes. The sensitized lymphocytes only produced a MIF if incubated with their 'own' specific antigen. The MIF remained active after heating at 56° C. for 30 minutes.

Dumonde, Howson, and Wolstencroft [25] have confirmed that specific MMI of purified macrophage populations occurred only upon the addition of sensitized lymphocytes (as little as 2 per cent) or of a MIF which was synthesizable by sensitized lymphocytes only in the presence of their specific antigen. They have furthermore found that the efficacy of sensitized peritoneal exudate cells in transferring local or systemic DH correlates with their content of lymphocytes and not macrophages [25].

These studies show, then, that in DH the lymphocytes become capable of actively synthesizing a soluble macrophage-immobilizing factor (probably protein in nature) when confronted by the specific antigen *in vitro*. The number of macrophages immobilized can be up to one hundred times the number of lymphocytes which produce the factor [22]. This provides an amplification mechanism for the cellular reaction to an antigen which might account for the abundance of macrophages often seen *in vivo* at the sites of cell-mediated reactions. It would also account for the earlier finding of Nelson and Boyden [26] that in animals having DH to various antigens (but not those having only Arthus hypersensitivity) the parenteral injection of the specific antigen caused marked clumping of macrophages in induced peritoneal exudates within one hour.

F. Potential Application of MMI to Clinical Studies

From the foregoing the MMI phenomenon emerges pretty clearly as a valuable *in vitro* demonstration of DH, but it has not been readily applicable for use in man because of the unavailability of peritoneal exudates or other macrophage-rich populations. However, Thor and Dray have been able to induce human lymph-node lymphocytes to migrate and to demonstrate specific MMI by cultivating them for 72 hours in tissue culture, and more recently these workers, with associates [27], have shown that the incubation with the appropriate antigens of separated human blood lymphocytes from delayed-hypersensitive individuals results in the appearance of a MIF which is highly effective in causing MMI of heterologous, viz., guinea-pig, peritoneal exudate cells. This finding appears to open up considerable new clinical vistas.

G. Other Reactions of Macrophages *in vitro* in Delayed Hypersensitivity

Infection by organisms which can survive and multiply *within* host macrophages results in the host developing a state of DH to antigens of the infecting organism [28]. The macrophages of such animals show another form of altered reactivity *in vitro*, namely an intrinsic enhanced microbicidal activity. This state, however, is non-specific and thus has little claim to be an *in vitro* counterpart of the specific *in vivo* phenomenon of DH.

Another *in vitro* reaction of macrophages sometimes associated with DH is that imparted to them by 'cytophilic antibody'. Boyden described such antibodies in the sera of guinea-pigs injected with sheep red blood-cells in CFA (which induced DH) but not in the sera of animals immunized with the red cells in incomplete Freund's adjuvant (and which had no DH) [29]. The antibodies imparted to normal macrophages the property of agglutinating to their surfaces sheep red blood-cells in rosette fashion and have been considered as possible mediators of DH (*see review by* Nelson and Boyden [30]). However, other workers have found a clear dissociation between the appearance of DH and cytophilic antibodies [31, 32], and in his monograph on DH Turk concludes that macrophage cytophilic antibodies are probably not involved in DH [33].

H. Summary

The cells carrying the 'immunological memory', accounting for the appearance of cell-mediated immune reactions *in vitro* upon re-exhibition of the sensitizing antigen, are to be found amongst the lymphocytes. On re-encountering the antigen they synthesize a soluble factor, probably a protein, which can immobilize relatively large numbers of macrophages in their vicinity. This mechanism accounts for the MMI phenomenon which a variety of different approaches have indicated to be a reliable *in vitro* measure of specific cell-mediated immunity. It also provides a possible explanation for the accumulation of large numbers of macrophages at the sites of cell-mediated reactions *in vivo*.

At the same time the response to the antigen may be further amplified by the transformation and replication of lymphocytes as described in the next section.

III. LYMPHOCYTE TRANSFORMATION

This section deals with a second way in which the lymphocytes of individuals capable of manifesting one or other type of cell-mediated reaction *in vivo* can be shown to react *in vitro*. The reaction consists of the transformation, induced by certain antigens or other stimulatory substances, of a proportion of the apparently mature lymphocytes of a sensitive individual into large primitive DNA-synthesizing blast cells which may proceed to mitosis and replication.

Many studies have now been performed on this phenomenon [*see* 34] and it has emerged that lymphocyte transformation *in vitro* occurs under three main sets of circumstances, the latter two of which certainly appear to represent true immune responses:—

A. Non-specific Stimulation: Certain substances (e.g., phytohaemagglutinin, staphylococcal filtrate, antilymphocyte serum) stimulate blast-cell transformation of many lymphocytes (50–70 per cent), of nearly all individuals of many species, by 72 hours.

B. Transformation as a Specific Secondary Immune Response: Specific antigens (e.g., tuberculin, tetanus toxoid, poliovirus vaccine) stimulate the transformation of about 5–30 per cent of lymphocytes (only of individuals previously sensitized to the antigen used) after about 5 days.

C. Transformation as a Primary Immune Response: Specific antigens (e.g., allogeneic or xenogeneic histocompatibility antigens (the 'mixed lymphocyte reaction')) stimulate the transformation of about 5–10 per cent of lymphocytes of previously unimmunized individuals, after about 5–7 days.

A. Non-specific Stimulation

1. PHYTOHAEMAGGLUTININ

In 1960 Nowell [35] made the startling observation that the addition of phytohaemagglutinin (PHA), an extract of the red bean, *Phaseolus vulgaris*, to cultures of normal human blood leucocytes to remove the red cells caused the appearance, after 72 hours' culture, of many large mononuclear cells of primitive appearance, and fairly numerous mitotic figures. This was surprising as blood leucocytes normally show no mitotic activity either *in vivo* or in culture, and until comparatively recently had been regarded simply as 'end-cells' merely awaiting senescence and death. This finding was immediately exploited to provide a new and relatively simple technique for the study of human chromosomes. However, it was simply the fact that lymphocytes could be 'brought to life' *in vitro* in this spectacular fashion which has proved of great importance to the immunologist.

PHA stimulates blast-cell transformation of human lymphoid cells obtained from lymph-nodes, spleen, thoracic duct, tonsils, and irregularly from the thymus (*see references in* [36]), and transformation has been obtained in many other species (*see references in* [36]). However, this is not a universal effect of PHA on all cells: blood-cells other than lymphocytes, for instance, are not stimulated to transform by PHA. Nevertheless, PHA has been reported to stimulate some mitosis of basal cells in human

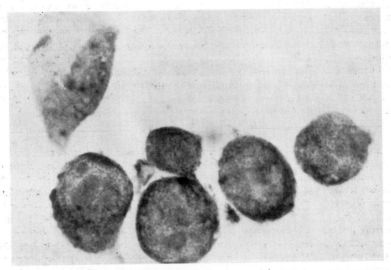

Fig. 54.—PHA-transformed blast cells. An untransformed lymphocyte (centre) and a macrophage (top left) are also present. Three-day PHA-culture of normal human lymphocytes. May-Grünwald Giemsa stain.

skin culture [37] and human carcinoma and rat fibroblast cultures [38] and of free-living amoebae [39]. This stimulation of cells not known to be capable of immune responses, and the fact that PHA stimulates the lymphocytes of virtually all individuals in a species without their having previously encountered it as an antigen, suggest that PHA-induced transformation is not in the nature of an immune response.

On the other hand, the resultant blast cells are very similar in their light and electron microscopic appearances to both the blast cells that appear *in vitro* in this fashion in more certainly immunologically specific responses (e.g., that to tuberculin, *see* p. 266) and to the large pyroninophilic 'immunoblasts' that arise in lymphoid tissues *in vivo* during the induction of cell-mediated immune responses.

The PHA blast cell, firstly, is usually large (up to 20–30 μ diameter) with deeply basophilic cytoplasm which is pyroninophilic and frequently has a paler perinuclear zone and small vacuoles. The nucleus is finely leptochromatic and contains one, two, or more nucleoli (*Fig.* 54). Electron microscopically [40, 41] the cytoplasm is seen to be rich in ribosomes, lying free or arranged in rosettes. Mitochondria are numerous and sometimes show increased cristae. A fairly well-developed Golgi apparatus is present but endoplasmic reticulum is usually very sparse.

Strikingly similar large mononuclear cells referred to as 'large lymphoid cells' [42] or 'hemocytoblasts' [43] have been described in the lymph-nodes draining primary skin allografts, in the spleen during graft-versus-host reactions, referred to as 'large pyroninophilic cells' [44], and in the lymph-nodes draining induction sites of contact sensitivity [45] and referred to as 'immunoblasts' [33]. These are, of course, all examples of primarily cell-mediated immune reactions. Oort and Turk [45] in fact found such immunoblasts to proliferate only if DH was being induced and not if only antibodies were being induced. The electron microscopic appearances of the immunoblasts in lymph-nodes draining skin-grafts [46, 47] or sites of skin sensitization to oxazolone [48] correspond very closely to those of PHA blast cells, and both are, of course, quite unlike those of the plasma cells associated with circulating antibody production with their abundant rough endoplasmic reticulum.

2. Metabolic Changes during Transformation

Since PHA-induced lymphocyte transformation is accompanied by the appearance of about 1–5 per cent of mitotic figures by the third day, it is not surprising that at 72 hours some 40–50 per cent of the cells can be shown to be synthesizing new DNA [49]. DNA synthesis starts after the first 24 hours. The addition of radioactive thymidine, which is exclusively utilized for the synthesis of new DNA, towards the end of the culture period provides a method of quantitating transformation alternative to morphological examination [49]. ^{14}C- or ^{3}H-labelled thymidine are usually added during the final hour of culture and subsequent auto-radiography shows the nuclei of about 10–30 per cent of the cells to be labelled (*Fig.* 55). Alternatively the radioactivity of the cultured cells or the extracted DNA may be measured in a scintillation counter. This method is less time-consuming than autoradiography and is now in widespread use, but is still not entirely free from shortcomings [50].

Studies using tritiated cytidine or uridine have shown that after a fall in RNA content during the first 30 minutes, its synthesis increases progressively during the culture period. The new RNA is largely non-ribosomal and therefore thought most likely to be 'messenger RNA' [51].

Despite the fact that the ultrastructural appearances of transforming and transformed lymphocytes might not suggest that they synthesize any significant amounts of protein for 'export' (cf. the paucity of endoplasmic reticular lamellae), several reports of such increased synthesis have appeared. Using immunofluorescence, immuno-electrophoresis, and auto-radiography, the addition of PHA has been reported to cause a mild (two-to threefold) [52] to manifold [53] increase in the synthesis of proteins, including the three immunoglobulins, IgG, IgA, and IgM. Hirschhorn et al. have calculated that 1 million transforming lymphocytes produced 10 μg. of gamma-globulin during 24 hours of culture. In contrast, the lymphocytes of agamma-globulinaemic patients, despite transforming normally in response to PHA, produced no gamma-globulin [54]. Several groups of workers, however, have been unable to demonstrate that PHA stimulates increased synthesis of immunoglobulins (see [55]).

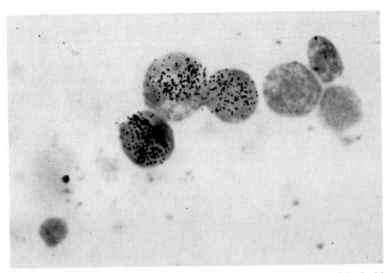

Fig. 55.—Auto-radiogram of 3-day PHA-culture which had been incubated with ³H-thymidine during the final hour of culture. Three 'blasts' show nuclear labelling. Stripping film, exposed 14 days. Counterstained with May-Grünwald Giemsa.

The energy for these various synthetic processes of transforming lymphocytes is apparently provided by anaerobic glycolysis: glycogen falls to very low levels in the blast cells while dehydrogenase enzymes (particularly lactic) increase [56] and lactate production rises. At the same time an increase in cytoplasmic lysosomes is accompanied by increased amounts of cytoplasmic hydrolytic enzymes [56, 57]. The uptake of labelled lipid precursors also increases [58].

3. POSSIBLE MECHANISMS OF NON-SPECIFIC STIMULATION; OTHER NON-SPECIFIC STIMULANTS

The mitogenic principle of PHA is a mucoprotein. It is absorbable by leucocytes but not by erythrocytes. However, prevention of leuco-agglutination by other means does not prevent PHA-induced transformation [59]. Moreover, many other non-specific and specific mitogens cause no leuco-agglutination.

Extracts of the American pokeweed [60] and several common legume seed extracts have been found to have mitogenic effects comparable to (e.g., lentils, broad beans, common beans) or much weaker than (e.g., common peas, chick peas) those of PHA [61]. In addition, two bacterial products have been found to have potent non-specific transformation- and mitosis-stimulating effects on the lymphocytes of most normal individuals. These are streptolysin S [62] and a factor present in filtrates of *Staphylococcus aureus* cultures [63]. Mitogenic stimulation by trypsin, chymotrypsin, and papain have also been reported [64].

The mechanism by which these non-specific stimulants (or for that matter the specific antigens to be discussed presently) trigger off the processes of transformation is not yet established. It has been suggested that PHA transformation might be a result of the release of lysosomal enzymes [65, 66], which increase during transformation. In support of this are cited the observations that streptolysin S and staphylococcal endotoxin have been shown to cause the release of lysosomal enzymes, and that PHA-induced transformation is prevented or inhibited by the prior addition of prednisolone or chloroquin, both of which drugs are said to 'stabilize' the lysosomal membrane. This theory has, however, been challenged [67].

An alternative theory that PHA-induced transformation, like that induced by specific antigens, is the result of an immunological reaction to a universally experienced antigenic stimulus [68] gains some support from the demonstrations that PHA is antigenic in animals and humans [69]. However, the curves of antibody production had the characteristics of a primary response, which argues against PHA transformation representing a secondary immune response to PHA.

One other stimulant of lymphocyte transformation which appears to be non-specific is heterologous antilymphocyte serum (ALS) [70, 71]. Grasbeck, Nordman, and de la Chapelle [70] compare this non-specific stimulatory effect to the parthenogenetic effects in sea-urchins of simple physical stimuli such as needle-pricks. They also cite a report of the induction of parthenogenesis in sea-urchin eggs by rabbit antisera to the eggs. In contrast, *homologous* antilymphocyte and in fact antiglobulin antisera stimulate lymphocyte transformation in an immunologically selective fashion and will be discussed later (p. 268).

4. CLINICAL CORRELATIONS WITH NON-SPECIFIC STIMULATION

The balance of the evidence cited seems to indicate that PHA-induced lymphocyte transformation is not the result of an immunological reaction. Nevertheless, it has emerged as a valuable *in vitro* measure of an individual's cellular immunological capabilities, since in a number of diseases the finding of reduced or absent PHA-induced lymphocyte transformation has correlated well with evidence of impaired cellular immune competence to reject allografts or to develop DH, e.g., to tuberculin or dinitrochlorobenzene, or by an increased susceptibility to certain infections.

Deficient cellular immunity *in vivo* without immunoglobulin or antibody deficiency has been found accompanied by impaired PHA-induced lymphocyte transformation in many cases of Hodgkin's disease [72] and in most cases of sarcoidosis, particularly during relapse [73]. In contrast, PHA-induced transformation has been normal in other cases of immunological deficiency where cellular immunity is intact and the deficiency is one of immunoglobulin production, as in the classic Bruton type of agammaglobulinaemia [54, 74]. We found this situation to obtain also in

11*

a case with normal immunoglobulin levels but deficient specific antibody formation [75]. In still other conditions deficiencies of both cellular immunity and immunoglobulins (and antibodies) are common, and in these, too, impaired PHA-induced lymphocyte transformation occurs, as in the 'Swiss type' of agammaglobulinaemia (thymic alymphoplasia) [76] and some cases of ataxia telangiectasia [77]. We have found this also to be the case in some patients with adult coeliac disease [78].

B. Transformation as a Specific Secondary Immune Response

The PHA-phenomenon has also proved valuable to the immunologist in leading directly to the discovery that transformation is also induced by certain antigens in immunologically specific fashion, which has provided a new *in vitro* test of specific cellular immune reactivity.

In 1963 Pearmain, Lycette, and Fitzgerald [68] considered the possibility that the PHA effect might be in the nature of an immunological response, and thus conceived the idea of testing whether the lymphocytes of individuals known to be hypersensitive to a specific antigen would be stimulated to a similar blastic transformation by the specific antigen *in vitro*. They cultured blood lymphocytes from individuals known to be hypersensitive to the tubercle bacillus (i.e., who were Mantoux positive) or non-sensitive (i.e., Mantoux negative), in the presence of tuberculin PPD. After 4–6 days of culture, transformation and mitosis of the Mantoux positive individuals' cells occurred, but not of the others. Since then many other antigens have been found to induce transformation and/or mitosis in this selective manner characteristic of a secondary immune response.

Within weeks of the tuberculin effect report Elves, Roath, and Israels [79] reported lymphocyte transformation induced by tetanus toxoid, typhoid–paratyphoid vaccine, diphtheria toxoid-antitoxin floccules, poliovirus vaccine, and small-pox vaccine lymph with fair correlation with the immunization histories of the lymphocyte donors. Hirschhorn et al. [80], at about the same time, similarly reported tuberculin, diphtheria toxoid, pertussis vaccine, and penicillin to stimulate lymphocyte mitosis in a manner completely in accordance with the subjects' previous sensitization histories.

In these and many other studies it has been found that transformation of lymphocytes by specific antigens is maximal after about 5–6 days, as compared to 3–4 days of culture in the case of PHA, and a much lower proportion of blast cells are stimulated (about 5–30 per cent) than by PHA or the other non-specific stimulants.

The specific-antigen-stimulated blast cells appear identical to PHA blast cells by light microscopy, although in electron microscopic studies differences have been reported [81]. They have been reported to synthesize immunoglobulins similarly to PHA blast cells but to a lesser degree [*see* 53]. They have even been reported by a few workers to synthesize specific antibodies when engendered by the specific antigen and, more markedly so, by PHA. PHA-stimulated lymphocytes of rheumatoid arthritic patients contained 'rheumatoid factor' in their cytoplasm [82]; cells of a patient with Hashimoto's disease stimulated by the addition of thyroglobulin, and more so by PHA, produced antithyroglobulin antibody [83]. This finding, however, could not be confirmed by others [55].

Recently Ripps and Hirschhorn [53] have found the cells of penicillin-sensitive patients to produce penicillin-binding substances on stimulation by penicillin and, more so, by PHA. Other workers, however, have been unable to demonstrate that PHA stimulates sensitized cells to produce antibodies [84].

1. AN INDEX OF DELAYED HYPERSENSITIVITY OR HUMORAL IMMUNITY? CLINICAL STUDIES IN ALLERGIES

It has been possible to test for both skin reactivity and lymphocyte transformation induced by the same specific antigen in allergic patients and drug hypersensitivity following initial reports of lymphocyte transformation induced by pollen extracts in patients with seasonal hay fever [85] or by the suspected drug in presumed drug-hypersensitivity reactions, e.g., to phenytoin sodium [86] or sulphonamide [87]. The results have been surprising and conflicting. In 10 patients with seasonal asthma or hay fever and skin sensitivity (of unspecified but presumably 'immediate' type) to grass pollen, Wiener and Brasch [88] reported transformation to be induced in all cases by the offending pollen extract. As Ricci, Rassaleva, and Ricca [89] have pointed out, this is an unexpected result as the bulk of the evidence indicates that lymphocyte transformation is a correlate of cellular immunity and in allergic patients DH to the allergen is not found, except rarely after desensitization treatment. In their studies Ricci et al. found no significant stimulation of transformation by pollen extract in 27 cases of pollenosis, including 12 that had had specific desensitization therapy.

Similarly, in drug sensitivity immediate skin hypersensitivity is the usual finding and yet lymphocyte transformation *in vitro* induced by the suspected drugs (including penicillin and sulphadimidine) has been reported in a small proportion of such cases [90]. Skin tests were not reported in these studies. Vischer [91] and Fellner et al. [92] found a striking correlation between the presence of immediate skin hypersensitivity and penicillin-induced lymphocyte transformation in 10 patients and no correlation with skin DH. Halpern, Ky, and Amache [93] found that the addition of a predetermined amount of the offending drug to the lymphocytes of nearly 100 patients in every case induced significant lymphocyte transformation regardless of whether skin tests showed immediate or delayed hypersensitivity. Normal and non-allergic individuals taking the same drugs gave negative results. Fellner et al. [92] do, however, draw the reader's attention to a recent animal study by Oppenheim, Wolstencroft, and Gell [94] in which the opposite correlation was found, namely with DH.

Animal studies

Oppenheim and his colleagues [94] induced pure DH to tuberculin PPD and albumin-orthanilic acid conjugate in guinea-pigs. Despite the absence of any detectable circulating antibodies, all draining lymph-node cells and about 40 per cent of spleen and peripheral leucocyte cultures underwent blast-cell transformation with these antigens *in vitro*. Moreover, induction of transformation was carrier specific as is DH *in vivo* [95], as mentioned earlier.

Mills [96] has similarly demonstrated a clear and convincing parallelism between lymph-node lymphocyte transformation and skin DH in guinea-pigs immunized with ovalbumin in complete Freund's adjuvant. Intravenously immunized animals developed antibodies but no lymphocyte reactivity to the antigens, and again transformation responses to DNP-protein conjugates were carrier specific whereas the antibodies induced were hapten specific.

2. The Transforming Lymphocyte acting as 'Antigen' in Specific Transformation

In all these instances of specific antigen-induced transformation it seems apparent that the added antigen combines with a specific receptor on or near the surface of the sensitized lymphocyte and that this interaction then triggers off the metabolic processes leading to transformation and mitosis. Even if the roles of the lymphocyte and the suspending medium are reversed it seems that some sort of specific immune complex can still be formed which is capable of triggering off the transformation process. Thus anti-rabbit leucocyte antibodies caused the transformation of some but not all other rabbits' lymphocytes [97], and similarly rabbit antibodies to various allotypes of rabbit gamma-globulin have stimulated transformation of rabbit lymphocytes but only those of the corresponding allotype [98]. The interaction, possibly with traces of the particular gamma-globulin allotype in or on the lymphocytes which leads to transformation, could occur within 15 minutes of adding the antibodies.

3. Transformation in the Investigation of Auto-immune Diseases

The exciting possibility that under certain circumstances lymphocytes might be shown to be reactive to autologous cellular antigens has particularly interested several workers. Such a finding would be suggestive of true cell-mediated *auto-immunity*, the very opposite of the normal state of 'horror autotoxicus' and in accordance with the considerable evidence suggesting that cell-mediated mechanisms rather than the numerous well-known auto-antibodies might have pathogenetic significance in a number of so-called 'auto-immune diseases' (*see* Chapter 12). However, in view of the obvious difficulties in obtaining samples of autologous tissue in sufficient quantity, most of such studies on human beings have perforce used as antigens allogeneic tissues obtained at operation or at autopsy.

In 1963 Hashem et al. [99] reported that the lymphocytes of 4 infants with severe eczema were stimulated to mitosis and transformation (up to 20 per cent) by extracts of their own skin. However, shortly thereafter they also reported comparable stimulation by extracts of autologous *lymphocytes* in infantile eczema and also in various other diseases of possibly auto-immune aetiology. One other report of lymphocyte transformation induced by autologous tissue has appeared: Tobias, Safran, and Schaffner [100] found 14–18 per cent of blast cells to be induced in the lymphocytes of 2 out of 4 patients with primary biliary cirrhosis and 1 of 2 with chronic active hepatitis after culture for 120 hours with homogenized fragments of their own biopsied liver tissue. Eight other patients with various other liver diseases gave negative results.

Autologous cerebrospinal fluid and, equally, allogeneic fluid were found by Fowler, Morris, and Whittey [101] to produce transformation of the lymphocytes of 6 multiple sclerosis patients but not of 9 controls. All these results still await confirmation.

In rabbits injected with allogeneic thyroglobulin in complete Freund's adjuvant, so as to induce allergic thyroiditis, Zavaleta and Stastny [102] found that the sensitized rabbits' lymphocytes responded *in vitro* to preparations of their own thyroglobulin (as shown by increased tritiated thymidine uptake). Sensitization with thyroglobulin without CFA produced neither thyroiditis, DH to thyroglobulin, nor lymphocyte responsiveness to thyroglobulin. As lymphocyte reactivity appeared several days before the usual time of appearance of the thyroiditis, the authors point out that the relationship between the two must still remain undecided.

Rather more attempts have been made to demonstrate organ-specific lymphocyte reactivity in human beings using allogeneic antigens, but not all have given positive results. Pipitone et al. [103] have reported that human liver ribosomal preparations stimulated significant transformation of the lymphocytes of 16 out of 23 patients with chronic hepatitis but not of patients with various other liver disorders. They later found a similar kidney preparation to stimulate transformation of the lymphocytes of patients with acute or chronic glomerulonephritis, or chronic pyelonephritis, but not other kidney diseases. Fractions of other organs did not stimulate the patients' lymphocytes [104].

Hoenig and Possnerova [105], on the other hand, found no significant blast-cell transformation of the lymphocytes of 7 patients with cirrhosis of the liver after 72 hours of culture with an extract of necropsied liver, although in 3 of them 'rare' mitoses occurred. Lehner [106] found that the lymphocytes of patients with recurrent aphthous ulcers but not those of normal controls were stimulated by homogenates of foetal oral mucosa and, to a lesser extent, skin. However, in view of his other finding that foetal liver homogenate caused stimulation of the lymphocytes of 16 per cent of 51 subjects without any liver disease, Lehner advocated caution in interpreting the above mentioned results of Tobias et al. [100] who included no controls without liver disease [107].

In another 'auto-immune' disease, myasthenia gravis, Housley and Oppenheim [108] could find no induction of lymphocyte transformation by homogenates of normal or myasthenic thymus, or of normal muscle. In lymphocyte studies on patients suffering from various diseases of possibly auto-immune nature of the gastro-intestinal tract, the present author has not obtained stimulation of transformation by either allogeneic tissue or dietary antigens. Thus the lymphocytes of pernicious anaemia patients were cultured with various preparations (crude and ultracentrifuged fractions) of 'normal' gastric mucosa obtained from gastrectomy specimens, and with intrinsic factor; cells from ulcerative colitis patients with similar mucosal preparations of various parts of the large and small bowel, and with the milk proteins to which circulating antibodies have been found in this disease [109], and cells from a few cases of regional ileitis, idiopathic steatorrhoea, and cirrhosis of the liver with the same antigens. In no instance was significant mitogenesis or blast-cell transformation found after 5 days of culture [110]. Similarly, Hinz, Perlmann.

and Hammarström [111] have failed to demonstrate selective stimulation of either blood lymphocytes or those of the colon-draining lymph-nodes of ulcerative colitis patients by either phenol–water or saline extracts of a colon antigen. Their patients' lymphocytes responded normally to PPD and PHA.

In sarcoidosis an increased spontaneous lymphocyte transformation rate which was further stimulated by Kveim antigen (prepared from sarcoidal human spleen) has been reported [112]. The response was unusually slow, requiring 8 days of culture, and thus conceivably a *primary* one to allogeneic histocompatibility antigens (*see below*), rather than necessarily specific to the 'sarcoidosis' antigens. Cowling, Quaglino, and Barret [113], in fact, found no response to Kveim antigen in sarcoidosis after 5 days of culture.

C. Transformation as a Primary Immune Response

In the previous section transformation of the lymphocytes of individuals having immunity (usually of cell-mediated type) to a variety of antigens was described as occurring in the manner of a specific secondary immune response. It has become apparent that lymphocyte transformation may also be stimulated by incubation with antigens encountered for the first time, constituting a visible primary cellular immune response *in vitro* analogous to the recently achieved induction *in vitro* of primary immune responses leading to specific antibody formation (*see* Chapter 4).

In 1965 Johnson and Russell [114] noticed an increased number of blastoid cells and mitoses amongst human lymphocytes cultured for 7 days in foetal calf serum as compared with others cultured in autologous plasma. This finding has been confirmed.

Even this response could conceivably be the manifestation of a secondary response to bovine serum proteins previously encountered in the diet, and there are few if any other reports of transformation occurring as the result of incubation of unsensitized lymphocytes with soluble antigens. On the other hand, abundant evidence now exists that foreign histocompatibility antigens can stimulate transformation and mitosis of lymphocytes in what is almost certainly a specific primary immune response of these cells *in vitro*.

1. HISTOCOMPATIBILITY–ANTIGEN-INDUCED TRANSFORMATION, AND ALLO-GRAFT DONOR SELECTION

The 'first set' rejection of allografts is probably largely a cell-mediated phenomenon (*see* Chapter 10); in fact humoral antibodies may even interfere with rejection, causing 'enhancement' of graft survival. It was therefore eminently reasonable to test whether the chief effector cells of rejection, the lymphocytes, would react *in vitro* to foreign histocompatibility antigens by transformation. In 1964 Bain, Vas, and Lowenstein [115] showed that this could occur by culturing together the lymphocytes of two unrelated individuals. After 5 days of incubation considerable numbers of transformed blast cells had appeared whereas mixed culture of the leucocytes of identical twins produced no such transformation.

The possible application of such a mixed-lymphocyte culture (MLC) as an *in vitro* measure of the degree of histo-incompatibility between individuals and thus as a guide to the selection of donors for organ grafting was immediately obvious since leucocytes are known to share at least some histocompatibility antigens with fixed tissues, e.g., skin. It was soon shown that a 'one-way' reaction could be obtained by stimulating one individual's lymphocytes (i.e., the prospective graft recipient's) with the other's histocompatibility antigens in a non-transformable form: e.g., lymphocytes disrupted by freezing and thawing, or rendered incapable of transformation by irradiation or mitomycin C, or as a monolayer of the blood macrophages.

Bain and Lowenstein later showed that more transformed cells arose in MLC's of two unrelated individuals than of two siblings, and in squirrel monkeys a very good inverse correlation was found between the survival times of skin-grafts between various pairs of animals and the transformation induced in their one-way MLC's [116]. After rejection the transformation responses were still greater.

Wilson's detailed studies of the MLC in rats [117] have led him to reaffirm that this is a primary *in vitro* immune reaction to histocompatibility antigens. In parent–F_1 hybrid MLC's, marker chromosomes showed that only the parental cells were stimulated. Lymphocytes of rats rendered tolerant at birth to certain transplantation antigens were specifically non-reactive in adulthood to cells containing these antigens, and neonatally thymectomized rats' lymphocytes non-reactive to allogeneic lymphocytes in adulthood in the MLC test.

In 8 volunteers amongst whom skin-grafts were exchanged Bach and Kisken [118] found excellent correlation between graft survival times and transformation induced in their one-way MLC's. However, Russell and his colleagues have so far found the MLC to be of little value in forecasting skin or renal allograft survival between pairs of unrelated individuals [119]. These workers, however, only used bidirectional MLC's in that study. Also relevant here are the reports that uraemic plasma contains an inhibitor of transformation [120] and the known depression in uraemia of such cell-mediated reactions as allograft rejection and DH as well as of humoral immunity.

Kasakura and Lowenstein have found a factor (released transplantation antigen) in MLC supernatants which stimulated blastogenesis of allogeneic (homologous) but not autologous lymphocytes after only 10 minutes of contact [121]. Gordon and MacLean have also found a mitogenic factor but concluded that it could not be preformed but was actively synthesized during MLC [122].

Recently the extraction and purification of strongly blastogenic histocompatibility antigens in soluble form from human lymphocyte cell-membranes has been reported [123]. Thus the keeping of complete 'kits' of freeze-dried human transplantation antigens for the typing of potential graft recipients and donors by one-way MLC's seems a possibility.

2. TRANSFER OF SPECIFIC LYMPHOCYTE REACTIVITY BY SOLUBLE FACTORS

Recently evidence has been presented of the existence of soluble substances which can impart to unsensitized lymphocytes the capacity to respond specifically to antigens by blast-cell transformation. Fireman et al. [124] have obtained such a dialysable 'transfer factor' from disrupted lymphocytes of tuberculin-positive individuals, and Dumonde and his colleagues [25] have found a similar non-sedimentable factor to be released into the supernatant fluid when lymphocytes of guinea-pigs with DH to bovine gamma-globulin are incubated with their specific antigen. Neither factor was itself blastogenic (i.e., in the absence of the antigen), unlike the mitogenic factors mentioned above which appear in MLC's.

Such 'mitogenic factors' would provide an amplification mechanism for the response of hypersensitive cells to antigen nearly but not quite analogous to the 'migration-inhibiting factor' discussed in the previous section. The latter, also produced by hypersensitive lymphocytes, acts upon normal 'bystander' cells (macrophages) even in the absence of the antigen. The former would provide an admirable explanation for the earlier observation [125] that in DH transferred passively to normal guinea-pigs by the intravenous injection of labelled hypersensitive lymphoid cells, only about 3 per cent of the lymphoid cells in the skin lesions were actually labelled, i.e., sensitized donor cells.

D. Summary

In this section the evidence has been marshalled that mature lymphocytes can transform *in vitro* into large 'blast' cells capable of replication. This change can be stimulated not only by a variety of non-specific mitogens which act regardless of whether or not the donor of the lymphocytes has had previous experience of them as antigens, but also by a large number of antigens which stimulate mitogenesis in a specific manner characteristic of a secondary immune response. Thus only the lymphocytes of donors who have previously encountered the antigen under test and developed hypersensitivity to it which is of delayed type (with one or two possible exceptions as in drug and pollen allergies) are stimulated by the antigen to transform *in vitro*. In addition, certain antigens, most importantly histocompatibility antigens, have been found capable of stimulating lymphocyte transformation as a primary response in genetically dissimilar cells, which holds promise as an *in vitro* test for organ-graft donor versus recipient testing. Very recently evidence has been obtained of the production by sensitized or transforming cells of soluble factors which can impart to unsensitized cells the capacity to undergo transformation in response to the addition of specific antigen.

IV. Specific Cell-mediated Cytotoxicity in vitro

In the previous two sections the demonstration of cell-mediated immunity *in vitro* by the eliciting of visible and measurable responses of immune-competent cells induced by their specific antigens was discussed. Here the converse situation is discussed: the demonstration *in vitro* of the immune powers of sensitized cells as shown by their ability to damage specifically cells in tissue culture bearing the appropriate antigens. Such cytotoxicity would provide a very realistic *in vitro* model of a successful cell-mediated immune reaction *in vivo* directed against living cells (e.g., allograft rejection, tumour immunity).

A. Cytotoxicity towards Histo-incompatible Cells

In 1960 Govaerts [126] first demonstrated that live (but not killed) thoracic duct lymphocytes obtained from dogs that had rejected kidney grafts produced cytopathic effects up to cell death within 24–48 hours on monolayer cultures of kidney-cells derived from the second kidney of the donor dog. The cultured cells were not damaged by lymphocytes from dogs that had received kidney grafts from a 'third-party' donor. Rosenau and Moon [127] then demonstrated that splenic lymphocytes from mice immunized with allogeneic fibroblasts had similar effects upon further cultures of these fibroblasts. They were unable to demonstrate the participation of any antibodies in this effect and it was, if anything, more efficient in the absence of complement. The close clustering of the sensitized lymphocytes about the target cells in the first 18 hours, not seen in the control tubes, suggested to Rosenau and Moon that actual cell-to-cell contact was a prerequisite for immune cytolysis.

Many subsequent studies have confirmed the reality of specific cell-mediated cytotoxicity and that it is usually preceded by close co-aggregation of the aggressor and target cells, and that humoral antibodies appear to play no part in the phenomenon and cannot transfer cytotoxic powers to normal cells.

Rosenau and Moon then showed that the cytolytic effects were strain specific and, later, that they were due to an intrinsic functional modification of the lymphocytes rather than to their simply adsorbing any coexistent cytotoxic serum antibodies [128]. Thus the cytotoxicity of immune sera was unaffected by X-irradiation or the addition of hydrocortisone, whereas irradiation completely abolished, and hydrocortisone suppressed, the cytotoxic effects of lymphocytes. Moreover, incubation of normal lymphoid cells with cytotoxic antisera did not impart cytotoxic activity to them.

Wilson, in 1963, showed that the lymphocytes of skin-grafted rats or mice became cytotoxic by the sixth or seventh day towards cultured allogeneic but not isogeneic kidney cells. The lymphocytes themselves appeared to emerge quite unscathed from the encounter and remote (thoracic duct) lymphocytes were as potent as the graft-draining lymph-node cells. Again complement and antibodies were shown to play no part in the specific cytolysis. He later showed [129] an inverse exponential relationship between target cell survival and the number of aggressor lymphocytes added, and calculated that about 1–2 per cent of the draining lymph-node cells were immunologically active. Non-immune lymphocytes could all easily be washed off the target monolayers, but after 6–8 hours of incubation a small percentage of sensitized lymphocyte populations could not be so removed, and these would inflict during the succeeding 40 hours of culture as much damage to the target cells as the total sensitized lymphocyte population left undisturbed throughout in parallel cultures [130]. Low doses of the immunosuppressive drug Imuran (azathioprine) not affecting the viability of the lymphocytes nevertheless inhibited their cytocidal effects.

B. Transfer of Cytotoxic Ability to Normal Cells

As in the other two *in vitro* models of cellular immunity already discussed (MMI and transformation), attempts have been made to transfer the ability to manifest such immunity to normal lymphocytes by means of a soluble factor obtained from the cytocidal cells. Wilson and Wecker using RNA [131] and Gerughty, Rosenau, and Moon [132], using ribosomes from sensitized lymphoid cells, have actually been able to impart to isogeneic non-sensitized lymphoid cells specific though weak cytotoxicity for the cultured allogeneic cells to which the original lymphoid cells were sensitized. RNase abolished the effect.

An *in vitro* model of the *in vivo* phenomenon of enhancement (*see* Chapter 10) has also been achieved by this technique which throws further light on the mechanisms involved. Erna Möller [133] found that the (complement-independent) cytotoxicity of immune mouse lymphocytes for allogeneic tumour cells was prevented if the target cells were first incubated, in the absence of complement, with antibodies which were cytotoxic for the target cells in the presence of complement—a demonstration of 'efferent' inhibition of cell-mediated immunity *in vitro*.

C. Cytotoxicity in Experimental Allergic Diseases

In 1962 Koprowski and Fernandes [134] found that draining lymphnode cells of rats injected with guinea-pig spinal cord in CFA, if collected shortly before the onset of the allergic encephalomyelitis, clustered tightly around puppy neuroglial cells in culture, causing their eventual lysis. Rats injected with the adjuvant only did not develop the disease, and their lymphocytes did not exhibit this 'contactual agglutination'. Similar results were obtained by Berg and Källén [135], and analogous demyelination of cultured trigeminal ganglion nerve-fibres by lymph-node cells of rats with experimental allergic neuritis has been reported by Winkler [136].

Lymph-node cells of rabbits immunized so as to develop immune thyroiditis were found by Rose et al. [137] to be cytotoxic for rat thyroid cell cultures (i.e., inhibited their uptake of radioactive iodine) whereas their sera were not. Non-specifically sensitized cells were also cytotoxic but rather less so than the thyroid-sensitized cells.

Björklund [138] similarly found the lymphocytes of some thyroid-CFA-sensitized rats to clump around and destroy cultured thyroid cells to a degree proportional to the histological severity of the thyroiditis in the lymphocyte donors. Ling et al. [139], however, were unable to confirm the results of these two studies using the same methods.

Holm [140] found that the lymphocytes of rats with experimental autoimmune nephrosis damaged rat-kidney monolayers whereas their sera did not. The organ specificity of the cytotoxicity, however, was not complete.

D. Cytotoxicity in Human 'Auto-immune' Diseases

The fact that many of the numerous organ-specific antibodies which have been demonstrated in human patients suffering from the so-called 'auto-immune diseases' have not been proved to play any pathogenic role has naturally stimulated efforts to demonstrate cell-mediated cytotoxicity *in vitro* in these diseases.

Perlmann and Broberger found, in 1963, that the circulating mononuclear cells of children with acute ulcerative colitis could damage cultured isotopically labelled foetal colon cells: significantly greater amounts of isotope were released than in the presence of normal blood mononuclears [141]. Cultured small intestinal, kidney, and liver cells were not affected. The anti-colon effect was suppressed if the mononuclears were preincubated with colon antigen extracts. The children's sera also contained colon-specific antibodies which were, however, not cytotoxic, nor did they impart to normal leucocytes incubated in the sera any anti-colon cytotoxicity. Cytotoxicity was apparent after only $2\frac{1}{2}$ hours, which is much earlier than in other studies of cell-mediated damage, this discrepancy perhaps being due to the greater sensitivity of their index of cell damage than mere morphological observation. Contrary to all the other demonstrations of cellular cytotoxicity *in vitro* mentioned, except that of Govaerts [126], complement was found necessary in this study. Watson, Quigley, and Bolt [142] were able to confirm the cytotoxicity of ulcerative-colitis-circulating lymphocytes for dispersed colon cells (as measured by the ability of viable cells to exclude a dye), but they found that complement was not required. Surprisingly they found a cell-free extract of the disrupted lymphocytes to be at least as potently cytotoxic, which also has not been the case in most other studies of cell-mediated cytotoxicity.

In multiple sclerosis antibodies to nervous system antigens have often been demonstrated, including factors capable of causing demyelination *in vitro*. In view of doubts about the pathogenicity of such antibodies, and the unquestionable role of cell-mediated immunity in experimental allergic encephalomyelitis, Berg and Källén [143] tested washed circulating mononuclear cells of multiple sclerosis patients for cytotoxic activity *in vitro*. In one-third of their cases these cells showed 'contactual agglutination' to neonatal rat glial cells in culture with subsequent destruction of the glial cells. Fibroblasts in the cultures remained intact; disruption of the leucocytes abolished their cytotoxicity. The leucocytes of normal or brain-damaged individuals were non-cytotoxic. It is interesting that cytotoxicity was not species-specific. However, in another suspected auto-immune disease, Hashimoto's thyroiditis, Ling et al. [139] could demonstrate no cytotoxic effects of patients' lymphocytes on cultured human thyroid cells.

On the other hand, there have been several reports of the lymphocytes of patients suffering from the various collagen diseases being cytotoxic to cultured human cells, mainly fibroblasts. In rheumatoid arthritis Braunsteiner, Dienstl, and Eibl [144] reported inguinal lymph-node cells to destroy human amnion cells within 3 hours. Hedberg [145] has concentrated upon the mononuclear cells actually present in the diseased joints. In about one-third of the cases these cells (but not blood lymphocytes) were cytotoxic within 24 hours to foetal fibroblasts and kidney cells. Thirteen cases of non-rheumatoid arthropathies gave negative results. However, Sukernik, Hanin, and Mosolov [146] found that in 19 out of 24 rheumatoid arthritic patients the separated blood lymphocytes clustered around and destroyed human embryo fibroblasts within 72 hours; normal lymphocytes were non-cytotoxic.

In systemic lupus erythematosus (SLE) Trayanova, Sura, and Svet-Moldavsky [147] found that the blood lymphocytes of all of 10 patients (and 2 with scleroderma) destroyed cultured foetal fibroblasts within 4–6 days. The lymphocytes of 6 out of 7 of these patients with lupoid kidney involvement also destroyed cultured foetal kidney cells. Control cells from normal or hypertensive patients were without effect on either the fibroblast or kidney cultures. Hedberg [145] had also found the synovial mononuclear cells of all of 3 cases of SLE to be cytotoxic to foetal fibroblasts.

E. Possible Macrophage-mediated Cytotoxicity

Granger and Weiser [148] have reported that peritoneal exudate cells, which are mainly macrophages, of mice immunized with mouse sarcoma from a different strain adhered specifically to monolayers of the sarcoma *in vitro* and then destroyed them. The authors concluded that this effect might be due to preformed specific antibody bound to the macrophage cell-membranes and that thereafter the intimate cell contact alone resulted in cell destruction as a non-specific but metabolically active process. However, the recent findings cited in the first section of this chapter seem relevant here, indicating that, at least in specific MMI, specificity is entirely lymphocyte-mediated, with macrophages then obediently playing a non-specific though active role. Thus it is not excluded that by analogy the 2–5 per cent of lymphocytes amongst Granger and Weiser's macrophage populations were in fact the mediators of the specificity of the macrophage adherence to target cells.

F. Relationship to the 'Allogeneic Inhibition' Phenomenon

The concept that cytotoxicity produced by either lymphocyte or macrophage-rich populations occurs in two stages (specific aggregation to target cells, followed by indiscriminate target-cell destruction) is reinforced by recent demonstrations of *in vitro* reactions (*see below*) corresponding to the *in vivo* phenomenon of 'Allogeneic Inhibition' [*see* 149]. Normal (unimmunized) lymphocytes do not aggregate upon nor cause lysis of allogeneic target cells, at least not within the 2–3 days usually taken by immune cells to cause lysis. However, when normal lymphoid cells were aggregated to allogeneic target renal cells [150] or sarcoma cells by non-specific agglutinins such as phytohaemagglutinin or heterologous anti-mouse-cell serum respectively, destruction of the target cells was caused within 18 and 48 hours respectively. That this was not simply a sort of non-specific 'strangulation' effect was shown by the fact that similar aggregation to isogenic target cells resulted in no cytotoxicity. However, the reaction could not be considered to be a conventional immune response either, since the lymphoid cells of F_1 hybrid mice, when co-aggregated with monolayers of embryonic cells of one of their parental strains, caused their destruction. Moreover, relatively high doses of irradiation, sufficient to abolish cell-mediated immunological reactions, did not abolish this effect. Thus this cytotoxic effect would appear to be simply the result of close confrontation with histo-incompatible cells [149].

Möller and Möller [149] suggest that such contactual cytotoxicity ('allogeneic inhibition') might be the basic effector mechanism of cell-mediated immune reactions as well as other processes such as the normal surveillance mechanism which eliminates any neoplastic (and antigenically altered) cells which might arise. In the former process the immunological specificity would be confined to causing the aggregation of the immune lymphocytes to their specific target cells, their lysis then following simply as the result of the contact between the antigenically dissimilar cells.

G. Cytotoxicity acquired as a Primary Immune Response *in vitro*

Although it is apparent from the controls included in many of the studies discussed that lymphocytes of normal individuals are not cytotoxic to allogeneic cells within the 48 hours or so during which sensitized cells can destroy target cells, it has been discovered that after several days of contact in culture normal cells can acquire the power to destroy xenogeneic and even allogeneic cells, without the aid of aggregating agents.

Ginsburg and Sachs [151] found that normal rat lymphocytes cultured on mouse or rat embryo fibroblast monolayers caused no cytopathic effects during the first 5 days. By this time many of the lymphocytes had transformed into large pyroninophilic cells and lysis of the mouse-cell target monolayers and even of some of the rat-cell monolayers began. The appearances of the transformed cells and the timing of their advent coincide closely with those of the blast cells that appear in histo-incompatible mixed lymphocyte cultures (*see* p. 270). Ginsburg regards this type of experiment as an *in vitro* graft-versus-host reaction induced as a primary response in normal lymphocytes. In support of this he was able to show that after 4–6 days of culture transfer of the lymphocyte suspensions, now rich in large transformed cells, to fresh monolayers from the same strain of mouse as the original monolayers, caused their complete lysis within only 19–24 hours. Moreover, on cells of other strains of mice the severity of the lysis correlated well with the degree of similarity between their antigens at the H2 locus and those of the original 'sensitizing' mouse-embryo fibroblasts [152]. Hirschhorn, Firschein, and Bach [153] reported similar destruction of human fibroblast monolayers by added normal unrelated human blood lymphocytes after 7–8 days of incubation, which they concluded was probably due to a primary immune response. Again, transfer of the lymphocytes at this stage to fresh fibroblast cultures caused their destruction after only 4 days, which was considered to be probably a secondary immune response.

These studies accord with those of Gordon, David-Fariday, and MacLean [154] in which the *in vitro* sensitization of leucocytes following their incubation with allogeneic leucocytes for 6 days was proved subsequently by their accelerated graft-rejecting ability *in vivo*.

H. Summary

The work discussed in this fourth section of the chapter has shown that the washed lymphoid cells of animals sensitized so as to develop cellular immunity towards particular cellular antigens can 'recognize' cells in tissue culture which contain these antigens and specifically aggregate tightly to them and cause their destruction. This is a humoral-antibody-, and probably complement-, independent function of the immune cells and it has been reported to be transferable to normal cells by RNA fractions of the immune cells. Reports of organ-specific cytotoxicity shown by the cells of patients suffering from certain diseases support the possibility that cellular immune, that is auto-immune, processes may be important in the pathogenesis of many of these diseases, as opposed to most of the numerous circulating antibodies which have been discovered.

It is now also apparent that normal lymphoid cells may become immunized by sufficiently protracted contact *in vitro* with disparate cells to acquire specific cytotoxicity for these cells, this change being accompanied by blast-cell transformation of the stimulated lymphocytes.

REFERENCES

1. LANDSTEINER, K., and CHASE, M. W. (1942), 'Experiments on Transfer of Cutaneous Sensitivity to Simple Compounds', *Proc. Soc. exp. Biol. Med.*, **49**, 688.
2. BLOOM, B. R., and CHASE, M. W. (1967), 'Transfer of Delayed Type Hypersensitivity. A Critical Review and Experimental Study in the Guinea Pig', *Prog. Allergy*, **10**, 151.
3. PATERSON, P. Y. (1966), 'Experimental Allergic Encephalomyelitis and Autoimmune Disease', *Adv. Immun.*, **5**, 131.
4. RICH, A. R., and LEWIS, M. R. (1928), 'Mechanism of Allergy in Tuberculosis', *Proc. Soc. exp. Biol. Med.*, **25**, 596.
5. ARONSON, J. D. (1931), 'The Specific Cytotoxic Action of Tuberculin in Tissue Culture', *J. exp. Med.*, **54**, 387.
6. CARPENTER, R. R. (1963), '*In vitro* Studies of Cellular Hypersensitivity. I, Specific Inhibition of Migration of Cells from Adjuvant Immunized Animals by Purified Protein Derivative and Other Protein Antigens,' *J. Immun.*, **91**, 803.
7. CARPENTER, R. R., and BRANDRISS, M. W. (1964), '*In vitro* Studies of Cellular Hypersensitivity. II, Relationship of Delayed Hypersensitivity, and Inhibition of Cell Migration of Picrylated Proteins', *J. exp. Med.*, **120**, 1231.
8. HEILMAN, D. H. (1963), 'Tissue Culture Methods for studying Delayed Hypersensitivity: A Review', *Tex. Rep. Biol. Med.*, **21**, 136.
9. GEORGE, M., and VAUGHAN, J. H. (1962), '*In vitro* cell Migration as a Model for Delayed Hypersensitivity', *Proc. Soc. exp. Biol. Med.*, **111**, 514.
10. ARONSON, J. D. (1933), 'Tissue Culture Studies on the Relation of the Tuberculin Reaction to Anaphylaxis and the Arthus Phenomenon', *J. Immun.*, **25**, 1.
11. RAFFEL, S. (1948), 'The Components of the Tubercle Bacillus, responsible for the Delayed Type of "Infectious Allergy"', *J. infect. Dis.*, **82**, 267.
12. WAKSMAN, B. H. (1959), in *Cellular and Humoral Aspects of the Hypersensitive States* (ed. LAWRENCE, H. S.), p. 123. New York: Hoeber.
13. DAVID, J. R., AL-ASKARI, S., LAWRENCE, H. S., and THOMAS, L. (1964), 'Delayed Hypersensitivity *in vitro*. I, The Specificity of Inhibition of Cell Migration by Antigen', *J. Immun.*, **93**, 264.
14. BENACERRAF, B., and LEVINE, B. B. (1962), 'Immunological Specificity of Delayed and Immediate Hypersensitivity Reactions', *J. exp. Med.*, **115**, 1023.
15. DAVID, J. R., LAWRENCE, H. S., and THOMAS, L. (1964), 'Delayed Hypersensitivity *in vitro*. The Specificity of Hapten Protein Complexes in the Inhibition of Cell Migration', *J. Immun.*, **93**, 279.
16. DAVID, J. R., and PATERSON, P. Y. (1965), '*In vitro* Demonstration of Cellular Sensitivity in Allergic Encephalomyelitis', *J. exp. Med.*, **122**, 1161.
17. AL-ASKARI, S., DAVID, J. R., LAWRENCE, H. S., and THOMAS, L. (1965), '*In vitro* Studies on Homograft Sensitivity', *Nature, Lond.*, **205**, 916.
18. DAVID, J. R., AL-ASKARI, S., LAWRENCE, H. S., and THOMAS, L. (1964), '*In vitro* Studies on Delayed Hypersensitivity and Homograft Immunity', *Ann. N.Y. Acad. Sci.*, **120**, 393.
19. PAAS, C. M. S., FLICK, J. A., KAPRAL, F. A., and RUDD, J. H. (1961), 'On the Persistence of Tuberculin Hypersensitivity in Guinea Pigs made Sensitive Passively', *Ann. Rev. resp. Dis.*, **83**, 372.
20. DAVID, J. R., LAWRENCE, H. S., and THOMAS, L. (1964), 'Delayed Hypersensitivity *in vitro*. II, Effect of Sensitive Cells on Normal Cells in the Presence of Antigen', *J. Immun.*, **93**, 274.
21. SVEJCAR, J., PEKAREK, J., and JOHANOVSKY, J. (1968), 'Studies on Production of Biologically Active Substances which inhibit Cell Migration in Supernatants and Extracts of Hypersensitive Lymphoid Cells incubated with Specific Antigen *in vitro*', *Immunology*, **15**, 1.
22. BLOOM, B. R., and BENNETT, B. (1966), 'Mechanism of a Reaction *in vitro* associated with Delayed Type Hypersensitivity', *Science, N.Y.*, **153**, 80.
23. BENNETT, B., and BLOOM, B. R. (1967), 'Studies on the Migration Inhibitory Factor associated with Delayed Type Hypersensitivity: Cytodynamics and Specificity', *Transplantation*, **5**, 996.

24. DAVID, J. R. (1966), 'Delayed Hypersensitivity *in vitro*: Its Mediation by Cell-free Substances formed by Lymphoid Cell-antigen Interaction', *Proc. nat. Acad. Sci. U.S.A.*, **56**, 72.
25. DUMONDE, D. C., HOWSON, W. T., and WOLSTENCROFT, R. A. (1967), 'The Role of Macrophages and Lymphocytes in Reactions of Delayed Hypersensitivity', in *Immunopathology*, 5th International Symposium, Punta Ala (Italy). Basel: Schwabe.
26. NELSON, D. S., and BOYDEN, S. V. (1963), 'The Loss of Macrophages from Peritoneal Exudates following the Injection of Antigens into Guinea Pigs with Delayed Hypersensitivity', *Immunology*, **6**, 264.
27. THOR, D. E., JUREZIZ, R. E., VEACH, S. R., MILLER, F., and DRAY, S. (1968), 'Cell Migration Inhibition Factor released by Antigen from Human Peripheral Lymphocytes', *Nature, Lond.*, **219**, 755.
28. MACKANESS, G. B. (1967), 'The Relationship of Delayed Hypersensitivity to Acquired Cellular Resistence', *Br. med. Bull.*, **23**, 52.
29. BOYDEN, S. V. (1964) 'Cytophilic Antibody in Guinea-pigs with Delayed Hypersensitivity', *Immunology*, **7**, 474.
30. NELSON, D. S., and BOYDEN, S. V. (1967), 'Macrophage Cytophilic Antibodies and Delayed Hypersensitivity', *Br. med. Bull.*, **23**, 15.
31. BLAZKOVEK, A. A., SORKIN, E., and TURK, J. L. (1965), 'A Study of the Passive Cellular Transfer of Local Cutaneous Hypersensitivity. II, The Possible Role of Cytophilic Antibody in Cutaneous Hypersensitivity Reactions', *Int. Archs Allergy appl. Immun.*, **28**, 178.
32. HOLTZER, J. D., and WINKLER, K. C. (1967), 'Experimental Delayed Type Allergy without Demonstrable Antibodies', *Immunology*, **12**, 701.
33. TURK, J. L. (1967), *Delayed Hypersensitivity*, p. 240. Amsterdam: North Holland.
34. LING, N. R. (1968), *Lymphocyte Stimulation*. Amsterdam: North Holland.
35. NOWELL, P. C. (1960), 'Phytohaemagglutinin: An Initiator of Mitosis in Cultures of Normal Human Leucocytes', *Cancer Res.*, **20**, 462.
36. ELVES, M. W. (1966), 'The Effect of Phytohaemagglutinin on Lymphoid Cells', in *The Biological Effects of Phytohaemagglutinin* (ed. ELVES, M. W.), p. 1. The Robert Jones and Agnes Hunt Orthopaedic Hospital Management Committee, Oswestry, England.
37. SARKANY, I., and CARON, G. A. (1965), 'Phytohaemagglutinin Induced Mitotic Stimulation of Epithelial Cells in Organ Culture in Adult Human Skin', *Br. J. Derm.*, **77**, 439.
38. IOACHIM, H. L. (1966), 'Effects of Phytohaemagglutinin *in vitro* in Cells other than Lymphocytes', *Nature, Lond.*, **210**, 919.
39. AGRELL, I. P. S. (1966), 'Phytohaemagglutinin as a Mitotic Stimulator on Free-living Amoebae', *Expl Cell Res.*, **42**, 403.
40. INMAN, D. R., and COOPER, E. H. (1963), 'Electron Microscopy of Human Lymphocytes stimulated by Phytohaemagglutinin', *J. cell. Biol.*, **19**, 441.
41. TANAKA, Y., EPSTEIN, L. B., BRECHER, G., and STOHLMAN, F., jun. (1963), 'Transformation of Lymphocytes in Cultures of Human Peripheral Blood', *Blood*, **22**, 614.
42. SCOTHORNE, R. J., and McGREGOR, I. A. (1955), 'Cellular Changes in Lymph Nodes and Spleen following Skin Homografting in the Rabbit', *J. Anat.*, **89**, 283.
43. ANDRÉ, J. A., SCHWARTZ, R. S., MITUS, W. J., and DAMESHEK, W. (1962), 'Lymphoid Responses to Skin Homografts. I, First and Second Set Responses in Normal Rabbits', *Blood*, **19**, 313.
44. GOWANS, J. L. (1962), 'The Fate of Parental Strain Small Lymphocytes in F_1 Hybrid Rats', *Ann. N.Y. Acad. Sci.*, **99**, 432.
45. OORT, J., and TURK, J. L. (1965), 'A Histological and Autoradiographic Study of Lymphnodes during the Development of Contact Sensitivity in the Guinea Pig', *Br. J. exp. Path.*, **46**, 147.
46. BINET, J. L., and MATHÉ, G. (1962), 'Optical and Electron Microscope Studies of "Immunologically Competent Cells" in Graft Reactions', *Nature, Lond.*, **193**, 992.
47. ANDRÉ-SCHWARTZ, J. (1964), 'The Morphological Response of the Lymphoid System to Homografts. III, Electron Microscopy Study', *Blood*, **24**, 113.
48. DE KARLSBAD, J. G., PETRIS, B., and TURK, J. L. (1966), 'The Ultrastructure of Cells Present in Lymphnodes during the Development of Contact Sensitivity', *Int. Archs Allergy appl. Immun.*, **29**, 112.

49. MacKinney, A. A., Stohlman, F., and Brecher, G. (1962), 'The Kinetics of Cell Proliferation in Culture of Human Peripheral Blood', *Blood*, **19**, 349.
50. Schellekens, P. T. A., and Eijsvogel, V. P. (1968), 'Lymphocyte Transformation *in vitro*. I, Tissue Culture Conditions and Quantitative Measurements', *Clin. exp. Immun.*, **3**, 571.
51. Cooper, H. L., and Rubin, A. D. (1966), 'Synthesis of Non-ribosomal R.N.A. by Lymphocytes. A Response to Phytohaemagglutinin Treatment', *Science, N.Y.*, **152**, 516.
52. Parenti, F., Franceschini, P., Forti, G., and Cepellini, R. (1966), 'The Effect of Phytohaemagglutinin on the Metabolism and Gamma Globulin Synthesis of Human Lymphocytes', *Biochim. biophys. Acta*, **123**, 181.
53. Ripps, C., and Hirschhorn, K. (1967), 'The Production of Immunoglobulins by Human Peripheral Blood Lymphocytes *in vitro*', *Clin. exp. Immun.*, **2**, 377.
54. Fudenberg, H. H., and Hirschhorn, K. (1964), 'Agammaglobulinaemia: The Fundamental Defect', *Science, N.Y.*, **145**, 611.
55. Greaves, M. F., and Roitt, I. M. (1968), 'The Effect of Phytohaemagglutinin and Other Lymphocyte Mitogens on Immunoglobulin Synthesis by Human Peripheral Blood Lymphocytes *in vitro*', *Clin. exp. Immun.*, **3**, 393.
56. Quaglino, D., and Hayhoe, F. G. J. (1965), 'Metabolic Changes in Short-term *in vitro* Cultures of Normal and Leukaemic Cells', in *Current Research in Leukaemia* (ed. Hayhoe, F. G. J.), p. 124. London: Cambridge University Press.
57. Gough, J., and Elves, M. W. (1967), 'Studies of Lymphocytes and their Derivative Cells *in vitro*', *Acta haematologica*, **37**, 42.
58. Kay, J. E. (1968), 'Phytohaemagglutinin. An Early Effect on Lipid Metabolism', *Nature, Lond.*, **219**, 172.
59. Börjeson, J., Chessin, L. N., and Landy, M. (1967), 'Dissociation of Leukagglutinating and Transforming Properties of Phytohaemagglutinin by the Coating of Lymphocytes with Vi Polysaccharide', *Int. Archs Allergy appl. Immun.*, **31**, 184.
60. Chessin, L. N., Borjeson, J., Welsh, P. D., Douglas, S. D., and Cooper, H. L. (1966), 'Studies on Human Peripheral Blood Lymphocytes *in vitro*. II, Morphological and Biochemical Studies on the Transformation of Lymphocytes by Pokeweed Mitogen', *J. exp. Med.*, **124**, 873.
61. Hashem, N., and Kabarity, A. (1966), 'Mitogenic Activity of Legumes and Other Vegetable Seeds on Peripheral Lymphocyte Cultures' (letter), *Lancet*, **1**, 1428.
62. Hirschhorn, K., Schreibman, R. R., Verbo, S., and Gruskin, R. H. (1964), 'The Action of Streptolysin S on Peripheral Lymphocytes of Normal Subjects and Patients with Acute Rheumatic Fever', *Proc. nat. Acad. Sci. U.S.A.*, **52**, 1151.
63. Ling, N. R., Spicer, E., James, K., and Williamson, N. (1965), 'The Activation of Human Peripheral Lymphocytes by Products of Staphylococci', *Br. J. Haemat.*, **11**, 421.
64. Mazzei, D., Novi, G., and Bazzi, C. (1966), 'Mitogenic Action of Papain' (letters), *Lancet*, **2**, 802.
65. Allison, A. V., and Mallucci, L. (1964), 'Lysosomes in Dividing Cells with Special Reference to Lymphocytes', *Lancet*, **2**, 1371.
66. Hirschhorn, K., and Hirschhorn, R. (1965), 'Role of Lysosomes in the Lymphocyte Response', *Lancet*, **1**, 1046.
67. Brecher, G., and Tanaka, Y. (1965), 'Lysosomes and Lymphocyte Response' (letter), *Lancet*, **2**, 595.
68. Pearmain, G., Lycette, R. R., and Fitzgerald, P. H. (1963), 'Tuberculin Induced Mitosis in Peripheral Blood Leukocytes', *Lancet*, **1**, 637.
69. Marshall, W. H., and Melman, S. (1966), 'Antibody Production in Sheep and Man against the Mitogenic Principle of the Bean Extract "Phytohaemagglutinin"', *Clin. exp. Immun.*, **1**, 189.
70. Grasbeck, R., Nordman, C., de la Chapelle, A. (1963), 'The Leucocyte-mitogenic Effect of Serum from Rabbits immunized with Human Leucocytes', *Acta med. scand.*, **175**, Suppl. 412, 39.
71. Holt, L. J., Ling, N. R., and Stanworth, D. R. (1966), 'The Effect of Heterologous Antisera and Rheumatoid Factor on the Synthesis of D.N.A. and Protein by Human Peripheral Lymphocytes', *Immunochemistry*, **3**, 359.
72. Hersch, E. M., and Oppenheim, J. J. (1965), 'Impaired *in vitro* Lymphocyte Transformation in Hodgkin's Disease', *New Engl. J. Med.*, **273**, 1006.

73. BUCKLEY, C. E., NAGAYA, H., and SIEKER, H. O. (1966), 'Altered Immunologic Activity in Sarcoidosis', *Ann. intern. Med.*, **64**, 508.
74. LING, N. R., and SOOTHILL, J. F. (1964), 'Lymphocytic Transformation', *Br. med. J.*, **2**, 1460.
75. BLECHER, T. E., SOOTHILL, J. F., VOYCE, M. A., and WALKER, W. H. C. (1968), 'Antibody Deficiency Syndrome; A Case with Normal Immunoglobulin Levels', *Clin. exp. Immun.*, **3**, 47.
76. MEUWISSEN, H. J., BACH, F. H., HONG, R., and GOOD, R. A. (1968), 'Congenital Thymic Dysplasia: Lymphocyte Stimulation Test', *J. Pediat.*, **72**, 177.
77. OPPENHEIM, J. J., BARLOW, M., WALDMAN, T. A., and BLOCK, J. B. (1966), 'Impaired in vitro Lymphocyte Transformation in Patients with Ataxia Telangiectasia', *Br. med. J.*, **2**, 330.
78. BLECHER, T. E., BRZECHWA-AJDUKIEWICZ, A., McCARTHY, C. F., and READ, A. E. (1969), 'Serum Immunoglobulins and Lymphocyte Transformation Studies in Coeliac Disease', *Gut*, **10**, 57.
79. ELVES, M. W., ROATH, S., and ISRAELS, M. C. G. (1963), 'The Response of Lymphocytes to Antigen Challenge in vitro', *Lancet*, **1**, 806.
80. HIRSCHHORN, K., BACH, F., KOLODNY, R. L., FIRSCHEIN, I. L., and HASHEM, N. (1963), 'Immune Response and Mitosis of Human Peripheral Blood Lymphocytes in vitro', *Science, N.Y.*, **142**, 1185.
81. MICHALOWSKI, A. (1963), 'Time-course of DNA Synthesis in Human Leucocyte Cultures', *Expl Cell Res.*, **32**, 609.
82. BARTFIELD, H., and JULIAR, J. F. (1964), 'Immunological Organization and Activity of Human Peripheral White Blood Cell Cultures', *Lancet*, **2**, 767.
83. FORBES, I. J. (1965), 'Specific and Non-specific Stimulation of Antibody Synthesis by Human Leucocytes in vitro', *Lancet*, **1**, 198.
84. GREAVES, M. F., and FLAD, H. D. (1968), 'Effect of Lymphocyte Stimulants on Specific Antibody Synthesis in vitro', *Nature, Lond.*, **219**, 975.
85. LYCETTE, R. R., and PEARMAIN, G. (1963), 'Further Observations of Antigen-induced Mitosis', *Lancet*, **2**, 386.
86. HOLLAND, P., and MAUER, A. M. (1964), 'Drug Induced in vitro Stimulation of Peripheral Leucocytes', *Lancet*, **1**, 1368.
87. CARON, G. A., and SARKANY, I. (1965), 'Lymphoblast Transformation in Sulphonamide Sensitivity', *Br. J. Derm.*, **77**, 556.
88. WIENER, S., and BRASCH, J. (1965), 'The Mitogenic Effect of Grass-pollen Extract', *Med. J. Aust.*, **1**, 148.
89. RICCI, M., RASSALEVA, A., and RICCA, M. (1966), 'Lymphocyte Reaction in Pollenosis', *Lancet*, **2**, 445.
90. SARKANY, I. (1967), 'Lymphocyte Transformation in Drug Hypersensitivity', *Lancet*, **1**, 732.
91. VISCHER, T. L. (1966), 'Lymphocyte Cultures in Drug Hypersensitivity', *Lancet*, **2**, 467.
92. FELLNER, M. J., BAER, R. L., RIPPS, C. S., and HIRSCHHORN, K. (1967), 'Response of Lymphocytes to Penicillin: Comparison with Skin Tests and Circulating Antibodies in Man', *Nature, Lond.*, **216**, 803.
93. HALPERN, B., KY, N. T., and AMACHE, N. (1967), 'Diagnosis of Drug Allergy in vitro with the Lymphocyte Transformation Test', *J. Allergy*, **40**, 168.
94. OPPENHEIM, J. J., WOLSTENCROFT, R. A., and GELL, P. G. H. (1967), 'Delayed Hypersensitivity in the Guinea Pig to a Protein–hapten Conjugate and its Relationship to in vitro Transformation of Lymphnode, Spleen, Thymus and Peripheral Blood Lymphocytes', *Immunology*, **12**, 89.
95. BENACERRAF, B., and GELL, P. G. H. (1959), 'Studies on Hypersensitivity. I, Delayed and Arthus-type Skin Reactivity to Protein Conjugates in Guinea Pigs', *Immunology*, **2**, 53.
96. MILLS, J. (1966), 'The Immunologic Significance of Antigen-induced Lymphocyte Transformation in vitro', *J. Immun.*, **97**, 239.
97. KNIGHT, S. C., and LING, N. R. (1967), 'Lymphocyte-transforming Activity of Homologous and Heterologous Antisera to Rabbit Leucocytes', *Immunology*, **12**, 537.
98. GELL, P. G. H., and SELL, S. (1965), 'Studies on Rabbit Lymphocytes in vitro. II, Induction of Blast Transformation with Antisera to Six IgG Allotypes and Summation with Mixtures of Antisera to Different Allotypes', *J. exp. Med.*, **122**, 813.

99. HASHEM, N., HIRSCHHORN, K., SEDLIS, E., and HOLT, L. E. (1963), 'Infantile Eczema: Evidence of Autoimmunity to Human Skin', *Lancet*, **2**, 269.
100. TOBIAS, H., SAFRAN, A. P., and SCHAFFNER, F. (1967), 'Lymphocyte Stimulation and Chronic Liver Disease', *Lancet*, **1**, 193.
101. FOWLER, I., MORRIS, C. E., and WHITTEY, T. (1966), 'Lymphocyte Transformation in Multiple Sclerosis induced by Cerebrospinal Fluid', *New Engl. J. Med.*, **275**, 1041.
102. ZAVALETA, A., and STASTNY, P. (1967), 'Immunological Memory to an Auto-antigen—The *in vitro* Response to Thyroglobulin', *Clin. exp. Immun.*, **2**, 543.
103. PIPITONE, V., NUMO, R., CARROZZO, M, and DE STASIO, G. (1965), 'Immunità cellulare ed epatopatie croniche', *Folia allergol.*, **12**, 450.
104. PIPITONE, V. (1967), 'Lymphocyte Stimulation and Liver Disease' (letter), *Lancet*, **1**, 849.
105. HOENIG, V., and POSSNEROVA, V. (1967), 'Cultivation of Peripheral Leucocytes in the Presence of Liver Antigen in Liver Cirrhosis', *Z. Immun-Allerg. Forsch.*, **133**, 199.
106. LEHNER, T. (1967), 'Stimulation of Lymphocyte Transformation by Tissue Homogenates in Recurrent Oral Ulceration', *Immunology*, **13**, 159.
107. LEHNER, T. (1967), 'Lymphocyte Stimulation and Liver Disease' (letter), *Lancet*, **1**, 332.
108. HOUSLEY, J., and OPPENHEIM, J. J. (1967), 'Lymphocyte Transformation in Thymectomized and Non-thymectomized Patients with Myasthenia Gravis', *Br. med. J.*, **2**, 679.
109. TAYLOR, K. B., and TRUELOVE, S. C. (1961), 'Circulating Antibodies to Milk Proteins in Ulcerative Colitis', *Br. med. J.*, **2**, 924.
110. BLECHER, T. E., in preparation.
111. HINZ, C. F., PERLMANN, P., and HAMMARSTRÖM, S. (1967), 'Reactivity *in vitro* of Lymphocytes from Patients with Ulcerative Colitis', *J. Lab. clin. Med.*, **70**, 752.
112. HIRSCHHORN, K., SCHREIBMAN, R. R., BACH, F. H., and SITZBACH, L. E. (1964), '*In vitro* Studies of Lymphocytes from Patients with Sarcoidosis and Lympho-proliferative Diseases', *Lancet*, **2**, 842.
113. COWLING, D. C., QUAGLINO, O. D., and BARRET, P. K. M. (1964), 'Effect of Kveim Antigen and Old Tuberculin on Lymphocytes, in Culture from Sarcoid Patients', *Br. med. J.*, **1**, 1481.
114. JOHNSON, G. J., and RUSSELL, P. S. (1965), 'Reaction of Human Lymphocytes in Culture to Components of the Medium', *Nature, Lond.*, **208**, 343.
115. BAIN, B., VAS, M. R., and LOWENSTEIN, L. (1964), 'The Development of Large Immature Mononuclear Cells in Mixed Leucocyte Cultures', *Blood*, **23**, 108.
116. MOYNIHAN, P., JACKSON, J. F., and HARDY, J. D. (1965), 'Lymphocyte Transfor-mation as an *in vitro* Histocompatibility Test', *Lancet*, **1**, 453.
117. WILSON, D. B., SILVERS, W. K., and NOWELL, P. C. (1967), 'Quantitative Studies on the Mixed Lymphocyte Interaction in Rats. II, Relationship of the Proliferative Response to the Immunologic Status of the Donors', *J. exp. Med.*, **126**, 655.
118. BACH, F. H., and KISKEN, W. A. (1967), 'Predictive Value of Results of Mixed Leucocyte Cultures for Skin Allograft Survival in Man', *Transplantation*, **5**, 1046.
119. RUSSELL, P. S., NELSON, S. D., and JOHNSON, G. J. (1966), 'Matching Tests for Histocompatibility in Man', *Ann. N.Y. Acad. Sci.*, **129**, 368.
120. KASAKURA, S., and LOWENSTEIN, L. (1967), 'The Effect of Uremic Blood on Mixed Leukocyte Reactions and on Cultures of Leukocytes with Phytohaemagglutinin', *Transplantation*, **5**, 283.
121. KASAKURA, S., and LOWENSTEIN, L. (1968), 'Effect of Length of Exposure to Cell-free Medium from Mixed Leucocyte Cultures on Blastogenesis in Leucocyte Cultures from Single Subjects', *Nature, Lond.*, **219**, 652.
122. GORDON, J., and MACLEAN, L. D. (1965), 'A Lymphocyte-stimulating Factor produced *in vitro*', *Nature, Lond.*, **208**, 795.
123. VIZA, D. C., DEGANI, O., DAUSSET, J., and DAVIES, D. A. L. (1968), 'Lymphocyte Stimulation by Soluble Human HL-A Transplantation Antigens', *Nature, Lond.*, **219**, 704.
124. FIREMAN, P., BOESMAN, M., HADDAD, Z. H., and GITLIN, D. (1967), 'Passive Transfer of Tuberculin Reactivity *in vitro*', *Science, N.Y.*, **155**, 337.
125. TURK, J. L. (1962), 'The Passive Transfer of Delayed Hypersensitivity in Guinea Pigs by the Transfusion of Isotopically Labelled Lymphoid Cells', *Immunology*, **5**, 478.

126. GOVAERTS, A. (1960), 'Cellular Antibodies in Kidney Homotransplantation', *J. Immun.*, **85**, 516.
127. ROSENAU, W., and MOON, H. D. (1961), 'Lysis of Homologous Cells by Sensitised Lymphocytes in Tissue Culture', *J. natn. Cancer Inst.*, **27**, 471.
128. ROSENAU, W., and MOON, H. D. (1966), 'Studies on the Mechanism of the Cytolytic Effect of Sensitized Lymphocytes', *J. Immun.*, **96**, 80.
129. WILSON, D. B. (1965), 'Quantitative Studies on the Behaviour of Sensitised Lymphocytes *in vitro*. I, Relationship of the Degree of Destruction of Homologous Target Cells to the Number of Lymphocytes and to the Time of Contact in Culture and Consideration of the Effects of the Iso-immune Serum', *J. exp. Med.*, **122**, 143.
130. WILSON, D. B. (1967), 'Lymphocytes as Mediators of Cellular Immunity: Destruction of Homologous Target Cells in Culture', *Transplantation*, **5**, 986.
131. WILSON, D. B., and WECKER, E. E. (1966), 'Quantitative Studies on the Behaviour of Sensitised Lymphoid Cells *in vitro*. III, Conversion of "Normal" Lymphoid Cells to an Immunologically Active Status with RNA derived from Isologous Lymphoid Tissues of Specifically Immunized Rats', *J. Immun.*, **97**, 512.
132. GERUGHTY, R. M., ROSENAU, W., and MOON, H. D. (1966), '*In vitro* Transfer of Immunity by Ribosomes', *J. Immun.*, **97**, 800.
133. MÖLLER, E. (1965), 'Antagonistic Effects of Humoral Iso-antibodies on the *in vitro* Cytotoxicity of Immune Lymphoid Cells', *J. exp. Med.*, **122**, 11.
134. KOPROWSKI, H., and FERNANDES, M. V. (1962), 'Autosensitisation Reaction *in vitro*. Contactual Agglutination of Sensitized Lymphnode Cells in Brain Tissue Culture accompanied by Destruction of Glial Elements', *J. exp. Med.*, **116**, 467.
135. BERG, O., and KÄLLÉN, B. (1963), 'White Blood Cells from Animals with Experimental Allergic Encephalomyelitis tested on Glia Cells in Tissue Culture', *Acta path. microbiol. scand.*, **58**, 33.
136. WINKLER, G. F. (1965) '*In vitro* Demyelination of Peripheral Nerve induced with Sensitized Cells', *Ann. N.Y. Acad. Sci.*, **122**, 287.
137. ROSE, N. R., KITE, J. H., DOEBBLER, T. K., and BROWN, R. C. (1963), '*In vitro* Reactions of Lymphoid Cells with Thyroid Tissue', in *Cell-bound Antibodies* (ed. AMOS, B., and KOPROWSKY, H.). Philadelphia: Wistar Institute Press.
138. BJÖRKLUND, A. (1964), 'Testing *in vitro* of Lymphoid Cells from Rats with Experimental Autoimmune Thyroiditis', *Lab. Invest.*, **13**, 120.
139. LING, N. R., ACTON, A. D., ROITT, I. M., and DONIACH, D. (1965), 'Interaction of Lymphocytes from Immunised Hosts with Thyroid and Other Cells in Tissue Culture', *Br. J. exp. Path.*, **46**, 348.
140. HOLM, G. (1966), '*In vitro* Cytotoxic Effects of Lymphoid Cells from Rats with Experimental Autoimmune Nephrosis', *Clin. exp. Immun.*, **1**, 45.
141. PERLMANN, P., and BROBERGER, O. (1963), '*In vitro* Studies of Ulcerative Colitis. II, Cytotoxic Action of White Blood Cells from Patients on Human Foetal Colon Cells', *J. exp. Med.*, **117**, 717.
142. WATSON, D. W., QUIGLEY, A., and BOLT, R. J. (1966), 'Effect of Lymphocytes from Patients with Ulcerative Colitis on Human Adult Colon Epithelial Cells', *Gastroenterology*, **51**, 985.
143. BERG, O., and KÄLLÉN, B. (1964), 'Effect of Mononuclear Blood Cells from Multiple Sclerosis Patients on Neuroglia in Tissue Culture', *J. Neuropath.*, **23**, 550.
144. BRAUNSTEINER, H., DIENSTL, F., and EIBL, M. (1964), 'Destructive Effect of Lymphnode Cells from Patients with Rheumatoid Arthritis in Tissue Culture', *Acta Haemat.*, **31**, 225.
145. HEDBERG, H. (1967), 'Studies on Synovial Fluid in Arthritis. II, The Occurrence of Mononuclear Cells with *in vitro* Cytotoxic Effect', *Acta med. scand.*, Suppl. 479.
146. SUKERNIK, R., HANIN, A., and MOSOLOV, A. (1968), 'The Reaction of Blood Lymphocytes from Patients with Rheumatoid Arthritis against Human Connective Tissue Cells *in vitro*', *Clin. exp. Immun.*, **3**, 171.
147. TRAYANOVA, T. G., SURA, V. V., and SVET-MOLDAVSKY, G. J. (1966), 'Destruction of Human Cells in Tissue Culture by Lymphocytes from Patients with Systemic Lupus Erythematosus', *Lancet*, **1**, 452.
148. GRANGER, G. A., and WEISER, R. S. (1966), 'Homograft Target Cells: Contact Destruction *in vitro* by Immune Macrophages', *Science, N.Y.*, **151**, 97.
149. MÖLLER, G., and MÖLLER, E. (1967), 'Humoral and Cell-mediated Effector Mechanisms in Tissue Transplantation', *Symp. Tissue Org. Transpl. Suppl., J. Clin. Path.*, **20**, 437.

150. HOLM, G., PERLMANN, P., and WERNER, B. (1964), 'Phytohaemagglutinin-induced Cytotoxic Action of Normal Lymphoid Cells on Cells in Tissue Culture', *Nature, Lond.*, **203**, 841.
151. GINSBURG, H., and SACHS, L. (1966), 'Destruction of Mouse and Rat Embryo Cells in Tissue Culture by Lymphnode Cells from Unsensitized Rats', *J. cell. comp. Physiol.*, **66**, 199.
152. GINSBURG, H. (1968), 'Graft versus Host Reaction in Tissue Culture. I, Lysis of Monolayers of Embryo Mouse Cells from Strains differing in the H_2 Histocompatibility Locus by Rat Lymphocytes sensitized *in vitro*', *Immunology*, **14**, 621.
153. HIRSCHHORN, K., FIRSCHEIN, I. L., and BACH, F. H. (1965), 'Immune Response of Human Peripheral Blood Lymphocytes *in vitro*', in *Histo-compatibility Testing*, Publication 1229, p. 131. Washington, D.C.: National Academy of Sciences.
154. GORDON, J., DAVID-FARIDAY, M. F., and MacLEAN, L. D. (1967), 'Transfer of Transplantation Immunity by Leukocytes sensitized *in vitro*', *Transplantation*, **5**, 1030.

CHAPTER 9

CELL-MEDIATED IMMUNITY AND DELAYED HYPERSENSITIVITY

By J. Verrier Jones

12

I. Introduction

WE have already seen that an animal which has recovered from a bacterial or virus infection is often protected against further infections with the same organism. In many cases serum from an immunized animal will confer immunity, for a limited period, on an unimmunized animal, and this immunity is produced by antibodies. However, some diseases, of which tuberculosis is an example, though conferring lasting immunity, produce no protective antibodies; immunity cannot be transferred passively by serum. A clue to the nature of this immunity came in 1890 (the year in which von Behring and Kitasato discovered antibodies), when Koch [1] described a remarkable form of hypersensitivity in tuberculous guinea-pigs. Animals which had carried a tuberculous infection for 4–6 weeks were reinoculated with tubercle bacilli. After 24 hours a dark indurated nodule appeared at the site of injection which spread to become a sloughing ulcer. This was quite different from the response to tubercle bacilli in an uninfected animal, where the inoculation site healed and remained unremarkable until 10–14 days, when a small nodule might develop.

Koch showed that this reaction, the *Koch phenomenon*, could be produced by killed tubercle bacilli and also by a cell-free extract of the bacteria (old tuberculin). Epstein [2], in the following year, pointed out that the reaction to old tuberculin could be produced in tuberculous children and was of value in establishing the diagnosis of tuberculosis. The clinical and epidemiological aspects of the tuberculin test were later developed by von Pirquet [3] and by Mantoux [4]. For many years there was confusion between immediate hypersensitivity reactions, such as the Arthus reaction (*see* Chapter 7), which can be produced by injecting antigens into animals with circulating antibodies, and the delayed hypersensitivity produced by tubercle bacilli. In 1925 Zinsser [5, 6] distinguished the two types of hypersensitivity and pointed out that the reaction to tubercle bacilli did not require the presence of circulating antibodies. The tuberculin reaction, because of its slow development, was known as 'delayed hypersensitivity'. Zinsser pointed out that it is by no means unique to tuberculin and can be demonstrated with a number of other bacterial antigens.

In 1926 Dienes and Schoenheit [7] showed that guinea-pigs could be induced to develop delayed hypersensitivity to egg albumin and to horse serum. The antigen was introduced directly into a tuberculous lesion, and the animals were tested 3–10 days later. In 1934 Jones and Mote [8] accidentally discovered that humans could also develop delayed hypersensitivity to foreign serum proteins. In the course of research into streptococcal allergy in patients with rheumatic fever they had occasion to inject rabbit peritoneal exudate intradermally in minute amounts (0·1 ml. of a 1/1000 dilution) and 57 out of their 70 patients developed delayed hypersensitivity to rabbit serum. They showed that this was transient and was followed by antibody production and the development of immediate hypersensitivity. This type of hypersensitivity, which was weaker and more transient than classic tuberculin hypersensitivity, became known as the 'Jones-Mote phenomenon'.

Landsteiner, who contributed so much to the study of antibodies, turned to delayed hypersensitivity and showed that simple chemical substances, such as dinitrochlorobenzene (DNCB) and picryl chloride, would produce delayed hypersensitivity in guinea-pigs [9]. They appear to act as haptens, interacting with cellular proteins in the epidermis. It was found that, like the tuberculin reaction, neither the delayed hypersensitivity to foreign proteins nor that to simple haptens could be transferred from a sensitized to an unsensitized animal by serum. In 1942, more than 50 years after the original description of delayed hypersensitivity by Koch, the means of transferring it was at last found. Landsteiner and Chase [10] showed that hypersensitivity to picryl chloride could be transferred, in guinea-pigs, by peritoneal exudate cells, and in 1945 Chase [11] succeeded in transferring tuberculin hypersensitivity in the same way.

The term 'cellular immunity' or 'cell-mediated immunity' is now used to describe those types of immunity in which antibodies cannot be demonstrated and which can be transferred by sensitized cells. Delayed hypersensitivity is one of the means of detecting cellular immunity. Apart from the conditions we have mentioned, cellular immunity is an important component in the rejection of grafts of foreign tissue (*see* Chapter 10) and in the development of some types of auto-immune disease (*see* Chapter 12). The whole topic of delayed hypersensitivity and cellular immunity has recently been reviewed, in an extensive monograph, by Turk [12]. Much of the material in this chapter derives from this readable and comprehensive book. An excellent, brief review by Uhr [13] covers similar ground in summary.

II. THE ELICITATION OF DELAYED HYPERSENSITIVITY

A. The Tuberculin Reaction and its Histology

The model for delayed hypersensitivity reactions is the tuberculin test (the Mantoux reaction). Old tuberculin is prepared (after the original recipe by Koch) by maintaining *Mycobacterium tuberculosis* in glycerin-broth culture for 6–8 weeks, concentrating it by boiling, and removing the bacteria by filtration. The filtrate is used in a dilution of 1/100, 1/1000, or 1/10,000, and 0·1 ml. (containing 100, 10, or 1 tuberculin units (t.u.) respectively) is injected intradermally. 'Purified protein derivative' (PPD) is a preparation of the active tuberculoprotein, obtained by precipitation from the culture filtrate with ammonium sulphate, and can be used instead of Old Tuberculin (OT).

After the intradermal injection of OT or PPD in a sensitive subject, there is no change for 2–4 hours. The skin then becomes pink in an area surrounding the injection, and an indurated lump develops gradually, reaching its maximum size in 48–72 hours, then fading gradually during the following week. Higher doses produce more rapid and more severe reaction, and may be associated with blistering and stripping of the epidermis and with petechial haemorrhages. A sensitive subject, for the purpose of this test, is one who has, or has recovered from, tuberculosis. Guinea-pigs can be rendered tuberculin-positive by infection with tuberculosis or by injection of killed tubercle bacilli in oil or wax [14].

The histology of the tuberculin reaction has been studied intensively for 60 years since it was first described by Auché and Augustrou [15], and it is noticeable that there is still disagreement over details. Dienes and Mallory [16] studied the histology of the tuberculin reaction in guinea-pigs and Gell and Hinde [17] in rabbits. The cellular responses are similar in most species: minor differences can generally be attributed to anatomical differences in the skin, which may be more or less cornified and more or less hairy.

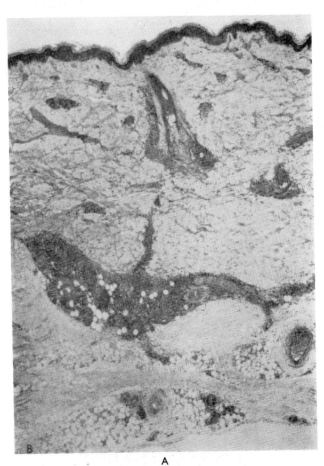

A

Fig. 56.—The tuberculin reaction. **A**, Skin from tuberculin-negative human subject inoculated 48 hours previously with 100 units PPD. **B**, Skin from tuberculin-sensitive human subject inoculated 48 hours previously with 10 units PPD. There is a dense infiltrate of mononuclear cells around the hair follicles, sweat-glands, sebaceous glands, and blood-vessels. **C**, Venule in deep plexus with mononuclear cells, mainly small lymphocytes. *Reproduced from J. H. Humphrey and R. G. White* (1964), '*Immunology for Students of Medicine*', *by kind permission of Blackwell Scientific Publications, Oxford.*

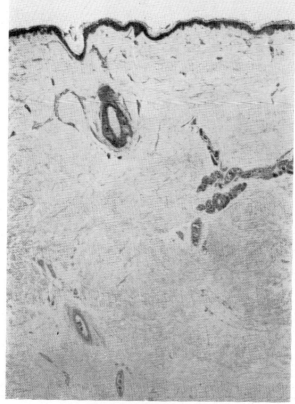

B

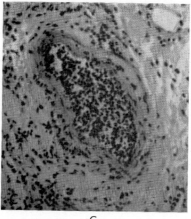

C

The earliest changes are those of inflammation: at 4 hours many of the small arteries, arterioles, capillaries, venules, and lymphatics are dilated and there is oedema of the dermis. Gell and Hinde, comparing the tuberculin reaction with the response to injected tuberculin in a control (unsensitized) animal, found that these changes were comparable in test and control animals, though in the test animal there was at this stage a slight serous exudate. At 4–6 hours in both guinea-pigs and rabbits there was a diffuse infiltration of the dermis with polymorphs. The dilated blood-vessels are full of polymorphs, and the endothelial and perithelial cells of the vessels themselves are hyperplastic. Around the vessels are collections of mononuclear cells. Most are phagocytic cells, derived either from circulating monocytes or from histiocytes in the tissues.

At 22–24 hours the picture has changed (*Fig.* 56). The test lesion is now clearly differentiated from the control. The vascular dilatation is subsiding and mononuclear cells greatly outnumber the degenerating polymorphs. Capillaries are plugged with leucocytes, and there is a dense infiltration of mononuclear cells surrounding the blood-vessels. Most of these are histiocytes, though there are a few lymphocytes. Whorls of lymphocytes are seen in the superficial dermis with occasional plasma cells. The infiltration with mononuclear cells spreads diffusely through the dermis, where the majority of cells are histiocytes.

Gell and Hinde [17] compared the tuberculin reaction with an acute inflammatory response produced by the injection of brain phospholipid. The main difference was that in both the 4-hour and 22-hour lesions polymorphs were the dominant cells. There was much less infiltration with mononuclear cells and lymphocytes were rare. Boughton and Spector [18] reviewed the tuberculin reaction in guinea-pigs in detail and in particular attempted to determine the origin of the mononuclear cells which form so striking a part of the cellular reaction. They found two peaks of leucocyte migration; the first, at 3 hours, was subsiding at 5 hours and occurred in non-sensitized as well as sensitized animals. The second peak occurred at 8 hours (in sensitized animals only) and was subsiding gradually at 24–28 hours. They pointed out that while mononuclear cells emigrating from blood-vessels will remain in the tissues for a number of days, polymorphs, once they have left the circulation, degenerate rapidly. This will partly account for the early predominance of polymorphs in the exudate and the later dominance of mononuclear cells. Spector and his co-workers [19, 20] studied the origin of cells in inflammatory granulomata by labelling mononuclear cells with tritiated thymidine, and by injecting colloidal carbon to mark phagocytes. Their conclusions are probably applicable to the lesions of hypersensitivity. They found that the mononuclear infiltrate at 12 hours was derived mainly from blood monocytes. This was followed by proliferation of cells in the blood-vessel walls and of histiocytes and macrophages in the tissue. They found that monocytes emigrate at a constant rate (2×10^5 cells per 24 hours) for a prolonged period.

The identification of the cells involved in delayed hypersensitivity is of considerable interest. We have seen that in antibody production the first cell to react with antigen after it has been processed by the macrophages is probably the lymphocyte. Subsequently lymphocytes, or their descendants, and the related plasma cells are the eventual antibody-forming units. It has been demonstrated that antibody-producing cells and their precursors, the antigen-reactive units, are probably unipotent and committed to a single antibody (*see* Chapter 4). Experiments have shown that lymphocytes will transfer delayed hypersensitivity from a sensitized to an unsensitized animal (*see* p. 304). If antibody-producing cells are unipotent it would be surprising if the lymphocytes involved in delayed hypersensitivity were not also unipotent. In order to test this it is necessary to have a clear picture of what part lymphocytes play in delayed hypersensitivity and what their origin is. In general, lymphocytes can be regarded as the immunologically specific cells in a delayed hypersensitivity

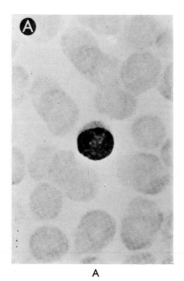
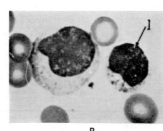

A   B

Fig. 57.—Agranular leucocytes of human blood. **A**, Lymphocyte. *Reproduced from W. Andrew (1966), 'Microfabric of Man', by kind permission of Yearbook Publishers, Chicago.* **B**, A monocyte from the peripheral blood, with a small lymphocyte (1) alongside. *Reproduced from S. J. Piliero, M. S. Jacobs, and S. Wischnitzer (1965), 'Atlas of Histology', by kind permission of Lippincott, Philadelphia.*

reaction, while the other cells mainly involved (macrophages and histiocytes) are phagocytic and seem not to be involved in an immunologically specific role.

It is important, then, to be able to distinguish lymphocytes from phagocytes in a delayed hypersensitivity reaction. This distinction is usually straightforward. Lymphocytes (*Fig.* 57A) are small, round cells, with scanty cytoplasm and a densely staining nuclei, showing a coarse pattern of chromatin. Histiocytes, by contrast, have an abundant cytoplasm containing occasional small granules. The nucleus is typically kidney-shaped and, because of its finely reticular chromatin, appears pale. However, Spector and Lykke [19], in their study of developing granulomata, described small round cells, which, although they had arisen from histiocytes, closely resembled lymphocytes morphologically. It is reasonable to conclude that not all small round cells are necessarily lymphocytes, and that in delayed hypersensitivity, as in political demonstrations, it is rather easy for bystanders to become confused with participants.

In addition to the cellular reaction in the dermis during delayed hypersensitivity, there are striking changes in the epidermis. In both the guinea-pig [16] and the rabbit [17] the epidermis becomes strikingly thickened within 24 hours of the injection of tuberculin. In the guinea-pig, where the epidermis is normally three cells deep, it may increase to ten cells, and in rabbits it may increase from two to six cells in depth.

If the tuberculin reaction is studied beyond 48 hours the lesion gradually comes to resemble a chronic inflammatory granuloma (*Fig.* 58), such as is

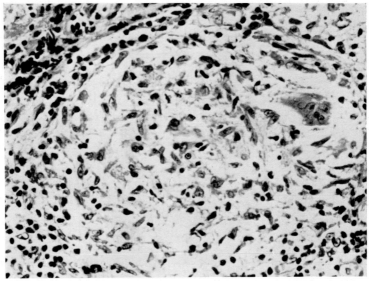

Fig. 58.—A granuloma from human skin. A whorl of epithelioid cells is seen, surrounded by lymphocytes. A multinucleate giant cell is seen to the right of the figure. (×375.)

seen in the course of a natural tuberculous infection [21]. The histiocytes develop into 'epithelioid' cells [22], which have very large ovoid nuclei, with pale chromatin and prominent nucleoli. The cytoplasm is copious and pale. At this stage giant cells begin to appear. These are enormous cells, with a number of quite distinct nuclei embedded in abundant pale cytoplasm. Spector and Lykke [19] showed that colloidal carbon, which is taken up by phagocytes and appears first in the macrophages, histiocytes, and epithelioid cells, is later seen in giant cells. It seems likely that these curious structures are formed by the amalgamation of a number of separate histiocytes possibly after ingesting polymorphs or lymphocytes, or even by cannibalism. Giant cells are also seen in granulomata produced in response to foreign materials such as liquid paraffin and may be associated with the removal of necrotic tissue [23, 24].

B. Delayed Hypersensitivity to Other Antigens and its Histology

1. Animals can be induced to develop delayed hypersensitivity to a wide range of antigens. Gell [25] studied the histology of delayed hypersensitivity reactions produced in the guinea-pig to proteins or hapten–protein complexes and showed that the histology was very similar to that of the tuberculin reaction. Goldberg, Kantor, and Benacerraf [26] used the electron microscope to study the delayed hypersensitivity reaction to ferritin in guinea-pigs. Ferritin particles are visible under the electron microscope, so that antigen could be localized exactly. They found ferritin in phagolysosomes in histiocytes. This localization did not appear to be immunologically specific. Ferritin was not bound to lymph-node cells from immunized animals; there was no evidence that sensitized lymphocytes carried cell-bound antibody.

2. Martins and Raffel [27] compared the histology of the typical delayed response to tuberculin with the weaker, transient Jones-Mote type of hypersensitivity, which can be produced with smaller doses of tuberculoprotein and which is usually followed by antibody production. They found that the cellular changes were similar in general outline to those seen in the typical tuberculin test, but that they developed rather more slowly. There were fewer lymphocytes and less tissue necrosis. In the later stages of the Jones-Mote reaction there were numerous plasma cells. They argued that the differences were sufficiently marked to suggest that the mechanisms for delayed hypersensitivity and the Jones-Mote reaction were different. However, Turk, Heather, and Diengdoh [28], using histochemical techniques to study the cellular infiltrates, were unable to find any striking differences between delayed hypersensitivity and the Jones-Mote reaction.

3. The third important type of delayed hypersensitivity is that developed to simple chemical compounds, such as dinitrochlorobenzene (DNCB) and picryl chloride. Unlike the antigens described previously, which are injected intradermally to elicit delayed hypersensitivity, the chemical allergens are effective when applied to the surface of the skin. This may partly account for the rather different histological pattern seen in the reaction to chemical sensitizers. Recent detailed accounts of the histology of the reaction to DNCB have been published by Flax and Caulfield [29], who included electron microscopic observations, Turk, Heather, and Diengdoh [28], who used histochemical methods to distinguish the various types of cell involved, and Ove Groth [30, 31, 32, 33], who used careful quantitative techniques of cell counting. The most striking difference between this reaction and reactions of the tuberculin type is the absence of the biphasic infiltration with polymorphs. DNCB in high concentrations may have a direct toxic effect on the skin, and the resulting tissue necrosis is often associated with some polymorph infiltration [34]; apart from this, lymphocytes are the dominant cells throughout. A second difference is that in contact sensitivity the proportion of macrophages is lower than in the tuberculin reaction. Otherwise the general pattern of the reaction to contact allergens is similar to the tuberculin response. Within

6–8 hours after application of the allergen there is oedema of the basal layers of the epidermis and a round-cell infiltration of the superficial dermis and the deeper layers of the epidermis. The oedema increases and the cellular infiltrate becomes more intense and more widespread up to about 12 hours. It then remains fairly constant, until the reaction begins to subside at 48–72 hours. Turk, Rudner, and Heather [35] showed that appearances in human skin were remarkably similar to those seen in the guinea-pig. In the later stages of the reaction in humans, epithelioid and giant cells may be seen.

III. The Induction of Delayed Hypersensitivity

A. Inducing Antigens

1. Tubercle Bacilli

We have discussed the histology of the tuberculin response and its analogues because delayed hypersensitivity is one of the indicators of cellular immunity, in the same way that the antigen–antibody reaction is an indicator of humoral immunity. A delayed hypersensitivity reaction can be defined as one having the gross and histological characteristics of the tuberculin test, and an antigen which provokes this reaction can be defined as a delayed hypersensitivity antigen. It is convenient to distinguish two separate aspects of delayed hypersensitivity. The introduction of antigen into a non-immunized animal leads to the *induction* of delayed hypersensitivity, while subsequent doses of antigen result in the *elicitation* of delayed hypersensitivity. In a sense, the induction phase corresponds to the primary phase of antibody production, while elicitation corresponds to the secondary response. Up to now we have been considering ways of *eliciting* delayed hypersensitivity. We can now consider the process of induction. In considering antibody production we looked first at the fate of administered antigen and its handling by the lymph-nodes. In parallel, we can now consider delayed hypersensitivity antigens and their fate, and the histological changes which follow their arrival in a lymph-node. A sharply defined difference between work in the two fields will soon become apparent. In antibody production we are dealing with a measurable effect, which challenges the development of techniques of increasing sensitivity. Since antibody can be quantitated it can be subjected to experimental investigation in a wide range of different conditions, which may either increase or diminish it. In delayed hypersensitivity we are considering the microscopic appearances of groups of cells and their changing configuration in time. Delayed hypersensitivity reactions are either present or absent. Quantitation has only limited applications and the outcome of the most sophisticated cellular manœuvres is often restricted to the observation of whether or not a guinea-pig develops pink spots. Despite the difficulty of quantitation, delayed hypersensitivity and cellular immunity are involved in some of the most challenging and rapidly advancing areas of present-day immunological research, and if some of the techniques are elementary they are all the more readily available.

What type of antigens will produce delayed hypersensitivity? We have already discussed the tuberculin reaction. It occurs in animals which have been infected with tubercle bacilli, but can also be produced by injecting killed mycobacteria in oil or a modified non-virulent strain, 'bacille Calmette-Guérin' (BCG) [14, 36]. Intradermal injections are more effective than subcutaneous injections. Just as there is a latent period in the induction of antibody production, so there is a latent period before delayed hypersensitivity can be demonstrated. For tubercle bacilli this is 4–5 days [36].

2. OTHER BACTERIA, FUNGI, AND PROTOZOA

The tuberculin reaction has been more extensively studied than any other natural delayed hypersensitivity reaction. Reactions of delayed hypersensitivity can, however, be induced by a number of other natural antigens. The leprosy bacillus (*Mycobacterium leprae*) is a close relative of the tubercle bacillus, and an antigen (lepromin) derived from the tissue of leprous patients will produce delayed hypersensitivity in some patients with leprosy. D'Arcy Hart and Rees [37] have described this reaction in detail and conclude that it is analogous with hypersensitivity to tuberculin.

A number of other bacteria have been shown to produce delayed hypersensitivity. *Salmonella typhi*, *Pfeifferella mallei*, and *Brucella abortus* are all effective; antigens derived from culture filtrates (typhoidin, mallein, and abortin) will produce delayed sensitivity in infected animals [12]. *Streptococcus viridans* also produces delayed hypersensitivity, and a nucleoprotein derived from pneumococci will evoke delayed hypersensitivity in animals previously injected with pneumococci [38]. Humans who have had diphtheria, or who have acquired active immunity as a result of inoculation with diphtheria toxoid, show a delayed hypersensitivity to diphtheria toxin. This interferes with the Schick test, which was of considerable epidemiological importance at the time when diphtheria was a major killing disease [39]. Injections of diphtheria toxoid, in adjuvant or combined with antibody, will produce a transient delayed hypersensitivity in guinea-pigs of the Jones-Mote type [40, 41].

A number of pathogenic fungi are known to produce delayed hypersensitivity in man and animals [42]. They include *Actinomyces bovis*, *Nocardia asteroides*, *Candida albicans*, *Cryptococcus neoformans*, *Blastomyces dermatitidis*, *Coccidioides immitis*, *Histoplasma capsulatum*, *Hormodendrum pedrosoi*, *Sporotrichum schenckii*, and *Trichophyton* spp. Cross-reactions between the fungal antigens are common.

Delayed hypersensitivity to protozoal antigens has rarely been shown convincingly. This may be because it is rarely looked for. Frenkel [43] found that humans infected with *Toxoplasma gondii* developed delayed hypersensitivity reaction to a saline extract of toxoplasma, and Montenegro [44] demonstrated a delayed hypersensitivity reaction to an extract of *Leishmania tropica* in patients with cutaneous leishmaniasis. In general, it is surprising to find that an enormous amount of effort has been devoted to studying the humoral aspects of immunity to protozoa, while hardly any attention has been paid to cellular aspects.

3. VIRUSES

Jenner gave the first description of delayed hypersensitivity in 1798 [45], when he described the effect of an intradermal inoculation of material from a small-pox lesion into the arm of a milkmaid who had previously recovered from cow-pox. Because of the cross-reactivity between the small-pox and cow-pox viruses, the girl, who had developed delayed hypersensitivity to cow-pox as a result of her infection, demonstrated delayed hypersensitivity to small-pox as well. Jenner not only described and defined the reaction, but also clearly recognized its relevance to immunity. 'Indeed', he writes, 'it becomes almost a criterion by which we can determine whether the infection will be received or not.' The production of delayed hypersensitivity by viruses as a whole has been reviewed by Allison [46]. Experimental studies have provided strong evidence that delayed hypersensitivity is important in the response to vaccinia and variola (small-pox); Pincus and Flick [47, 48] found that delayed hypersensitivity to inactivated virus developed 4 days after primary vaccination. An antigen from mumps virus will produce a delayed hypersensitivity reaction in those who have had mumps and gives a useful indication of immunity. Herpes simplex virus has also been reported to cause delayed hypersensitivity [49]. The duration of delayed hypersensitivity to virus infections has not been studied systematically. Natural infections with measles or small-pox are followed by a prolonged period of immunity (and presumably of delayed hypersensitivity) while the protection afforded by small-pox vaccination declines over 5–10 years.

4. PROTEIN ANTIGENS

Foreign proteins can also be used to produce delayed hypersensitivity (the Jones-Mote phenomenon). In 1929 Dienes and Schoenheit [50] showed that guinea-pigs would develop delayed hypersensitivity to ovalbumin and horse serum if the antigen was injected into a tuberculous focus. Dienes and Mallory [51] later showed that delayed hypersensitivity could be produced in uninfected guinea-pigs and rabbits by the intra-peritoneal injection of 5 mg. of egg-white or 0·1 ml. of horse serum. The reaction was stronger in the infected than in uninfected animals, but not qualitatively different. A positive reaction was detected at 3 days in infected animals and at 6 days in uninfected animals. They did not establish the duration of the latent period, but it must have been less than 3 days. Uhr et al. [40] showed that diphtheria toxoid and ovalbumin produced delayed hypersensitivity in guinea-pigs when injected intra-dermally in the form of antigen–antibody complexes in antibody excess, and Salvin [41] showed that diphtheria toxoid or ovalbumin was effective if injected with Freund's incomplete adjuvant. Salvin found negative skin reactions in animals tested 3 days after injection of antigen. At 4 days delayed hypersensitivity was demonstrated, which persisted for up to 25 days. The latent period for diphtheria toxoid was related to the dose. With smaller doses the latent period could be as long as 6 days. During the period of delayed hypersensitivity, reactivity could be transferred from sensitized to non-sensitized animals by lymph-node cells In Salvin's experiments (*Fig.* 59) delayed hypersensitivity was followed by antibody production, and tuberculin-type skin reactions were replaced by Arthus reactions (*see* Chapter 7) after a variable time, depending on the dose of antigen. With smaller doses of antigen (0·03 μg. ovalbumin) delayed hypersensitivity lasted for about 13 days, before being replaced by antibody production. With larger doses (0·3 μg. ovalbumin) the change-over took place at 8 days. With very small doses of diphtheria toxoid (0·01 Lf) delayed hypersensitivity continued to the end of the experiment (25 days) and there was no antibody production. If tubercle bacilli were injected with diphtheria toxoid, delayed hypersensitivity to toxoid was more marked and persisted longer before being overtaken by antibody production.

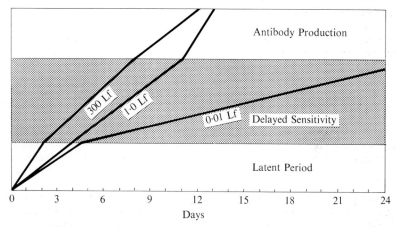

Fig. 59.—Guinea-pigs were injected with three doses of diphtheria toxoid in incomplete Freund's adjuvant and tested at intervals for delayed hypersensitivity and antibody production. The smallest dose (0·01 Lf) produced delayed hyper-sensitivity only. The largest dose (300 Lf) produced transient delayed hyper-sensitivity followed by sustained antibody production. *After Salvin.*

Raffel and Newel [52], following up the work of Uhr et al. [40], confirmed that transient delayed hypersensitivity could be induced by antigen–antibody complexes injected intradermally. After 2–3 weeks most animals had lost this hypersensitivity. They showed that a similar degree of hypersensitivity could be induced with the same amount of antigen in incomplete adjuvant and, like Salvin, found that delayed hyper-sensitivity was gradually followed by antibody production. In animals tested 20 days after sensitization it was found that the greater responses were in those stimulated with larger amounts of antigen, while those given smaller doses of antigen had often lost all reactivity. They were the first to suggest the term 'Jones-Mote reactivity' to describe this early, transient form of delayed hypersensitivity and suggested that it was qualitatively different from tuberculin-type hypersensitivity. This point is discussed in more detail in connexion with the histology of the lesions (p. 293).

Sell and Weigle [53] confirmed that delayed hypersensitivity could be produced when guinea-pigs were injected with bovine gamma-globulin (BGG) in the form of antigen–antibody complexes in incomplete adjuvant. Antibody production and the Arthus reaction appeared at day 12, and, interestingly, a delayed reaction reappeared in some animals after 24 and

27 days. They also showed that delayed hypersensitivity could be blocked if antigen were given intravenously before the intradermal test dose.

In summary: when delayed hypersensitivity to protein antigens is induced there is a latent period of about 3 days, the length of which varies inversely with the dose of antigen. This is followed by a period of delayed hypersensitivity which may last for a few days or several weeks. The duration of this period is also related inversely to the dose of antigen. It is terminated, in many cases, by a phase of antibody production, when delayed hypersensitivity may be masked by the Arthus reaction. Finally, if the animals are studied for longer periods delayed hypersensitivity may reappear.

5. CONTACT ALLERGENS

Landsteiner, who had studied in detail the specificity of antibodies produced against chemical haptens, found that simple molecules were also capable of producing delayed hypersensitivity. With Jacobs [54, 55] he tested substituted benzene compounds, including p-nitroso-dimethylaniline and various nitrochlorobenzenes, and found that some were strong sensitizers while other structurally similar compounds were ineffective. He showed that those substances which produced sensitization had reactive chloro- and nitro-groups which were labile when treated with alkali, and that they also readily formed substitution compounds with aniline. He suggested that this reactivity enabled them to combine more readily with proteins in the skin, and that the hapten–protein complex then behaved as an antigen. This view has been confirmed by later work. Eisen, Orris, and Belman [56] found that the ability of dinitrophenyl compounds to elicit delayed hypersensitivity correlated with their ability to combine with proteins in vivo and in vitro. Epstein [57] found a similar correlation with the ability of dinitrophenyl compounds to induce delayed hypersensitivity.

After they have been painted on the skin both dinitrochlorobenzene (DNCB) and dinitrofluorobenzene (DNFB) lose their halogen atoms and are converted into dinitrophenyl groups. In this form they are bound in the epidermis, principally to the ε-amino groups of the lysine residues in cellular proteins [58].

While protein antigens will produce delayed hypersensitivity best if injected intradermally with adjuvant, the chemical allergens are effective after a single application to the skin. DNCB can be applied in various ways: 0·002 ml. of a 50 per cent solution in acetone is recommended by Turk [12] for sensitizing guinea-pigs, while Aisenberg [59] has used 0·1 ml. of 10 per cent DNCB in humans. Oxazolone (2-ethoxymethylene-5-oxazolone) is effective in guinea-pigs if 0·2 ml. of a 10 per cent solution in ethanol is applied to the ear. A single application in each case will produce delayed hypersensitivity within 5 days.

Not many workers have reported quantitative studies of the effect of varying the dose of chemical allergens on the latent period and duration of hypersensitivity. Frey [60] showed that after a dose of 0·1 ml. of 0·1 per cent DNCB, guinea-pigs became sensitized in 4–10 days. The sensitivity lasted for 30–90 days; it may have been artificially lengthened by the frequent small doses of DNCB used in testing. Epstein and Kligman (61)

studied the effect of sensitizing humans with varying doses of DNCB and
p-nitrosodimethylaniline (NDMA). They found that 5 per cent of their
subjects were sensitized with 0·0005 molar DNCB and none with the
same strength of NDMA. With 0·05 molar solutions, 91 per cent were
sensitized to DNCB and 80 per cent to NDMA. There is very little
evidence available on the rate of decay of delayed hypersensitivity to
chemical allergens in humans.

In summary, delayed hypersensitivity can be induced by infection with
tuberculosis or other bacterial, viral, fungal, or protozoal agents, by
intradermal injection of foreign proteins and toxins (with or without
adjuvants), and by epidermal contact with chemical allergens. Though
there are differences in detail between the effects of these agents, there are
enough similarities for us to consider them as a group, and to conclude
that we are dealing with a branch of immunology as important and as
far-reaching as the humoral immunity resulting from antibody production.

B. The Role of the Skin and Lymph-nodes

When antigen is injected into or painted on the skin of an unsensitized
animal it is rapidly carried to the draining lymph-nodes. It has been
shown that the development of delayed hypersensitivity can be prevented
by removal of an area of skin within 16 hours of the application of a
chemical allergen [62]. If the skin is removed more than 16 hours after
the application of antigen, sensitization is not prevented [63]. Freund and
Lipton [64] examined the production of allergic encephalomyelitis in
guinea-pigs by injecting an emulsion of spinal cord in adjuvant. The
development of clinical and histological evidence of encephalomyelitis is a
sensitive indicator of delayed hypersensitivity, and in this system sensitization could not be prevented if the injection site was excised after only
1 hour.

Frey and Wenk [62] studied the role of the skin site in the induction of
delayed hypersensitivity by using an area of skin which was linked to the
guinea-pig only by a vascular pedicle. Lymphatic drainage was completely
severed. They found that DNCB applied to this isolated skin fragment
failed to sensitize the animals; this implies that for effective sensitization
it is necessary for antigen to travel via lymphatics from the skin to the
draining lymph-node. Lymphatic connexions are not, however, necessary
for the *expression* of delayed hypersensitivity. Frey and Wenk found that
isolated skin fragments would develop delayed hypersensitivity if the
animal had previously been sensitized in the normal way. The cells
responsible for the expression of delayed hypersensitivity are therefore in
circulation, and reach the site of a delayed hypersensitivity reaction by
escaping from the local blood-vessels.

The next step, then, in following the induction of delayed hypersensitivity
is to study the changes in the draining lymph-node. These have been
extensively investigated by Turk [12]. Gallone, Radici, and Riquier [65]
had briefly described lymph-node changes accompanying the rejection of
skin homografts, but it was Scothorne and McGregor [66] who first
published a detailed account of lymph-node histology during graft
rejection. They exchanged skin-grafts from the dorsum of the ear in
rabbits and studied the preauricular node. They found that changes were

seen as early as 2 days after grafting and were confined to the first draining node on the side of operation. Nodules appeared at the corticomedullary junction and contained numerous large (15 μ diameter) cells, which were round or ovoid, with prominent nucleoli, a pale nucleus, and vacuolated cytoplasm staining strongly with pyronin (*Fig.* 60A). These cells have been termed 'large pyroninophilic cells'; Dameshek [67] has called them 'immunoblasts' and it has now been found that they appear in lymph-nodes which are being stimulated by a delayed hypersensitivity antigen.

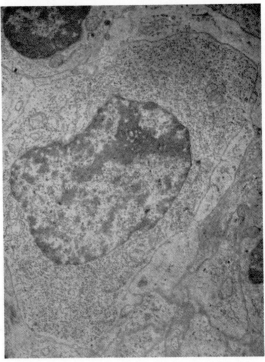

Fig. 60.—Electron micrograph of immunoblast. There is a large nucleus with loosely arranged chromatin. There are clusters of ribosomes in the cytoplasm. The endoplasmic reticulum is scanty. *Reproduced from S. de Petris, J. G. Karlsbad, B. Pernis, and J. L. Turk* (1966), '*International Archives of Allergy and Applied Immunology*', *vol.* 29, p. 112, *by kind permission of Karger, Basel.*

Oort and Turk [68] studied the changes in the structure of guinea-pig lymph-nodes during the induction of delayed hypersensitivity to oxazolone. Two days after sensitization the nodes developed active follicles in the cortex, which compressed the medulla and which were quite distinct from the germinal follicles which appear during antibody production. Oort and Turk called these 'paracortical areas' and showed that they contained large numbers of immunoblasts. Four days after sensitization the para-cortical areas occupied a large portion of the medulla and contained even more immunoblasts. At 6 days immunoblasts had decreased in numbers and were replaced by small lymphocytes. Labelling with ³H-thymidine suggests that the small lymphocytes are the descendants of immuno-blasts. The morphology of the lymph-node contrasted sharply with the appearances seen after the subcutaneous injection of 10 μg. of pneumo-coccal polysaccharide. This antigen induces antibody production, but no delayed hypersensitivity. Fifteen days after injection germinal centres began to appear in the cortex and plasma cells accumulated in the medulla. The 'paracortical areas' did not develop and there were no immunoblasts (*Fig.* 61). Turk suggested that these two alternative patterns

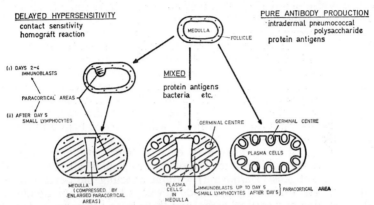

Fig. 61.—Diagram to represent the contrast between lymph-node changes during antibody production and those during delayed hypersensitivity. *Reproduced from J. L. Turk (1967), 'Delayed Hypersensitivity', by kind permission of North-Holland Publishing Company.*

of lymph-node stimulation are fundamental to the two types of immuno-logical response and pointed out that in the response to natural antigens, in bacterial or viral infections, the changes will be a mixture of the 'para-cortical area–immunoblast' pattern and the 'germinal centre–plasma cell pattern', depending on the proportion of cellular and humoral immunity evoked by a particular antigen.

Immunoblasts appear to play an important part in delayed hyper-sensitivity, and it is therefore relevant to consider their nature and role in more detail. Studies with the electron microscope [69, 70] have shown that they have large round nuclei (*Fig.* 60), with one or several prominent nucleoli. There are very numerous ribosomes in clusters of 4–6. The presence of polyribosomes indicates that they are synthesizing protein. The synthesis of large amounts of protein for export from the cell is usually associated with the presence of an abundant endoplasmic reticulum, as in plasma cells (*see* Chapter 4). It is, therefore, interesting that immuno-blasts contain no endoplasmic reticulum or, at most, a few strands. It seems likely that immunoblasts are manufacturing protein which is largely retained within the cell. The nature of this protein will be an important key to our understanding of the mechanism of delayed hypersensitivity. Some form of immunoglobulin molecule might be expected, but so far none has been demonstrated.

13

Before we can discuss the role of immunoblasts we need to know where they come from and where they go. The origin of immunoblasts was studied by Gowans et al. [71]. They injected a suspension of rat small lymphocytes into irradiated mice. Spleens from the mice were examined up to 60 hours later and showed numerous immunoblasts, all of which had originated from rat cells. Porter and Cooper [72] injected lymphocytes from male rats into newborn female rats. Again the immunoblasts were found to have originated from donor cells. There is therefore strong evidence that immunoblasts can develop from donor cells in allogeneic hosts; it is also highly likely that they are formed from small lymphocytes.

The fate of immunoblasts is less certain. On the fourth day after sensitization, when immunoblasts are at their maximum, lymph-node cells become capable of transferring sensitivity to an unsensitized recipient. Immunoblasts leave the lymph-node 5 days after sensitization, and if the sensitized node is removed at or after this stage the animal retains its sensitization. Immunologically competent cells must have left the gland, to settle and proliferate in other centres. Both these observations are compatible with the theory that immunoblasts are immunologically competent cells, but direct experiments will be needed before this can be more than a plausible guess.

To sum up, in the induction of delayed hypersensitivity the site of application can be excised after 16 hours (for chemical allergens) or after 1 hour (for antigens in adjuvant) without affecting the development of sensitivity. The draining lymph-node develops large pyroninophilic cells in the enlarging paracortical areas, and these leave the node at about the same time as generalized delayed hypersensitivity begins to develop. The large pyroninophilic cells (immunoblasts) are probably formed from small lymphocytes, and are likely to be immunologically competent cells, which, in turn, transform into the small lymphocytes which participate in delayed hypersensitivity reactions.

IV. ANTIGENIC SPECIFICITY IN DELAYED HYPERSENSITIVITY

We saw that, in antibody production, there is a close correlation between antigens used to evoke a primary response and those capable of combining with the antibody produced or eliciting a secondary response. The degree of specificity involved in the secondary response closely resembles that of the antigen–antibody reaction. The specificity of delayed hypersensitivity has also been studied in detail. The corresponding experimental situation is to sensitize an animal with one antigen and then test with related antigens to find those which will elicit delayed hypersensitivity. Experiments of this kind suggest that specificity in delayed hypersensitivity is rather broader than in antibody production. The antigenic determinants seem to involve a larger portion of the molecule, and the mechanism is less sensitive to small changes in the antigen.

Benacerraf and Gell [73] were the first to draw attention to the difference in specificity between antibody and delayed hypersensitivity. Guinea-pigs were injected with a hapten, the picryl group, attached to a carrier protein, bovine gamma-globulin (pic-BGG), and developed both antibodies and delayed hypersensitivity. The antibodies not only reacted with the whole molecule pic-BGG, but also with the hapten, when it was conjugated to another carrier protein such as guinea-pig gamma-globulin (pic-GPGG). The antibodies failed to react with the unconjugated carrier protein, BGG. This type of specificity, directed against the whole antigen or against the hapten alone, is known as hapten specificity (*Table XXI*). By contrast, delayed hypersensitivity was directed against the whole molecule pic-BGG or against the unconjugated carrier protein, BGG, but not against the hapten when it was conjugated to another carrier protein. This is carrier specificity (*Table XXI*). In a number of systems it has been confirmed that hapten specificity is typical of antibody while carrier specificity is typical of delayed hypersensitivity.

Table XXI.—DELAYED HYPERSENSITIVITY. THE SPECIFICITY OF ANTIBODY PRODUCTION AND DELAYED HYPERSENSITIVITY

IMMUNIZATION WITH	SPECIFICITY	TYPE OF SENSITIZATION	
		Antibody	Delayed Hyper-sensitivity
Carrier/Hapten	Carrier/Hapten	+	+
	Carrier	−	+
	Hapten	+	−

Most haptens obey this rule; an exception is *p*-azobenzene arsonate (*p*-ABA). Leskowitz in an extensive series of investigations [74, 75] showed that this hapten, when linked to polytyrosine, produced a delayed hypersensitivity which had no carrier specificity. Sensitized guinea-pigs, in fact, showed hapten specificity, developing delayed hypersensitivity to *p*-ABA linked to guinea-pig serum albumin. However, *p*-ABA appears to be unique; related haptens, such as azobenzoates and azosulphonates, show typical carrier specificity. Several explanations for the curious behaviour of *p*-ABA are considered by Gell and Wolstencroft [76]; none is completely satisfactory. The arsenic atom itself may, by its affinity for sulphydryl groups, increase the binding strength of the hapten.

The phenomenon of carrier specificity indicates that delayed hypersensitivity is directed against a greater area of the antigen than antibody. While antibody, reacting against a small area of antigen, is capable of recognizing the hapten alone, delayed hypersensitivity, reacting against a much larger area, can only recognize the hapten and the adjacent areas of the protein molecule to which it is attached. Apart from the special case of *p*-ABA, there is no clear indication of how large the 'combining site' involved in delayed hypersensitivity may be.

The specificity of antibodies is such that they can distinguish between *o*-, *m*-, and *p*-forms of the same compound (*see* Chapter 2). Silverstein and Gell [77] studied the specificity of delayed hypersensitivity in guinea-pigs sensitized to *o*-azobenzene sulphonate conjugated to guinea-pig serum albumin: 12 out of 12 animals showed delayed hypersensitivity to the sensitizing *o*-isomer, but 9 and 7 also reacted to the *m*- and *p*-isomers. Similar observations by other workers have confirmed that the delayed hypersensitivity system is less able to discriminate between related compounds than the antibody system.

It was originally thought that the contrasts in specificity between antibody and delayed hypersensitivity were so great that they must represent fundamental differences in mechanism. However, recent studies have shown that antibodies formed early in the antibody response have specificities similar to delayed hypersensitivity. Borek and Silverstein [78] sensitized guinea-pigs with *p*-aminobenzoate and *p*-nitroaniline, coupled to guinea-pig albumin or ovalbumin. The earliest antibodies formed showed carrier specificity (as in delayed hypersensitivity). It was only the later antibodies that showed the more typical hapten specificity.

In summary, the specificity of delayed hypersensitivity shows marked differences from the specificity of late antibody. Delayed hypersensitivity is directed against a larger antigenic determinant and is carrier specific, and (generally) not hapten specific. It is also less sensitive to minor changes in the chemical structure of antigen. However, early antibody shares many of these features with delayed hypersensitivity, and the differences are probably less fundamental than was originally supposed.

V. TRANSFER OF DELAYED HYPERSENSITIVITY BY CELLS

Zinsser and Mueller [79] clarified the difference between the tuberculin reaction and anaphylaxis by pointing out that while the latter could be transferred to an unsensitized animal by serum from an immune animal, the former could not. Before and after Zinsser there have been numerous claims to transfer tuberculin reactivity [12] with cell-free extracts. The earlier claims must be regarded with suspicion because of the possibility that the agent used for transfer also contained antigen; the recipients would then have demonstrated active rather than passive immunity. Landsteiner and Chase [10] showed that delayed hypersensitivity to picryl chloride could be transferred from a sensitized to an unsensitized animal by living peritoneal exudate cells. Chase [11] later showed that tuberculin sensitivity could be transferred in the same way. Subsequent investigations have confirmed that delayed hypersensitivity can be transferred by peritoneal exudate cells, lymph-node cells, spleen mononuclear cells, and peripheral blood leucocytes [12]. An important technical point is that earlier work on cell transfer was carried out in guinea-pigs which were either genetically dissimilar or, at best, from a closed colony. It is only recently that studies have been performed in fully histocompatible (syngeneic) animals. This point is important, since lymphoid cells injected into a non-histocompatible (allogeneic) animal will either be destroyed by the recipient animal or react against it in a graft–host reaction (*see* Chapter 10).

Bauer and Stone [80] were the first to compare in detail the effects of passive transfer of tuberculin hypersensitivity in syngeneic (Strain 13) and allogeneic (Hartley, random-bred) guinea-pigs. They took lymphoid cells from animals 9–14 days after immunization with mycobacteria in Freund's adjuvant, and found that a small cell transfer (1×10^8 or 1×10^9) of lymphoid cells, which produced little or no hypersensitivity in allogeneic animals, was effective in sensitizing syngeneic animals. While earlier work, in non-inbred animals [81, 82], involved a large cell-transfer and showed a short latent period (2–3 days) and a short duration (7 days) of hypersensitivity, the experiments of Bauer and Stone produced, in syngeneic animals, a much longer period of hypersensitivity (up to 50 days) after a longer latent period (5–30 days). Chase [83] later found that tuberculin hypersensitivity could persist for 200–500 days after transfer of cells in inbred guinea-pigs. The importance of studying transfer of delayed hypersensitivity in histocompatible (syngeneic) animals has not been sufficiently emphasized. In view of the complicating factors introduced by host-versus-graft and graft-versus-host reactions, it is impossible to extrapolate from experiments in non-histocompatible strains to delayed hypersensitivity in the intact animal.

This point becomes particularly important when we consider what part specifically immunized cells play in the transfer reaction. The work of Metaxas and Metaxas-Buehler [82] suggested that, although there might be a latent period of 1–2 days before hypersensitivity could be elicited after the intraperitoneal injection of sensitized lymphoid cells, the latent period could be abolished if sensitized cells were administered intra-venously. This is an important observation, since it suggests that sensitized donor cells are capable of participating directly in a delayed hyper-sensitivity reaction. Najarian and Feldman [84] studied this problem by injecting lymphoid cells from guinea-pigs sensitized to tubercle bacilli (TB) or to dinitrofluorobenzene (DNFB) intravenously into unsensitized recipents. In each transfer either the TB-sensitive cells or the DNFB-sensitive cells were labelled with tritiated thymidine. Unsensitized animals, which had received both sets of cells, were then tested with PPD and with DNFB. When TB cells were labelled and DNFB cells were unlabelled, the PPD test site contained more radioactivity than the DNFB test site. Conversely, when DNFB cells were labelled and TB cells unlabelled, the radioactivity was greater in the DNFB test site. This strongly suggested that sensitized donor cells accumulated specifically at a test site in response to the appropriate antigen. The authors comment, however, that even when the transfer was highly successful only a small number (about 10 per cent) of cells at the reaction site were donor cells. The remainder were cells from the unsensitized host.

Other workers have reported findings at variance with those of Najarian and Feldman. McCluskey, Benacerraf, and McCluskey [85] sensitized guinea-pigs with picrylated bovine gamma-globulin (pic-BGG), parachlorobenzoyl chloride (PCBC), or diphtheria toxoid. Transfer experiments similar to those of Najarian and Feldman's were performed, in which unsensitized donors were transfused with two sets of cells, each sensitized to a different antigen and either labelled or unlabelled. When the recipients were tested with both antigens, 4 per cent of the infiltrating mononuclear cells were labelled, and there was no difference between the two test sites; these experiments failed to show that sensitized, labelled lymphoid cells collected specifically at the test site. Turk and Oort [86] also failed to show a specific accumulation of sensitized labelled lymphoid cells in delayed hypersensitivity test sites and Prendergast [87] failed to show specific lymphocytic infiltration in skin-homografts in rabbits.

The implications of this work are rather important since they cast doubt on the immunological specificity of the cells involved in delayed hypersensitivity. If we accept, with the majority of workers, that when sensitized cells are transferred to an unsensitized recipient the majority of cells accumulating in a test site are of recipient origin, and that those few donor cells which do accumulate do so with no pretence to immunological specificity, then we are forced to question the degree of immunological commitment of lymphocytes in delayed hypersensitivity. But studies in antibody production (*see* Chapter 4) point to the lymphocyte as a totally committed cell, capable of only a single, unique immunological response. Moreover, it seems that such cells are probably derived by selection from a precommitted population. The resemblances between delayed hypersensitivity and antibody production are more impressive than the differences. It would be uneconomical to postulate two completely separate mechanisms in the immune response, but it is not easy to reconcile the picture of the uniquely competent antibody-producing cell with the uncommitted lymphocyte which blunders into delayed hypersensitivity reactions, apparently by accident.

However, there are a number of important limitations in experiments on lymphocyte transfer. In the first place, the detailed interpretation of the cytology of delayed hypersensitivity is important. Two main types of cell participate in the reaction: the lymphocytes, some of which might reasonably be expected to be immunologically committed, and the group of phagocytic cells (macrophages, histiocytes, and epithelioid cells), which engulf antigen and tissue debris and whose function is not immunologically determined. But Spector and Lykke [19] demonstrated that many of the small round cells which would be regarded as lymphocytes on morphological grounds are, in fact, derived from histiocytes. It is therefore reasonable to expect that the lymphocytes described in transfer experiments are diluted with uncommitted 'pseudo-lymphocytes' derived from the scavenger cells.

In the second place, *in vitro* studies (*see* Chapter 8) have shown that the reaction of immunized lymphocytes with their specific antigen liberates a substance which immobilizes macrophages. This substance, acting *in vivo*, is presumably responsible for the striking accumulation of phagocytes at the site of a delayed hypersensitivity reaction. A single immunized lymphocyte will immobilize up to 100 macrophages *in vitro*, and assuming that the *in vivo* effect is similar in magnitude, we need not expect to find that more than 1 per cent of the cells in a delayed hypersensitivity reaction are immunologically committed.

The third and perhaps the most important point is that very little of the work on the specificity of lymphocytes involved in the transfer of delayed hypersensitivity has been carried out between histocompatible strains. If lymphocytes from one strain of animal are injected into another non-histocompatible strain, the recipient animal will treat their surface antigens as foreign and mount a host-versus-graft reaction (*see* Chapter 10). It seems likely that a number of the recipient lymphocytes found at the site of delayed hypersensitivity reactions in transfer experiments are reacting against foreign lymphocytes and are quite indifferent to the delayed hypersensitivity antigen.

How should we interpret transfer experiments with these reservations in mind? First, there is no doubt that the majority of small round cells taking part in delayed hypersensitivity are of recipient origin. But this may be partly because some are recipient lymphocytes reacting against foreign cells and partly because some are small round cells of the phagocytic series, masquerading as lymphocytes. Secondly, although a number of workers have failed to show that immunized lymphocytes 'home' on their specific antigen, this may be because only a very small number (less than 1 per cent) of committed lymphocytes are needed to initiate a delayed hypersensitivity reaction. To identify this small number of committed cells is beyond the power of resolution of most experimental work so far.

Recent work in syngeneic systems has thrown some light on the origin of the recipient cells involved in transferred delayed hypersensitivity reactions. Lubaroff and Waksman [88, 89] transferred tuberculin sensitivity between rats and found that recipient bone-marrow cells were essential for the reaction. The bone-marrow cells gave rise to macrophages and histiocytes at the site of the reaction.

We can now summarize the evidence on the way in which lymphocytes are involved in delayed hypersensitivity. In the *induction* phase, antigen drains in the lymphatics to the regional lymph-nodes. There, in the paracortical areas, immunoblasts are formed, probably from lymphocytes. We know that there is a steady circulation of lymphocytes through the lymph-node. We do not know whether the antigen, on arrival in the node, stimulates uncommitted lymphocytes which are already there or whether antigen is trapped and held until the arrival of specifically committed lymphocytes from the circulation. The immunoblasts leave the regional node, presumably to settle in other nodes and in the spleen. They are likely to be immunologically committed and to transform into immunologically competent lymphocytes. A subsequent application of antigen to the same animal will elicit delayed hypersensitivity. It is probable that lymphocytes are in continual circulation through the peripheral tissues from blood to lymph, 'searching' for antigen [90, 91], and it may well be that the encounter of an appropriately committed lymphocyte with the administered antigen is a matter of chance. Once a sensitized lymphocyte and its antigen have come together, a factor is released which will immobilize up to 100 phagocytic cells. At least one other pharmacological agent, the lymph-node permeability factor, is known to be released. This increases vascular permeability and facilitates the escape of leucocytes from the capillaries. These two agents will amplify and accelerate the process by which lymphocytes and macrophages accumulate [92].

In discussing antibody production we distinguished the primary and secondary responses, but pointed out that these are both experimental artefacts, and that the natural stimulus of infection would lead to a gradual change from the production of less efficient to more efficient antibody. In the same way it is convenient to consider separately the process of induction of delayed hypersensitivity to a new antigen, and its elicitation, when the antigen is reintroduced. However, in the course of a natural infection the two processes will proceed simultaneously, as part of a continuous cycle of defence.

VI. The Role of Humoral Factors in the Transfer of Delayed Hypersensitivity

Lawrence [93] showed that delayed hypersensitivity to tuberculin and to streptococcal antigens could be passively transferred in humans. Leucocytes from a sensitized donor were injected intradermally into an unsensitized recipient, and antigen was injected into the same skin area at various intervals afterwards. A typical delayed hypersensitivity reaction developed if the antigen was injected 18 hours or more after the lymphocytes. In some subjects the hypersensitivity to tuberculin lasted for several months. Streptococcal hypersensitivity developed in the same way, but lasted only 10 days. This phenomenon is known as 'local passive transfer' of delayed hypersensitivity. In 1955 Lawrence [94] found that intact cells were not necessary for this transfer. An extract of peripheral blood leucocytes from sensitized subjects was prepared by freezing and thawing the cells, or by disrupting them in distilled water, and was injected intradermally into unsensitized subjects. When antigen was injected into the same site, delayed hypersensitivity could be demonstrated which reached a maximum at about 1 week and persisted for up to 6 months. Lawrence termed the agent involved 'transfer factor' and studied its properties in detail. He found that it was resistant to RNAse. DNAse, and trypsin. It did not appear to be an immunoglobulin and had a molecular weight of less than 10,000. There are a number of technical points which make it difficult to accept work on transfer factor without reservations. First, the peripheral leucocytes used in these experiments include a certain number of macrophages, and it is known that these cells contain fragments of antigen in a highly immunogenic form (*see* Chapter 4). This may have been sufficient to produce active sensitization of the recipents. Secondly, in many experiments, recipients were skin tested with antigen to establish that they were negative before the experiments were performed. This small test dose may itself have been sufficient to produce sensitization. Finally, even subjects who were negative on skin-testing may have shown a very low (subliminal) level of immunity as a result of previous exposure to the antigen. They would then react with a 'secondary response' to very small amounts of antigen in the transfer fluid. For these reasons, and because it has so far been impossible to demonstrate transfer factor in animal experiments, there must remain some doubt about its significance in man. The arguments are developed more fully by Turk [12] and Uhr [13].

Recently [95] it has been claimed that if BCG-sensitized guinea-pigs are treated with X-irradiation, plasma taken 3–5 days later is capable of transferring delayed hypersensitivity to tuberculoprotein to unsensitized animals. If this work in confirmed, it may indicate that a 'transfer factor' (possibly some kind of antibody) is liberated from lymphocytes when the guinea-pig is irradiated.

VII. Antibody and Delayed Hypersensitivity

There has been a great deal of discussion on the relationship between delayed hypersensitivity and antibody production. It will be useful, first, to summarize the differences between delayed hypersensitivity and antibody production and then to discuss the types of antibody which have been implicated [96].

First, it has been repeatedly shown that animals can develop delayed hypersensitivity at a stage when no circulating antibodies can be detected [97]. This might, however, indicate that delayed hypersensitivity is a more sensitive indicator of immunity than the methods for detecting antibody. Secondly, antigenic specificity in delayed hypersensitivity differs from that of antibody. We have already discussed this point (p. 303 and Chapter 8) and have concluded that the differences are not absolute and that specificities sometimes overlap. Finally, antibody production and delayed hypersensitivity are affected differently by a number of factors; these have been discussed in Chapter 4. They include X-irradiation, anti-lymphocytic serum, immunological paralysis, and immune deviation.

So far the differences, though striking, are not sufficient to prove that antibody *cannot* be involved in delayed hypersensitivity. We will now consider briefly some of the types of antibody which have been implicated in delayed hypersensitivity.

A. Macrophage Cytophilic Antibodies

The relationship between cytophilic antibodies and delayed hypersensitivity has been reviewed by Nelson and Boyden [98]. If guinea-pigs are injected with sheep erythrocytes in Freund's complete adjuvant, a type of antibody is produced which will adhere to macrophages when these are allowed to form a monolayer on a glass slide. These antibodies can be detected by adding a suspension of sheep erythrocytes to the coated macrophages. Rosettes of erythrocytes will adhere to macrophages which have taken up cytophilic antibody. Cytophilic antibodies against other antigens can be detected by using erythrocytes coupled to antigen as an indicator. Since an antibody involved in delayed hypersensitivity would be likely to be cell-bound, cytophilic antibodies have been suggested for the role. Nelson and Boyden review the evidence: delayed hypersensitivity and cytophilic antibodies are produced by similar stimuli. In mice there is a reasonable correlation between the level of circulating cytophilic antibodies and the degree of delayed hypersensitivity. In guinea-pigs, however, the correlation is less satisfactory, and cytophilic antibodies cannot be detected during the early or late stages of delayed hypersensitivity. A serious objection to the association of cytophilic antibodies and delayed hypersensitivity is that the former can be transferred in serum from one animal to another, while the latter cannot. Nelson and Boyden conclude that the evidence is not sufficient to associate cytophilic antibodies with delayed hypersensitivity.

B. High-affinity Antibodies

In 1962 Karush and Eisen [99] put forward a provocative theory to link antibody with delayed hypersensitivity. They suggested that if antibody of exceptionally high affinity for antigen were formed it would form a stable complex with antigen when levels in the circulation were too low to be detected. High-affinity antibody would not be effective on passive transfer of serum because of the very small amount free in serum. Transfer of living lymphoid cells would be effective, because they would synthesize antibody continuously. Karush and Eisen calculated that antibody with an intrinsic association constant (K_A) of the order of 1×10^{10} litres per mole would be required to produce this effect, and antibodies with a K_A of this order have been described. It would be very difficult to disprove this theory, since the amount of free antibody involved is too small to be detected by conventional methods. Eisen was unable to transfer delayed hypersensitivity with large amounts of serum containing antibody to dinitrophenyl with a K_A of 10^9 [100]. For the present, we must regard this as an attractive theory for which there is as yet no experimental evidence.

C. The Role of Antibody in Delayed Hypersensitivity

There are two possible ways in which antibody could be involved in delayed hypersensitivity: (1) in the recognition of antigen by sensitized lymphocytes, and (2) in the cytotoxic effect of sensitized lymphocytes.

If we assume that delayed hypersensitivity lymphocytes are committed in the same way as antibody-producing cells, then we must postulate some mechanism by which the lymphocyte recognizes antigen. The most economical agent for recognizing antigen is antibody, and it has been supposed that the precursors of antibody-forming cells carry antibody bound to the cell surface (*see* Chapter 4). If we apply the same arguments to delayed hypersensitivity, we should expect to be able to detect antibody on the surface of cells engaging in delayed hypersensitivity, or at least to show that such cells are capable of binding antigen. Experiments in this field are inconclusive; Turk [101] found that lymph-node cells from guinea-pigs sensitized with picryl-bovine serum albumin would take up bovine serum albumin *in vitro*. Peltier and Kourilsky [102], in similar experiments, failed to detect any uptake of antigen by sensitized lymphocytes. Other experiments are discussed by Turk [12]. There are two dangers in work of this kind: it is difficult to be certain that an animal is reacting only with delayed hypersensitivity, and that there are no antibody-producing cells. Furthermore, free antibody can be taken up non-specifically on the surface of lymphocytes; the presence of antibody on a cell surface is no proof of its manufacture within the cell. Despite the difficulties, the search will continue for antigen-reactive units on the cells of sensitized lymphocytes, and it would certainly simplify theories of immunity if these could be shown to be antibodies.

It is known that lymphocytes which have been sensitized against cellular antigens can destroy the sensitizing cells *in vitro* (*see* Chapter 8). Do lymphocytes produce cell damage by liberating antibody of a special type, which is active only over short distances, and not detectable by conventional means? Some recent experiments by Ruddle and Waksman [103–105] suggest another interesting possibility; they showed that the reaction of sensitized lymphocytes with their antigen *in vitro* resulted in the liberation of a cytotoxic substance which destroyed embryo fibroblasts in tissue culture. It may be that the immunologically specific reaction of lymphocyte and antigen releases a cytotoxic 'effector' substance which is not itself immunologically specific. There is no evidence that antibody plays a part in delayed hypersensitivity at this level.

VIII. THE ROLE OF THE THYMUS IN DELAYED HYPERSENSITIVITY

Miller [106] and Parrott [107] have recently reviewed the role of the thymus in immunity. Neonatal thymectomy impairs the ability of animals to reject homografts and to develop delayed hypersensitivity. If adult animals are thymectomized, delayed hypersensitivity reactions may be lost slowly [108] or, if thymectomy is combined with irradiation, rapidly. After neonatal thymectomy, many antibody-producing systems are left intact, though some (such as the haemolysin-forming cells in the mouse) are depressed [109]. There is, then, evidence that in the neonatal period delayed hypersensitivity is largely dependent on the thymus, while antibody production is only partly thymus-dependent. Parrott studied the morphology of lymphoid tissues from neonatally thymectomized animals and found that lymphocytes are depleted from the mid- and deep cortex of lymph-nodes and from the areas of the spleen surrounding the central arterioles. These have become known as 'thymus-dependent' areas, and in lymph-nodes they are the areas which are involved in delayed hypersensitivity. Lymph-nodes from thymectomized mice fail to develop immunoblasts in the paracortical areas, though germinal centres and plasma cells are formed normally.

In the chicken there is a dual control of the immune system. The thymus appears to regulate homograft rejection and 'cellular immunity', while antibody production is controlled by the hindgut bursa of Fabricius [110]. Attempts have been made to extrapolate from chickens to humans and to find an equivalent for the bursa of Fabricius in the appendix and Peyer's patches [111]. Differences between species are so great, however, that at present such analogies seem rather fanciful. We can, however, accept that in mammals and probably in humans an intact thymus is important (especially in the neonatal period) for the development of delayed hypersensitivity. The thymus itself seems to be populated by cells from the bone-marrow and to export lymphocytes which, in turn, populate the thymus-dependent areas of spleen and lymph-nodes [107]. There is some evidence that the thymus produces a humoral substance which affects the development of the lymphoid system [112]. Failure of development of the thymus in man is often associated with inability to develop delayed hypersensitivity [113].

IX. FACTORS AFFECTING DELAYED HYPERSENSITIVITY

A number of adjuvants are known which increase delayed hypersensitivity, while factors, such as immunological paralysis, X-irradiation, and cytotoxic drugs, will depress both delayed hypersensitivity and antibody production. These have been considered in Chapter 4.

A few diseases are known in man which depress delayed hypersensitivity, without affecting antibody production. Hodgkin's disease, a malignant condition of the lymphoid system, is associated with complete absence of all delayed hypersensitivity reactions [59]. In sarcoidosis, a chronic granulomatous disease of unknown cause, delayed hypersensitivity to natural antigens and the ability to develop contact allergy to DNCB are often lost [114]. Some cases of Crohn's disease (a granulomatous disorder of the intestines) show a similar deficiency [115]. Some patients with lepromatous leprosy fail to react to DNCB [116]. There is no convincing explanation for this failure of delayed hypersensitivity.

X. Delayed Hypersensitivity and Immunity

There is a temptation for immunologists to regard delayed hypersensitivity as a fascinating plaything, fashioned perhaps as a challenge to investigative ingenuity. To be realistic, we must try to fit it into its biological background. The first problem is whether delayed hypersensitivity really helps animals and men in combating infection. This may seem a strange question to ask in connexion with a major aspect of the immune response. It is important to bear in mind, however, that, although we think of the immune system as protecting the host against unwanted invaders, there is a number of circumstances where the immune response can be harmful. These include serum sickness and the allergies (examples of immediate hypersensitivity, *see* Chapter 7), as well as the auto-immune diseases (*see* Chapter 12). It is not impossible, then, that delayed hypersensitivity might be a harmful aberration on the part of the immune mechanism.

There is some evidence that this is not so. Arnason and Waksman [117] have reviewed the relationship of tuberculin hypersensitivity to immunity. The correlation is striking. In animals, the unrestricted growth of tubercle bacilli is arrested at the stage at which delayed hypersensitivity develops. Young adults with a positive tuberculin test are less susceptible to reinfection with tuberculosis. In Hodgkin's disease, in which delayed hypersensitivity is lost, there is an increased risk of fatal disseminated tuberculosis [59]. The histological features of delayed hypersensitivity seem designed to bring the infecting bacilli in contact with immune lymphocytes, and with macrophages which will engulf and destroy them. There are, however, some anomalies. Guinea-pigs which have been rendered tuberculin-positive can be desensitized by injecting increasing amounts of old tuberculin over several months [118]. Even when they have been completely desensitized, so that they no longer react to an intradermal injection of 100 mg. of old tuberculin, they are still resistant to reinfection with tubercle bacilli. Raffel [119] also showed that guinea-pigs which have been made tuberculin-positive by injections of a wax fraction from tubercle bacilli have no increased resistance to tuberculosis. *In vitro* experiments throw some light on this paradox. Lurie [120] showed that while tubercle bacilli would multiply freely in the macrophages of normal rabbits, their multiplication was suppressed in immune macrophages (*see* Chapter 8). Suter [121] confirmed this observation with guinea-pig macrophages *in vitro*. The resistance of macrophages appears to be non-specific once it is established [122], though Mackaness [123] has shown that the events leading up to it are immunologically specific.

In summary, in tuberculosis delayed hypersensitivity usually develops in parallel with immunity, but cellular immunity can be present in the absence of delayed hypersensitivity. The position in other bacterial and virus diseases seems to be similar. Since it is accepted that the immune macrophage is an important agent in protection against tuberculosis, it is reasonable to suppose that delayed hypersensitivity, which is an efficient method for bringing aggressive macrophages rapidly into contact with antigen, may be a first-line defence. If the first line is destroyed by desensitization, the battle is not over. The conflict moves deeper into the host's defensive system.

REFERENCES

1. KOCH, R. (1890), 'Weitere Mitteilungen ueber ein Heilmittel gegen Tuberkulose', Dt. med. Wschr., 16, 1029.
2. EPSTEIN, A. (1891), 'Ueber die Anwendung Koch'scher Injectionen im Säuglings- und ersten Kindesalter', Prag. med. Wschr., 16, 13.
3. VON PIRQUET, C. (1907), 'Tuberkulindiagnose durch cutane Impfung', Berl. klin. Wschr., 44, 644.
4. MANTOUX, C. (1910), 'L'Intradermo-réaction à la Tuberculine et son Interprétation clinique', Presse méd., 18, 10.
5. ZINSSER, M. (1924), 'Bacterial Allergy and Tissue Reactions', Proc. Soc. exp. Biol., Med., 22, 35.
6. ZINSSER, H., and MUELLER, J. H. (1925), 'On the Nature of Bacterial Allergies', J. exp. Med., 41, 159.
7. DIENES, L., and SCHOENHEIT, E. W. (1926), 'Local Hypersensitiveness in Tuberculous Guinea Pigs', Proc. Soc. exp. Biol. Med., 24, 32.
8. JONES, T. D., and MOTE, J. R. (1934), 'The Phases of Foreign Protein Sensitization in Human Beings', New Engl. J. Med., 210, 120.
9. LANDSTEINER, K. (1947), The Specificity of Serological Reactions. Cambridge, Mass.: Harvard University Press.
10. LANDSTEINER, K., and CHASE, M. W. (1942), 'Experiments on Transfer of Cutaneous Sensitivity to Simple Compounds', Proc. Soc. exp. Biol. Med., 49, 688.
11. CHASE, M. W. (1945), 'The Cellular Transfer of Cutaneous Hypersensitivity to Tuberculin', Proc. Soc. exp. Biol. Med., 59, 134.
12. TURK, J. L. (1967) Delayed Hypersensitivity. Amsterdam: North-Holland.
13. UHR, J. W. (1966), 'Delayed Hypersensitivity', Physiol. Rev., 46, 359.
14. FREUND, J., CASALS, J., and HOSMER, E. P. (1938), 'Sensitization and Antibody Formation after Injection of Tubercle Bacilli and Paraffin Oil', Proc. Soc. exp. Biol. Med., 37, 509.
15. AUCHÉ, B., and AUGUSTROU, F. (1910), 'Les Lesions cutanées de l'Intradermoréaction', C. r. Séanc. Soc. Biol., 68, 330.
16. DIENES, L., and MALLORY, T. (1932), 'Histological Studies of Hypersensitive Reactions. Part I, The Contrast between the Histological Responses in the Tuberculin (Allergic) Type and the Anaphylactic Type of Skin Reactions', Am. J. Path., 8, 689.
17. GELL, P. G. H., and HINDE, I. T. (1951), 'The Histology of the Tuberculin Reaction and its Modification by Cortisone', Br. J. exp. Path., 32, 516.
18. BOUGHTON, B., and SPECTOR, W. G. (1963), 'Histology of the Tuberculin Reaction in Guinea-pigs', J. Path. Bact., 85, 371.
19. SPECTOR, W. G., and LYKKE, A. W. J. (1966), 'The Cellular Evolution of Inflammatory Granulomata', J. Path. Bact., 92, 163.
20. SPECTOR, W. G., LYKKE, A. W. J., and WILLOUGHBY, D. A. (1967), 'A Quantitative Study of Leucocyte Emigration in Chronic Inflammatory Granulomata', J. Path. Bact., 93, 101.
21. LAPORTE, R. (1934), 'Histo-cytologie des Réactions locales d'Hypersensibilité chez le Cobaye (Réactions allergiques à la Tuberculine et Réactions anaphylactiques)', Annls Inst. Pasteur, Paris, 53, 598.
22. EPSTEIN, W. L. (1967), 'Granulomatous Hypersensitivity', Prog. Allergy, 11, 36.
23. KOLIN, A., JOHANOVSKY, J., and PEKÁREK, J. (1965), 'Histological Manifestations of Cellular (Delayed) Hypersensitivity. I, Alternative Component in Tuberculin Skin Reaction in Guinea Pigs', Z. Immunitäts-Allergieforsch., 128, 117.
24. KOLIN, A., JOHANOVSKY, J., and PEKÁREK, J. (1965), 'Histological Manifestations of Cellular (Delayed) Hypersensitivity. II, Regressive Changes of the Subcutaneous Musculature in the Skin Test to Ovalbumin in Guinea-pigs', Int. Archs Allergy appl. Immun., 26, 167.
25. GELL, P. G. H. (1958), 'Experimental Allergic Lesions in Animals with Special Reference to Histological Appearances', Int. Archs Allergy appl. Immun., 13, 112.

26. GOLDBERG, B., KANTOR, F. S., and BENACERRAF, B. (1962), 'An Electron Microscopic Study of Delayed Sensitivity to Ferritin in Guinea-pigs', *Br. J. exp. Path.*, **43**, 621.
27. MARTINS, A. B., and RAFFEL, S. (1964), 'Cellular Activities in Hypersensitive Reactions. I, Comparative Cytology of Delayed "Jones-Mote" and Arthus Reactions', *J. Immun.*, **93**, 937.
28. TURK, J. L., HEATHER, C. J., and DIENGDOH, J. V. (1966), 'A Histochemical Analysis of Mononuclear Cell Infiltrates of the Skin with Particular Reference to Delayed Hypersensitivity in the Guinea Pig', *Int. Archs Allergy appl. Immun.*, **29**, 278.
29. FLAX, M. H., and CAULFIELD, J. B. (1963), 'Cellular and Vascular Components of Allergic Contact Dermatitis. Light and Electron Microscopic Observations', *Am. J. Path.*, **43**, 1031.
30. GROTH, O. (1964), 'The Epidermal Infiltration of Lymphoid Cells in Allergic Contact Dermatitis. A Quantitative Approach in Guinea-pigs', *Acta derm. vener., Stockh.*, **44**, 1.
31. GROTH, O. (1964), 'The Selection of Lymphoid Cells in Allergic Contact Dermatitis of Guinea-pigs', *Acta derm. vener., Stockh.*, **44**, 21.
32. GROTH, O. (1967), 'Cell Proliferation in Epidermis during the Development of Contact Reactions as revealed by Autoradiography after Injection of Thymidine-H^3. 1, The Epithelial Cells', *Acta derm. vener., Stockh.*, **47**, 397.
33. GROTH, O. (1967), 'Cell Proliferation in Epidermis during the Development of Contact Reactions as revealed by Auto-radiography after Injection of Thymidine-H^3. 2, The Lymphoid Cells', *Acta derm. vener., Stockh.*, **47**, 403.
34. MIESCHER, G. (1962), in *Handbuch der Haut- und Geschlechtskrankheiten* (ed. JADASSOHN, J.), vol. 2, Part I, p. 1. Berlin: Springer-Verlag.
35. TURK, J. L., RUDNER, E. J., and HEATHER, C. J. (1966), 'A Histochemical Analysis of Mononuclear Cell Infiltrates of the Skin. II, Delayed Hypersensitivity in the Human', *Archs Allergy appl. Immun.*, **30**, 248.
36. BOQUET, A., and BRETEY, J. (1934), 'Développement et Évolution de la Sensibilité à la Tuberculine chez le Cobaye', *Annls Inst. Pasteur, Paris*, **52**, 252.
37. HART, P. D'ARCY, and REES, R. J. W. (1967), 'Lepromin and Kveim Antigen Reactivity in Man, and their Relation to Tuberculin Reactivity', *Br. med. Bull.*, **23**, 80.
38. JULIANELLE, L. A. (1930), 'Reactions of Rabbits to Intracutaneous Injections of Pneumococci and their Products. IV, The Development of Skin Reactivity to Derivatives of Pneumococcus', *J. exp. Med.*, **51**, 625.
39. COPEMAN, S. M., O'BRIEN, R. A., EAGLETON, A. J., and GLENNY, A. T. (1922), 'Experiences with the Schick Test and Active Immunization against Diphtheria', *Br. J. exp. Path.*, **3**, 42.
40. UHR, J. W., SALVIN, S. B., and PAPPENHEIMER, A. M. (1957), 'Delayed Hypersensitivity. II, Induction of Hypersensitivity in Guinea-pigs by Means of Antigen–antibody Complexes', *J. exp. Med.*, **105**, 11.
41. SALVIN, S. B. (1958), 'Occurrence of Delayed Hypersensitivity during the Development of Arthus Type Hypersensitivity', *J. exp. Med.*, **107**, 109.
42. SALVIN, S. B. (1963), 'Immunologic Aspects of the Mycoses', *Prog. Allergy*, **7**, 213.
43. FRENKEL, J. K. (1948), 'Dermal Hypersensitivity to *Toxoplasma* Antigens (Toxoplasmins)', *Proc. Soc. exp. Biol. Med.*, **68**, 634.
44. MONTENEGRO, J. (1926), 'Cutaneous Reaction in Leishmaniasis', *Archs Derm. Syph.*, **13**, 187.
45. JENNER, E. (1798), *An Inquiry into the Causes and Effects of the Variolae Vaccinae.* London.
46. ALLISON, A. C. (1967), 'Cell-mediated Immune Responses to Virus Infections and Virus-induced Tumours', *Br. med. Bull.*, **23**, 60.
47. PINCUS, W. B., and FLICK, J. A. (1963), 'Inhibition of the Primary Vaccinial Lesion and of Delayed Hypersensitivity by an Antimononuclear Cell Serum', *J. infect. Dis.*, **113**, 15.
48. PINCUS, W. B., and FLICK, J. A. (1963), 'The Role of Hypersensitivity in the Pathogenesis of Vaccinia Virus Infection in Humans', *J. Pediat.*, **62**, 57.
49. ROSE, H. M., and MOLLOY, E. (1947), 'Cutaneous Reactions with the Virus of Herpes Simplex', *Fedn Proc. Fedn Am. Socs exp. Biol.*, **6**, 432.

50. DIENES, L., and SCHOENHEIT, E. W. (1929), 'The Reproduction of Tuberculin Hypersensitiveness in Guinea-pigs with Various Protein Substances', *Am. Rev. Tuberc.*, **20**, 92.
51. DIENES, L., and MALLORY, T. (1932), 'Histological Studies of Hypersensitivity Reactions', *Am. J. Path.*, **8**, 689.
52. RAFFEL, S., and NEWEL, J. M. (1958), 'The "Delayed Hypersensitivity" induced by Antigen–antibody Complexes', *J. exp. Med.*, **108**, 823.
53. SELL, S., and WEIGLE, W. O. (1959), 'The Relationship between Delayed Hypersensitivity and Circulating Antibody induced by Protein Antigens in Guinea Pigs', *J. Immun.*, **83**, 257.
54. LANDSTEINER, K., and JACOBS, J. (1935), 'Studies on the Sensitization of Animals with Simple Chemical Compounds', *J. exp. Med.*, **61**, 643.
55. LANDSTEINER, K., and JACOBS, J. (1936), 'Studies on the Sensitization of Animals with Simple Chemical Compounds', *J. exp. Med.*, **64**, 625.
56. EISEN, H. N., ORRIS, L., and BELMAN, S. (1952), 'Elicitation of Delayed Allergic Skin Reactions with Haptens: The Dependence of Elicitation on Hapten Combination with Protein', *J. exp. Med.*, **95**, 473.
57. EPSTEIN, S. (1960), 'Role of Dermal Sensitivity in Ragweed Contact Dermatitis', *Archs Derm.*, **82**, 48.
58. EISEN, H. N., and TABACHNICK, M. (1958), 'Elicitation of Allergic Contact Dermatitis in the Guinea Pig. The Distribution of Bound Dinitrobenzene Groups within the Skin and Quantitative Determination of the Extent of Combination of 2,4-Dinitrochlorobenzene with Epidermal Protein *in vivo*', *J. exp. Med.*, **108**, 773.
59. AISENBERG, A. C. (1962), 'Studies on Delayed Hypersensitivity in Hodgkin's Disease', *J. clin. Invest.*, **41**, 1964.
60. FREY, J. R. (1951), 'Quantitative Untersuchungen bei epidermaler Sensibilisierung von Meerschweinchen mit Dinitrochlorobenzol', *Dermatologica*, **102**, 1.
61. EPSTEIN, W. L., and KLIGMAN, A. M. (1958), 'The Interference Phenomenon in Allergic Contact Dermatitis', *J. invest. Derm.*, **31**, 103.
62. FREY, J. R., and WENK, P. (1957), 'Experimental Studies on the Pathogenesis of Contact Eczema in the Guinea-pig', *Int. Archs Allergy*, **11**, 81.
63. TURK, J. L., and STONE, S. H. (1963), 'Implications of the Cellular Changes in Lymph Nodes during the Development and Inhibition of Delayed Type Hypersensitivity', in *Cell-bound Antibodies* (ed. AMOS, B., and KOPROWSKI, H.), p. 51. Philadelphia: Wistar Institute.
64. FREUND, J., and LIPTON, M. M. (1955), 'Experimental Allergic Encephalomyelitis after the Excision of the Injection Site of Antigen-adjuvant Emulsion', *J. Immun.*, **75**, 454.
65. GALLONE, L., RADICI, G., and RIQUIER, G. (1952), 'La Reazione dei Linfogangli regionali agli Omoinnesti de Pelle', *Archo atti Soc. ital. Chir.*, **2**, 329.
66. SCOTHORNE, R. J., and McGREGOR, I. A. (1955), 'Cellular Changes in Lymph Nodes and Spleen following Skin Homografting in the Rabbit', *J. Anat.*, **89**, 283.
67. DAMESHEK, W. (1963), ' "Immunoblasts" and "Immunocytes"—An Attempt at a Functional Nomenclature', *Blood*, **21**, 243.
68. OORT, J., and TURK, J. L. (1965), 'A Histological and Autoradiographic Study of Lymph Nodes during the Development of Contact Sensitivity in the Guinea-pig', *Br. J. exp. Path.*, **46**, 147.
69. ANDRÉ-SCHWARTZ, J. (1964), 'The Morphological Responses of the Lymphoid System to Homografts. III, Electron Microscopy Study', *Blood*, **24**, 113.
70. DE PETRIS, S., KARLSBAD, G., PERNIS, B., and TURK, J. L. (1966), 'The Ultrastructure of Cells present in Lymph Nodes during the Development of Contact Sensitivity', *Int. Archs Allergy appl. Immun.*, **29**, 112.
71. GOWANS, J. L., McGREGOR, D. D., COWEN, D. M., and FORD, C. E. (1962), 'Initiation of Immune Responses by Small Lymphocytes', *Nature, Lond.*, **196**, 651.
72. PORTER, K. A., and COOPER, E. H. (1962), 'Transformation of Adult Allogeneic Small Lymphocytes after Transfusion into Newborn Rats', *J. exp. Med.*, **115**, 997.
73. BENACERRAF, B., and GELL, P. G. H. (1959), 'Studies on Hypersensitivity. I, Delayed and Arthus-type Skin Reactivity to Protein Conjugates in Guinea Pigs', *Immunology*, **2**, 53.

316 BASIC IMMUNOLOGY

74. LESKOWITZ, S. (1963), 'Immunochemical Study of Antigenic Specificity in Delayed Hypersensitivity. II, Delayed Hypersensitivity to Polytyrosine-azobenzenearsonate and its Suppression by Haptens', *J. exp. Med.*, **117**, 909.
75. LESKOWITZ, S., and JONES, V. E. (1965), 'Immunochemical Study of Antigenic Specificity in Delayed Hypersensitivity. III, Suppression of Hapten-specific Delayed Hypersensitivity by Conjugates of Varying Size', *J. Immun.*, **95**, 331.
76. GELL, P. G. H., and WOLSTENCROFT, R. A. (1967), 'Delayed Hypersensitivity and Desensitization to Chemical Haptens: Antigenic Specificity of Delayed Hypersensitivity', *Br. med. Bull.*, **23**, 21.
77. SILVERSTEIN, A. M., and GELL, P. G. H. (1962), 'Delayed Hypersensitivity to Hapten–protein Conjugates. II, Antihapten Specificity and the Heterogeneity of the Delayed Response', *J. exp. Med.*, **115**, 1053.
78. BOREK, F., and SILVERSTEIN, A. M. (1965), 'Specificity of Guinea-pig Antibodies and Delayed Hypersensitivity', *Nature, Lond.*, **205**, 299.
79. ZINSSER, H., and MUELLER, J. H. (1925), 'On the Nature of Bacterial Allergies', *J. exp. Med.*, **41**, 159.
80. BAUER, J. A., jun., and STONE, S. H. (1961), 'Isologous and Homologous Lymphoid Transplants. I, The Transfer of Tuberculin Hypersensitivity in Inbred Guinea Pigs', *J. Immun.*, **86**, 177.
81. KIRCHHEIMER, W. F., and WEISER, R. S. (1947), 'The Tuberculin Reaction. I, Passive Transfer of Tuberculin Sensitivity with Cells of Tuberculous Guinea Pigs', *Proc. Soc. exp. Biol. Med.*, **66**, 166.
82. METAXAS, M. N., and METAXAS-BUEHLER, M. (1955), 'Studies on the Cellular Transfer of Tuberculin Sensitivity in the Guinea Pig', *J. Immun.*, **75**, 333.
83. CHASE, M. W. (1963), 'Persistence of Tuberculin Hypersensitivity following Cellular Transfer between Genetically Similar Guinea Pigs', *Fedn Proc. Fedn Am. Socs exp. Biol.*, **22**, 617.
84. NAJARIAN, J. S., and FELDMAN, J. D. (1963), 'Specificity of Passively Transferred Delayed Hypersensitivity', *J. exp. Med.*, **118**, 341.
85. MCCLUSKEY, R. T., BENACERRAF, B., and MCCLUSKEY, J. W. (1963), 'Studies on the Specificity of the Cellular Infiltrate in Delayed Hypersensitivity Reactions', *J. Immun.*, **90**, 466.
86. TURK, J. L., and OORT, J. (1963), 'A Histological Study of the Early Stages of the Development of the Tuberculin Reaction after Passive Transfer of Cells labelled with (^{3}H) Thymidine', *Immunology*, **6**, 140.
87. PRENDERGAST, R. A. (1964), 'Cellular Specificity in the Homograft Reaction', *J. exp. Med.*, **119**, 377.
88. LUBAROFF, D. M., and WAKSMAN, B. H. (1968), 'Bone Marrow as Source of Cells in Reactions of Cellular Hypersensitivity. I, Passive Transfer of Tuberculin Sensitivity in Syngeneic Systems', *J. exp. Med.*, **128**, 1425.
89. LUBAROFF, D. M., and WAKSMAN, B. H. (1968), 'Bone Marrow as Source of Cells in Reactions of Cellular Hypersensitivity. II, Identification of Allogeneic or Hybrid Cells by Immunofluorescence in Passively Transferred Tuberculin Reactions', *J. exp. Med.*, **128**, 1437.
90. MEDAWAR, P. B. (1965), 'Transplantation of Tissues and Organs: Introduction', *Br. med. Bull.*, **21**, 97.
91. GOWANS, J. L. (1965), 'The Role of Lymphocytes in the Destruction of Homografts', *Br. med. Bull.*, **21**, 106.
92. SPECTOR, W. G., and WILLOUGHBY, D. A. (1968), *The Pharmacology of Inflammation*. London: English Universities Press.
93. LAWRENCE, H. S. (1949), 'The Cellular Transfer of Cutaneous Hypersensitivity to Tuberculin in Man', *Proc. Soc. exp. Biol. Med.*, **71**, 516.
94. LAWRENCE, H. S. (1954), 'The Transfer of Generalized Cutaneous Hypersensitivity of the Delayed Tuberculin Type in Man by Means of the Constituents of Disrupted Leucocytes', *J. clin. Invest.*, **33**, 951.
95. DUPUY, J. M., PEREY, D. Y. E., and GOOD, R. A. (1969), 'Passive Transfer, with Plasma, of Delayed Allergy in Guinea Pigs', *Lancet*, **1**, 551.
96. SZENBERG, A., and WARNER, N. L. (1967), 'The Role of Antibody in Delayed Hypersensitivity', *Br. med. Bull.*, **23**, 30.
97. BENACERRAF, B., and GELL, P. G. H. (1959), 'Studies on Hypersensitivity. III, The Relation between Delayed Reactivity to Picryl Group of Conjugates and Contact Sensitivity', *Immunology*, **2**, 219.

98. NELSON, D. S., and BOYDEN, S. V. (1967), 'Macrophage Cytophilic Antibodies and Delayed Hypersensitivity', *Br. med. Bull.*, **23**, 15.
99. KARUSH, F., and EISEN, H. N. (1962), 'A Theory of Delayed Hypersensitivity', *Science, N.Y.*, **136**, 1032.
100. EISEN, H. N. (1966), unpublished work, quoted by UHR, J. W. [13].
101. TURK, J. L. (1960), 'Some Quantitative Aspects of the Uptake of Antigens *in vitro* by the Lymphocytes of Hypersensitive Guinea Pigs', *Int. Archs Allergy*, **17**, 338.
102. PELTIER, A. P., and KOURILSKY, R. (1966), 'Étude de la Fixation d'Antigène protéique par les Cellules ganglionnaires de Cobayes en État d'Hypersensibilité retardée pure', *Annls Inst. Pasteur. Paris*, **110**, 813.
103. RUDDLE, N. H., and WAKSMAN, B. H. (1968), 'Cytotoxicity mediated by Soluble Antigen and Lymphocytes in Delayed Hypersensitivity. I, Characterization of the Phenomenon', *J. exp. Med.*, **128**, 1237.
104. RUDDLE, N. H., and WAKSMAN, B. H. (1968), 'Cytotoxicity mediated by Soluble Antigen and Lymphocytes in Delayed Hypersensitivity. II, Correlation of the *in vitro* Response with Skin Reactivity', *J. exp. Med.*, **128**, 1255.
105. RUDDLE, N. H., and WAKSMAN, B. H. (1968), 'Cytotoxicity mediated by Soluble Antigen and Lymphocytes in Delayed Hypersensitivity. III, Analysis of Mechanism', *J. exp. Med.*, **128**, 1267.
106. MILLER, J. F. A. P. (1966), 'The Function of the Thymus in Immunity', *Hosp. Med.*, **1**, 199.
107. PARROTT, D. M. V. (1968), 'The Thymus, Delayed Hypersensitivity and Autoimmunity', *Proc. R. Soc. Med.*, **61**, 863.
108. MILLER, J. F. A. P. (1965), 'Effect of Thymectomy in Adult Mice on Immunological Responsiveness', *Nature, Lond.*, **208**, 1337.
109. MILLER, J. F. A. P., and MITCHELL, G. F. (1968), 'Cell to Cell Interaction in the Immune Response. I, Hemolysin-forming Cells in Neonatally Thymectomized Mice reconstituted with Thymus or Thoracic Duct Lymphocytes', *J. exp. Med.*, **128**, 801.
110. WARNER, N. L., and SZENBERG, A. (1964), 'Immunologic Studies of Hormonally Bursectomized and Surgically Thymectomized Chickens. Dissociation of Immunologic Responsiveness', in *The Thymus in Immunobiology* (ed. GOOD, R. A., and GABRIELSEN, A. E.), p. 395. New York: Hoeber.
111. COOPER, M. D., PEREY, D. Y., MCKNEALLY, M. F., GABRIELSEN, A. E., SUTHERLAND, D. E. R., and GOOD, R. A. (1966), 'A Mammalian Equivalent of the Avian Bursa of Fabricius', *Lancet*, **1**, 1388.
112. OSOBA, D. (1965), 'The Effects of Thymus and Other Lymphoid Organs enclosed in Millipore Diffusion Chambers on Neonatally Thymectomized Mice', *J. exp. Med.*, **122**, 633.
113. FULGINITI, V. A., HATHAWAY, W. E., PEARLMAN, D. S., BLACKBURN, W. R., REIQUAM, C. W., GITHENS, J. H., CLAMAN, H. N., and KEMPE, C. H. (1966), 'Dissociation of Delayed Hypersensitivity and Antibody-Synthesizing Capacities in Man. Report of Two Sibships with Thymic Dysplasia, Lymphoid Tissue Depletion and Normal Immunoglobulins', *Lancet*, **2**, 5.
114. JONES, J. VERRIER (1967), 'The Development of Sensitivity to Dinitrochlorobenzene in Patients with Sarcoidosis', *Clin. exp. Immunol.*, **2**, 477.
115. JONES, J. VERRIER, HOUSLEY, J., ASHURST, P. M., and HAWKINS, C. F. (1969), 'Development of Delayed Hypersensitivity to Dinitrochlorobenzene in Patients with Crohn's Disease', *Gut*, **10**, 52.
116. WALDORF, D. S., SHEAGREN, J. N., TRAUTMAN, J. R., and BLOCK, J. B. (1966), 'Impaired Delayed Hypersensitivity in Patients with Lepromatous Leprosy', *Lancet*, **2**, 773.
117. ARNASON, B. G., and WAKSMAN, B. H. (1964), 'Tuberculin Sensitivity. Immunologic Considerations', *Adv. Tuberc. Res.*, **13**, 1.
118. ROTHSCHILD, H., FRIEDENWALD, J. S., and BERNSTEIN, C. (1934), 'The Relation of Allergy to Immunity in Tuberculosis', *Bull. Johns Hopkins Hosp.*, **54**, 232.
119. RAFFEL, S. (1955), 'The Mechanism involved in Acquired Immunity to Tuberculosis', in *Experimental Tuberculosis*, p. 261. Ciba Foundation Symposium. London: Churchill.
120. LURIE, M. B. (1942), 'Studies on the Mechanism of Immunity in Tuberculosis: The Fate of Tubercle Bacilli ingested by Mononuclear Phagocytes derived from Normal and Immunized Animals', *J. exp. Med.*, **75**, 247.

121. SUTER, E. (1953), 'Multiplication of Tubercle Bacilli within Mononuclear Phagocytes in Tissue Cultures derived from Normal Animals and Animals vaccinated
with BCG', *J. exp. Med.*, **97**, 235.
122. ELBERG, S. S., SCHNEIDER, P., and FONG, J. (1957), 'Cross-immunity between
Brucella melitensis and *Mycobacterium tuberculosis*. Intracellular Behavior of
Brucella melitensis in Monocytes from Vaccinated Animals', *J. exp. Med.*, **106**,
545.
123. MACKANESS, G. B. (1964), 'The Immunological Basis of Acquired Cellular
Resistance', *J. exp. Med.*, **120**, 105.

CHAPTER 10

TRANSPLANTATION IMMUNOLOGY

BY M. O. SYMES

I. Introduction

II. The fate of grafts

III. The mechanism of the homograft reaction
   A. Historical aspects
      1. Athrepsia
      2. Innate resistance
      3. Individuality differential
   B. Active immunity
      1. Second-set reaction
      2. Adoptive immunity
   C. Factors influencing the intensity of the homograft reaction

IV. Methods for abrogating the homograft reaction
   A. Irradiation
   B. Cytotoxic drugs
   C. Thymectomy
   D. Chronic thoracic duct drainage
   E. Antilymphocytic serum
      1. Immunosuppressive properties *in vivo*
      2. Dangers of administration
      3. Properties *in vitro* and assay of potency
      4. Mechanism of action

V. Specific immunological tolerance

VI. Graft-versus-host reactions
   A. Conditions for occurrence
   B. Clinical and pathological features
   C. Pathogenesis
   D. Prevention of graft-versus-host reactions
   E. The measurement of graft-versus-host reactions

I. INTRODUCTION

THIS chapter is concerned with describing the natural outcome, and its modification, when transplants of tissues or organs are made between two subjects which stand in a variety of genetic relationships to one another.

This genetic relationship between the subject providing the graft, the 'donor', and the recipient, the 'host', is fundamental in determining the fate of the graft. It is therefore necessary, at the outset, to define the possible circumstances that may exist.*

A graft may be made between two sites on the same subject and would then be referred to as an 'autograft'. In describing a given tissue transplanted under these conditions, one might for example refer to an 'autoplastic' kidney.

A graft transferred between separate subjects of identical genetic constitution, such as human uniovular twins, or members of a given inbred† animal colony, is referred to as an 'isogenic graft'. Thus one may speak of an isogenic kidney.

A graft between two genetically unrelated members of the same animal species is known as an 'allograft', the appropriate adjective being 'allogeneic'.

Finally, a graft made between two animals of different species is referred to as an 'xenograft', and the corresponding adjective is 'xenogeneic'.

A further point concerns the siting of the graft. When a graft is transplanted to its physiological situation it is referred to as 'orthotopic'; when to another situation 'heterotopic'.

II. THE FATE OF GRAFTS

Autografts and isogenic grafts are normally accepted and survive permanently, whilst allogeneic grafts and xenogeneic grafts are, after a brief latent period, rejected by a process called the 'homograft reaction'.‡

---

* The terms used to describe different grafts have been selected from among those suggested in the revised terminology for *Transplantation* [1].

† An inbred animal is one arising as the progeny of a brother × sister cross of litter mates, where such breeding has been maintained for at least the twenty preceding generations.

‡ The term 'homograft reaction' denotes the process by which allografts and xenografts are rejected.

The macroscopic and microscopic features of this reaction vary for different tissues, but the essential items, following initial vascularization, are invasion of the graft by host round cells, in the first instance mainly small lymphocytes with subsequent necrosis of the graft and its replacement by host granulation tissue.

For a description of specific examples of the homograft reaction the reader is referred to Medawar [2], who described the rejection of allogeneic grafts of rabbit skin, and Woodruff [3] for a description of the rejection of allogeneic renal transplants in dogs.

The survival times of allogeneic grafts vary with the species as shown in *Table XXII*. This refers to skin-grafts where survival is measured as the time taken for complete destruction of the surface epithelium.

Table XXII

Species	Graft Survival Time (Days)
Mouse [4]	
Strain combination WU→CBA	8·5
CBA →A	11
Rats [5]	13–14
Guinea-pigs [6]	5–17
Pigs [7]	11–14
Cattle [8]	9
Man	14–21
	Sometimes up to 6 weeks

III. THE MECHANISM OF THE HOMOGRAFT REACTION

A. Historical Aspects

A number of mechanisms have been held to account for the homograft reaction. These have been reviewed [9].

1. ATHREPSIA

This hypothesis held that transplants were rejected owing to the inability of the host to supply their specific nutritional requirements.

2. INNATE RESISTANCE

Transplants were said to be rejected by a humoral mechanism analogous to the reaction to incompatible erythrocytes, and it was suggested that if the donor and host were completely consanguineous, transplant rejection would not occur. However, it was demonstrated [10] that in man allogeneic skin transplants were rejected when the donor and host showed, as far as could be determined, total blood-group compatibility.

3. INDIVIDUALITY DIFFERENTIAL

All tissues and organs of a given subject were said to possess a common and peculiar chemical identity, known as an individuality differential. On transplantation this differential evoked both a cellular reaction and a toxic effect by the host against the donor tissue, with resulting destruction of the latter.

B. Active Immunity

Two pieces of evidence have firmly established the concept that a state of active immunity is responsible for the homograft reaction. First, the demonstration of heightened reactivity by the host to a second transplant of tissue from the same donor. Second, the finding that such heightened reactivity may be adoptively transferred to a host, which has never previously rejected a transplant of the given tissue, by injection of immunologically competent cells from a host which has. It is therefore necessary to consider this evidence in greater detail.

1. SECOND-SET REACTION

Using rabbits, it was demonstrated [2, 11] that if allogeneic skin was transplanted for a second time between the same donor–host pair, the second transplant was rejected more rapidly than the first. If, however, the second skin transplant was from a different allogeneic donor, its rejection was not accelerated to the same degree, and, indeed, it sometimes survived for as long as the first transplant.

Histologically the second-set reaction against skin-grafts differs from that to primary grafts in that second grafts from the same donor, made to a given host, fail to become vascularized and in consequence undergo ischaemic necrosis, whilst the host mononuclear cell reaction is confined to the graft bed.

This second-set reaction to skin has also been found in all other animal species so far examined, including man. In addition to free grafts, the second-set reaction was also manifest against organs transplanted by vascular anastomosis, e.g., kidneys [12, 13]. These observations have been extended by the finding that in dogs a second-set reaction to an allogeneic skin-graft may be evoked by a previous lung transplant from the same donor and vice versa [14]. This active immunity has been demonstrated to persist, albeit at a diminishing level, for at least 120 days [15], using mice.

2. ADOPTIVE IMMUNITY

This term was coined by Medawar to denote the transfer of immunity by immunologically competent cells rather than by serum. This apart, the fundamental distinction between the two methods lies in the capacity of the cells to survive in suitable (isogenic) hosts and thus confer long-lasting immunity. The technique of adoptive immunization may be explained thus. An animal of strain A is immunized by a graft of normal or malignant tissue from a donor of strain B. Immunologically competent strain-A cells (usually spleen or lymph-node cells) from the host are then transferred to a second animal either isogenic or allogeneic with respect to the primary host. If this second host is now challenged with a graft of strain B it will show a second-set response thereto. This accelerated response in the second host persists longer if the latter is isogenic with the primary host, thus permitting the transferred cells to survive.

It was found [15] that when regional lymph-node or splenic cells, from CBA mice which had received A-strain skin-grafts 11–30 days previously, were transferred intraperitoneally to further CBA-strain hosts, the latter showed accelerated (second-set) rejection of a first A-strain skin-graft.

Furthermore, specific immunological tolerance (conferred by neonatal injection of donor immunologically competent cells) of A-strain skin by CBA mice was abolished by injection of both CBA lymph-node cells draining the site of an A-strain skin-graft and normal lymph-node cells [16]. The immune cells acted more rapidly, but the fact that the non-immune cells were also effective shows that the phenomenon is not dependent on active immunization of the donor of the transferred cells.

C. Factors influencing the Intensity of the Homograft Reaction

Having established that the homograft reaction is a manifestation of active immunity, it is pertinent to consider the factors which might influence the intensity of the reaction.

The most obvious of these is the degree of genetic disparity between donor and host, and an example of its effect may be seen in the different times of rejection for skin-grafts in the two mouse combinations listed in *Table XXII*.

Three sites, the anterior chamber of the eye, the testis, and the brain, in the mammalian body are privileged, in that otherwise susceptible tissues placed therein are not destroyed by the homograft reaction. It was found that provided they did not become vascularized, skin allografts survived indefinitely in the anterior chambers of rabbit eyes [17] as did thyroid tissue in thyroidectomized hosts [18]. In the latter case, however, vascularization of the graft did not adversely affect its survival.

The testis has been described as a favourable site for allografts of pituitary gland, thyroid, and kidney, whilst allogeneic transplants of ovary showed prolonged survival in the brains of guinea-pigs [19].

The common property showed by these immunologically privileged sites is thought to be their absence of a lymphatic drainage.

There remains the question of the type of tissue transplanted. In pigs orthotopic allogeneic transplants of liver, performed with appropriate vascular anastomoses, were found to be relatively insusceptible to the homograft reaction [20, 21], and one liver survived 2 years in a recipient which received no immunosuppressive treatment. On the other hand, orthotopic skin-grafts made between the same breeds of pig as above were rejected within 14 days [7]. Delayed rejection of liver allografts in pigs has been confirmed in a further study [22]. The antigenicity of several normal tissues has been arranged in the following order: Lymphoid tissue > kidney > liver [23].

IV. Methods for Abrogating the Homograft Reaction

There is a variety of ways in which the immunologically competent cells of a host may be rendered incompetent and each has been exploited in turn in an attempt to overcome the barrier of the homograft reaction, with the ultimate aim of transplanting tissues and organs in man.

The immunologically competent cells may be destroyed by irradiation or radiomimetic drugs, removed as in chronic thoracic duct drainage, or prevented from developing by thymectomy in certain species of neonate.

In addition to these methods, in which the end-point is a relative absence of competent cells, a more subtle technique has recently come to the fore. This involves preoccupation of the host's immunologically competent cells by an antigen, which being an heterologous leucocyte antibody has a special ability to coat these cells.

A. Irradiation

Ionizing radiations damage immunologically competent cells during mitosis. An increased survival of allogeneic skin-grafts in rabbits, when the latter were given 250 R whole-body irradiation on the day before grafting, was demonstrated [24]. A similar effect of 450 R, given to mice 4–5 days before skin-grafting, has been observed [25], but attempts to influence the time of rejection of allogeneic kidney transplants, following 100 and 225 R respectively, were unsuccessful [12, 26]. Attempts to produce permanent survival of grafts by further increase in the dose of irradiation has led to death of the host from damage to the haemopoietic tissue or the gut.

This problem is well illustrated by an instance in which a kidney was transplanted from a brother to a sister following administration of 200 R whole-body irradiation 2 days prior to operation and 50 R 11 days postoperatively [27]. The patient died 30 days after operation from overwhelming infection secondary to a severe leucopenia, and at autopsy the kidney was found to be in excellent condition.

B. Cytotoxic Drugs

These may be divided into three classes: alkylating agents, antimetabolites, and miscellaneous (*Table XXIII*).

Table XXIII.—Some Cytotoxic Agents used for Immunosuppression

Alkylating Agents	Antimetabolites	Miscellaneous
Nitrogen mustard	Methotrexate (Amethopterin)	Actinomycin C
L-Phenylalanine mustard (Melphalan)	6-Mercaptopurine	Cortisone and analogues
Cyclophosphamide	Azathioprine (Imuran)	

The alkylating agents all contain labile alkyl groups and react by transferring this group in place of such biologically important groups as amino, sulphydryl, carboxyl, hydroxyl, and phosphate. The result is alkylation of nucleoproteins with disorganization of mitosis and morphological changes in the chromosomes.

The antimetabolites are so called because they are analogues of various DNA and RNA precursors and in excess are thus able to antagonize DNA and RNA synthesis competitively. Methotrexate is an analogue of folic acid and thus blocks its conversion to folinic acid by the enzyme folic acid reductase. The effect of methotrexate on DNA synthesis may thus be by-passed by administration of folinic acid, the citrovorum factor.

6-Mercaptopurine is a purine analogue, its molecule being very similar to that of adenine and hypoxanthine, of which it is an antagonist in RNA synthesis.

Imuran is a precursor of 6-mercaptopurine into which it is broken down by the liver after administration. The actions of Imuran and 6-mercaptopurine are therefore similar.

Attention has been drawn [28] to the great importance of the time at which drug therapy is begun in relation to the antigenic challenge. Irradiation and the alkylating agents are most effective if given 1 or 2 days before antigenic challenge, whilst the antimetabolites methotrexate, 6-mercaptopurine, and Imuran (azathioprine) act best if given after the antigen. It may be noted, however, that melphalan is unique in being effective whether given before or after the antigen.

The mechanism of inhibition of the immune response has been reviewed by Berenbaum [28, 29]. Five factors may be considered.

1. Immunosuppression is a by-product of general host toxicity. However, a number of drugs, e.g., the antibiotics and alkaloids, are not immunosuppressive even when given in near lethal dosage. Furthermore, it is difficult to explain the importance of timing of administration in relation to antigenic challenge on the basis of general toxicity.

2. Inhibition of antigen uptake: Irradiation does not interfere with phagocytosis and in addition such interference could not explain the action of drugs effective after antigenic challenge.

3. Inhibition of cell proliferation acting alone: Here again it is difficult to reconcile the hypothesis with the temporal relation between administration of inhibitor and antigenic challenge.

4. Destruction of lymphoid cells: Some agents, e.g., irradiation, melphalan, and cyclophosphamide, cause a rapid fall in the peripheral blood lymphocytes and necrosis of lymphoid tissue. However, the antimetabolites depress the immune response without a similar destructive effect. Also, this hypothesis is difficult to reconcile with the differences in timing of drug administration for optimal effect.

5. Differential sensitivity of immunologically competent cells: Antigenic challenge of a host results in both proliferation and differentiation of immunologically competent cells. These cells show changes in their sensitivity to individual drugs at the several stages of both these processes and it is upon this basis that the relation between the timing of drug and antigen administration may best be explained. For example, the alkylating agents, with their profound effect on cell proliferation, are most effective if given before antigenic stimulation, whilst antimetabolites, which interfere with antibody synthesis, are best administered after transplantation.

Much confusion exists as to the relative efficacy of individual drugs, but certain statements would seem justified.

Methotrexate is especially useful in suppressing graft-versus-host disease (see p. 338) in rodents [30–32]. Furthermore, by using folinic acid to effect a delayed rescue from the toxic effects of methotrexate, it was possible to give massive doses of the latter to guinea-pigs, without overt toxicity [33]. The folinic acid did not affect the immunosuppressive potency of the methotrexate and hence about half the allogeneic skin-grafts, made to guinea-pigs thus treated, survived permanently. Apart from this finding, however, long-term survival of grafts has rarely been obtained without serious toxicity so that the value of immunosuppressive therapy with cytotoxic drugs would appear dubious.

At a clinical level the most favoured drug, but for no clear reason, is Imuran [*see*, for example, 34].

C. Thymectomy

It was originally supposed that the thymus did not participate in immunological reactions because antibody was not demonstrable in the normal organ, plasma cells were not seen in the thymus even after intense antigenic stimulation, and thymectomy in adult mice had no significant effect on antibody production.

However, it was demonstrated [35] that in three strains of mice thymectomy, at between 1 and 16 hours after birth, resulted in the persistence of a neonatal lymphocyte/polymorph ratio (i.e., $\simeq 1.0$), absence of germinal centres in the spleen, and prolonged tolerance to allogeneic skin-grafts made at 6 weeks of age. Similar tolerance of skin-grafts was not seen in mice thymectomized within 1 day of birth and restored with isogenic thymus grafts from animals nearing the end of their gestation period.

Also thymectomy in adult mice delayed or inhibited the recovery of immune competence which followed sublethal whole-body irradiation [36, 37]. A similar finding in mice using allogeneic tumour transplants in place of skin-grafts as indicators of the homograft reaction has also been reported [38]. It was shown that immune reactivity could be restored by grafting isogenic or allogeneic thymus from newborn or 1-month-old donors, although the newborn thymus was more effective.

When melphalan was substituted for irradiation, in similar experiments, no effect of thymectomy in potentiating the survival of allogeneic tumour transplants was seen, even when the thymus was removed 49 days beforehand [39].

The ability of thymus grafts to restore immunological reactivity in thymectomized hosts could theoretically depend on migration of immunologically competent cells from the grafts, migration of host precursor cells to the graft, in which environment they are able to develop immunological competence, or elaboration by the thymus graft of a soluble substance which enables the differentiation of immunologically competent cells from their precursors. In the latter case no cell migration would be necessary.

It was shown that the homograft reaction, against allogeneic skin-grafts, could be restored, in neonatally thymectomized mice, by grafts of embryonic or neonatal thymus placed in a cell-impermeable diffusion chamber which was implanted intraperitoneally on the seventh day of life [40]. Histologically, at 6 weeks after implantation, no evidence was found for leakage of lymphocytes from the diffusion chamber, a finding confirmed by cytological examination of the lymphoid tissues in restored mice, which were shown to consist exclusively of host cells. The diffusion chamber itself contained only epithelial and reticular cells, lymphoid cells being completely absent. These results suggested that the epithelial-reticular cells elaborated a humoral substance which enabled the host lymphoid tissue to become immunologically competent.

Furthermore, reactivity to allogeneic skin-grafts could be partly restored in neonatally thymectomized mice by implantation for 1 week of thymus grafts which had been irradiated *in vitro* with 500 R, a dose sufficient to destroy all but the epithelial-reticular tissue [41]. Again no evidence of thymus donor-type cells was found in the restored hosts, by cytological examination for marker chromosomes.

The impairment of immunological reactivity following neonatal thymectomy has been correlated with the resultant wasting syndrome and deficiency of small lymphocytes in the lymphoid tissues. However, it was found [42] that this wasting disease did not occur in germ-free mice thymectomized at birth. Subsequently the impairment of reactivity to allogeneic skin-grafts, whilst still present, was found to be of lesser degree in neonatally thymectomized germ-free mice, as opposed to normal mice [43]. Therefore it was held that whilst some degree of immunological impairment is a primary consequence of neonatal thymectomy, other factors, such as bacterial contamination, endotoxins, and competing antigens, are also operative in normal mice to produce depression of the immunological response.

So far this discussion has been confined to mice. The consequences of thymectomy in higher mammals have been far less exciting.

In dogs no increased survival of allogeneic renal transplants was observed when thymectomy was combined with administration of immunosuppressive drugs [44, 45]. The value of the findings in [44] is limited by there being no interval between thymectomy and the start of immunosuppressive-drug therapy. Thus no time was allowed for any immunological consequences of thymectomy to become fully manifest. However, in further experiments with dogs there was an interval of 1 month between thymectomy and sublethal whole-body irradiation and a further month between irradiation and challenge with an allogeneic skin-graft [46]. Again there was no prolongation of graft survival by comparison with that in untreated dogs.

In man Starzl [45] performed thymectomy concomitant with allogeneic renal transplants. Supporting immunosuppressive therapy was given using radiomimetic drugs. He found no decrease in the need for drug therapy or in the number of 'rejection crises' suffered by his patients and concluded that the value of thymectomy was not proved.

It would thus seem that the usefulness of thymectomy as a means of abrogating the homograft response is confined to rodents, and the results cited above provide an interesting example of species variation.

D. Chronic Thoracic Duct Drainage

Allogeneic skin-graft survival was prolonged in rats depleted of small lymphocytes by chronic thoracic duct drainage [47]. This finding received support from the observation [48] that when a thoracic duct fistula was maintained in rats for 5 days prior to skin-grafting, the mean survival time of the allogeneic grafts was 13 days, as compared with 8 days in untreated controls.

E. Antilymphocytic Serum

1. IMMUNOSUPPRESSIVE PROPERTIES *in vivo*

Interest in the potentialities of antilymphocytic serum as an immuno-suppressive agent stemmed from the concept that, as the lymphocyte played a crucial role in the destruction of foreign grafts, so an antiserum, raised in an xenogeneic host by immunization with lymphocytes of the potential recipient species, might be effective in suppressing homograft immunity.

This hypothesis was first investigated by Woodruff, Woodruff, and Forman [*see* 9], without any encouraging results. However, Woodruff and Anderson [48, 49] were subsequently able to obtain a profound suppression of homograft immunity and have thus opened perhaps the most exciting era, to date, in transplantation immunology. They immunized rabbits with three intraperitoneal injections of rat thoracic duct lymphocytes, given at weekly intervals, and bled them 10 days thereafter. Further bleedings were at a similar interval after subsequent single injections of lymphocytes. The resulting rabbit anti-rat lymphocyte serum was administered intraperitoneally to rats bearing allogeneic skingrafts. A number of therapeutic regimens was employed, but the maximum effect was obtained by 'combining pretreatment in the form of either the creation of thoracic duct fistula or administration of antilymphocytic serum in high dosage with long continued administration of antilymphocytic serum in smaller dosage after grafting'. An indication of the magnitude of the effect is given by the finding that among 7 animals, treated according to the above method, the survival time for allogeneic grafts was greater than a mean of 91 days, whilst in untreated animals the corresponding figure was 8 days. Although an initial lymphopenia and histologically evident damage to the lymphoid tissue resulted from the therapy, in animals where antiserum administration was continued with resulting survival of allografts the latter occurred in spite of a return of the peripheral lymphocyte count to normal. This finding suggested that destruction of lymphocytes alone was not responsible for the immunosuppressive effect.

Subsequent studies have confirmed and extended the above finding. In mice [50] daily dosage of rabbit anti-mouse lymphocyte serum for 7 days prior to skin-grafting was capable of producing prolonged survival of both first- and second-set allografts and also xenogeneic grafts of rat skin. The active principle resided in the gamma-globulin fraction of the serum.

Thymectomy in adult mice potentiated the immunosuppressive effect of rabbit anti-mouse lymphocyte serum, given for 7 days before skin-allografting [51].

The optimal time for administration of antiserum in relation to challenge with an allogeneic skin-graft has been investigated [52]. Antiserum was most effective when it followed antigenic challenge. Also the degree of immunosuppression was proportional to dosage and duration of treatment. In addition, the antiserum was found to be very effective in depressing the second-set reaction to skin allografts, although after a finite course of treatment rejection eventually took place.

In the above [52] an antiserum prepared against mouse thymocytes was used. The reasons for this were that antithymocyte serum was more effective than antilymphocyte serum [53], and thymectomy coupled with antiserum administration resulted in a greater degree of immunosuppression [51]. It is thought that antithymocyte serum may perform an 'immunological' thymectomy.

In dogs [54] a striking prolongation of renal allograft survival was found following the daily administration of horse anti-dog lymphocyte serum, by intravenous injection, commencing the day before kidney grafting.

In a further study [55] it was reported that horse anti-dog lymphocyte serum was poorly tolerated by the intravenous route, but when given as a daily subcutaneous injection prolonged the survival of renal allografts. Two dogs from a series of 10 lived for more than 250 days after operation.

In a preliminary experiment horse anti-pig leucocyte serum, prepared by immunizing horses with pig mesenteric lymph-node cells, was effective in prolonging the survival of skin allografts [56]. In pigs which received daily intravenous injections of 1·5 ml. serum per kg. of body-weight from the day of grafting, skin-graft rejection was found to begin on day 18 as compared with day 8 for pigs receiving no treatment or normal horse serum.

In monkeys subcutaneous injection of both antithymocyte and to a lesser extent antilymphocyte serum, prepared in rabbits, was effective in prolonging the survival of allogeneic skin-grafts [57]. IgG obtained from the serum was also effective. It is of interest to note that an allogeneic monkey antilymphocyte serum (cynomolgus anti-Rhesus) was only able to produce a slight prolongation of skin-allograft survival, even when given in high doses.

Clinical studies have to date been limited. However, Starzl et al. [58] have administered a horse anti-human lymphocyte globulin prepared against human spleen cells, and consisting of gamma-globulin, T-equine-globulin, and beta-globulin, for 6 days before and 4 months after renal allografting in 20 patients. The injections were by the intramuscular route. Imuran and prednisone were also given to the patients. Nineteen of the patients were alive and well up to 9 months postoperatively, despite the fact that the doses of Imuran and steroids given were less than in any previous series of renal transplants performed by Starzl and his group.

Purified IgG globulin from rabbit anti-human lymphocyte serum was tested in 5 volunteers [59]. Three subcutaneous injections were given, two before and one after skin allografting. A modest prolongation of skin-graft survival was observed.

Recently the *in vivo* potency of human antileucocyte sera has been assayed by its ability to prolong the survival of skin-allografts in chimpanzees [60]. The rationale of this procedure is that man and chimpanzee share a significant number of major histocompatibility antigens. Using this assay it was found that an antiserum raised in a horse, against human peripheral blood lymphocytes, was more immuno-suppressive and less toxic than one raised against spleen cells.

In a further study, antisera raised in horses against human blood lymphocytes were again found to be more potent, as judged by the cyto-toxic titre *in vitro*, than antisera against spleen cells [61].

2. DANGERS OF ADMINISTRATION

Although antilymphocyte serum is so profound a suppressant of the homograft reaction that it has been termed the 'magic bullet', its administration particularly in man is not without risk. The dangers encountered are:—

a. Anaemia: However antilymphocyte serum is prepared there is always some erythrocyte contamination of the immunizing injections. This results in the production of haemagglutinins and if antisera with this activity are administered they result in severe anaemia of the recipient. The haemagglutinin titre can be reduced to safe levels by prior absorption, *in vitro*, of the antiserum with packed erythrocytes of the potential recipient species [*see*, for example, 54].

b. The administration of foreign protein is obviously liable to induce either acute anaphylaxis or serum sickness (*see* Chapter 7). This danger is highlighted by the observation [62] that antilymphocyte serum does not suppress immunity to itself. The use of IgG rather than whole serum is a necessary precaution in man. None the less, mild reactions have been encountered following administration of IgG, obtained from anti-leucocyte serum, to man [58, 59].

c. Two kinds of renal injury can theoretically follow administration of heterologous antilymphocyte serum. The first is a Masugi-type nephritis wherein there is binding of anti-kidney antibody to glomerular antigen shortly after the beginning of antiserum administration [63]. Using fluorescein-labelled antibodies it can be shown that there are secondary accumulations of host gamma-globulin and β_1C complement. The presence of anti-kidney antibody in antilymphocyte serum may initially cause surprise, but it is known that there is considerable antigenic overlap between the several types of nucleated cell for a given species. This is demonstrated by the finding [64] that the anti-white cell titre of an anti-dog serum could be markedly reduced by prior absorption against dog liver or kidney tissue.

The other type of renal lesion, which arises secondary to serum sickness, results from the deposition of peripherally formed soluble antigen–antibody complexes in the microcirculation of the glomeruli, where they provoke a secondary inflammatory reaction. An associated accumulation of host gamma-globulin and β_1C complement again occurs. Such a lesion has been found in antiserum-treated dogs [64].

Both the above lesions are difficult to reverse since the globulin deposits have been shown to persist for a long period [65].

d. Pain, oedema, and tenderness at the site of injection of antiserum have been reported in man [58, 59]. Such reactions may be accompanied by fever.

3. PROPERTIES *in vitro* AND ASSAY OF POTENCY

There is no way of predicting, from activity *in vitro*, the power of a given sample of antilymphocyte serum to suppress the homograft reaction. However, a number of *in vitro* properties have been employed to give a rough guide to this.

a. Leuco-agglutination: A suspension of leucocytes from an animal of the species against which the antiserum is directed is incubated with serial doubling dilutions of the antiserum under test. The highest serum dilution at which agglutination of leucocytes is present, as assessed microscopically after 2 hours' incubation at room temperature, is known as the 'leuco-agglutinin titre'. The reaction is independent of the presence of complement.

b. Cytotoxicity: Incubation for $1\frac{1}{2}$ hours at 37° C. is carried out with an equal volume of leucocyte suspension and serial doubling dilutions of serum. Exogenous complement must be added if the serum under test has previously been decomplemented. At the end of the incubation period a sample of the leucocytes is diluted with 0·165 per cent trypan blue in a haemocytometer tube and the percentage of stained and unstained cells determined. The titre is recorded as the highest dilution of antiserum giving a predetermined percentage of stained (or dead) cells. This percentage has been taken as 10 [66]. It will be clear that control tubes containing leucocytes+complement+normal serum, leucocytes+complement, and leucocytes alone must be included. Using these reactions, it was shown [66] that absorption with red cells to reduce the haemagglutinin titre of the antiserum did not reduce its effect on leucocytes. In addition, it was found that the antiserum was species specific: rabbit anti-rat serum had no effect on dog leucocytes, and sheep anti-dog serum none on rat leucocytes. On the other hand, the antiserum did not show intraspecies specificity in that horse–anti-beagle serum was equally effective against both beagle and mongrel dog leucocytes. Finally, freezing and thawing or freeze drying with reconstitution in distilled water did not reduce the leucoagglutinin or cytotoxic titres of the antiserum against the appropriate leucocytes.

c. By first treating rat thoracic duct lymphocytes *in vitro* with rabbit anti-rat lymphocyte serum and subsequently, after washing, with goat anti-rabbit globulin serum, conjugated with fluorescein, it was shown [66] that the rat lymphocytes became coated with rabbit globulin.

d. In the *absence* of complement, rabbit anti-human leucocyte sera have mitogenic activity when added to human leucocytes in tissue culture [67, 68]. The explanation of this finding is thought to be the presence of specific receptors on the cell membranes of the lymphocytes from which a biochemical message is transmitted to the nucleus, following stimulation of the receptor by the antiserum.

4. MECHANISM OF ACTION

The mechanism by which antileucocyte sera suppress the homograft reaction is unknown, but there are a number of hypotheses with varying amounts of evidence to support them. The subject has been reviewed [52, 69].

The first mode of action may be by destruction of lymphocytes. The administration of antilymphocyte serum has been observed to produce a lymphopenia in a variety of species: mice, rats, dogs, monkeys, and man. The effect is greatest after the initial injections of antiserum and depression of the homograft response has been observed to outlast the lymphopenia. Furthermore, a far more profound depletion of lymphocytes was found following the creation of a chronic thoracic duct fistula than is observed following administration of antiserum [47]. On the other hand, the effect of antiserum on the homograft reaction was much more marked.

In view of the particular effectiveness of antithymocytic sera (*see above*), it has been suggested that the antisera may act through the production of damage to the thymus. This, however, is difficult to reconcile with the relatively small immunosuppressive effect of adult thymectomy.

A more attractive hypothesis is that the antiserum acts as a competitive antigen which having a specific affinity for lymphocytes effectively pre-empts the available immunologically competent cells, leaving none free to respond to other antigens. One way in which pre-emption might be assisted would be for the antiserum to act as a mitogenic agent *in vivo* as it does *in vitro* (*see above*), and so transform a significant proportion of the immunologically competent cells to a more primitive and hence incompetent state. It must be remembered, however, that transformation *in vitro* only occurs in the absence of complement, a situation which does not occur *in vivo*.

Antilymphocyte sera may act by coating the cell membranes of lympho-cytes, as has been shown to occur [66] (*see above*). In this way the recognition of antigen may be prevented. Further experiments [70] demonstrated that the immunological competence of C57B1-strain lymph-node cells, as shown by their ability to produce a graft-versus-host reac-tion on injection into newborn A-strain animals, was impaired by exposure of the cells to antilymphocyte serum *in vivo* or *in vitro*. Reactivity could, however, be restored by *in vitro* exposure of the treated lymph-node cells to trypsin, a finding which favours the cell-coating hypothesis of ALS action.

The latter two mechanisms of action would account for the non-specific suppression of the homograft reaction (e.g., to both allogeneic and xenogeneic grafts) produced, which may be contrasted with the specific suppression associated with specific immunological tolerance.

V. Specific Immunological Tolerance

Specific immunological tolerance has been defined [3] as 'a state of reduced or absent reactivity to a particular antigen (or group of antigens), which would ordinarily evoke a specific reaction, in consequence of previous exposure of the organism to the same, or a closely related antigen (or group of antigens)'.

The existence of this type of tolerance was predicted by Burnet and Fenner [71, 72] as a consequence of their attempt to explain non-reactivity to effete 'self'-antigens (in the form of breaking down or damaged body tissues) as opposed to foreign antigens. They held that 'self'-antigens possessed 'self-marker' components able to forestall an immunological reaction. The ability to recognize these markers developed in embryo, so that exposure to a foreign antigen during this period would result in a specific non-reactivity to the antigen during later life.

The first demonstration of specific immunological tolerance was the finding, by serological tests, that the blood of synchorial cattle twins consists of a mixture of erythrocytes from the two individuals con-cerned [73]. Subsequently it was shown [74] that this erythrocyte chimaerism persisted longer than the life of the erythrocytes exchanged in utero. Therefore, haemopoietic precursor cells must also have been exchanged.

Skin-allografts made between cattle twins similar to the above survived permanently [75], whilst an orthotopic renal transplant made between a pair of such twins functioned for 5 months [76].

When skin was transplanted between two human twins, who were blood-group chimaeras, the grafts survived in good condition for a year [77].

It will be clear that the basis for the examples of tolerance described above is the exchange of antigen, in the form of cells, between the subjects concerned, during intra-uterine life. This exchange occurred by accident, but a similar situation was soon deliberately reproduced [16, 78, 79]. Sixteen-day embryo CBA mice were injected with 0·01 ml. of a suspension of cells from the testis, kidney, or spleen of A-strain mice. Those mice which survived received A-strain skin-grafts at 8 weeks of age. The majority of such grafts survived longer than in untreated animals. Furthermore, the tolerance so induced was specific in that it did not extend to third-party, AU-strain skin.

The story was carried a stage further by the observation [80] that rats of the Wistar strain, injected subcutaneously on the day of birth with an allogeneic spleen suspension from rats of the 'hooded' strain, showed a high degree of tolerance to 'hooded' skin when challenged therewith in adult life. A similar injection of spleen cells made at 2 weeks after birth was also capable of inducing partial tolerance to skin-grafts. Furthermore, the level of tolerance so induced could be markedly increased by administration of cortisone to the prospective spleen-cell recipients for the first 14 days of life.

In similar experiments [81] A-strain mice received an intravenous injection of 4–10 million CBA-strain spleen cells within 24 hours of birth. The majority of the mice showed a high level of tolerance to CBA-strain skin when challenged at 8 weeks of age. The proportion of such mice showing tolerance was reduced to 50 per cent when the spleen-cell injection was postponed to the fourth day of life, and the phenomenon did not occur when the cell injection was made on day 7. It was found that lymph-node or spleen-cell suspensions, prepared from tolerant mice, could induce immunity to skin of donor (CBA) strain, if injected into mice isogenic with the tolerant animals (A-strain). This afforded evidence that the tolerant animals were indeed chimaeras.

It would seem from the above that there is a critical period after birth, different for differing animal species, during which exposure to an antigen results in tolerance. Further evidence in support of this idea has been provided by work [5, 82] in chickens where a first transplant which had been in place for a considerable period of time may continue to survive, without gross change in its appearance, whilst a second transplant from the same donor is rejected. This finding also serves to illustrate the phenomenon of partial tolerance, for if tolerance had been complete the second graft would have been accepted as readily as the first. Partial tolerance is the result of exposure during the critical period to an inadequate quantity of antigen for the induction of complete tolerance. Tolerance may be abolished by the adoptive transfer of immunologically competent cells from a non-tolerant donor isogenic with the tolerant host (*see* p. 323).

The results cited above would permit of explanation on a qualitative or quantitative basis. Either there is a qualitative change in the reactivity of an animal to antigen, ranging from tolerance to immunity, with increasing age, or alternatively at a given age the development of tolerance or immunity is a function of the quantity of antigen used for challenge. It was found [83] that A-strain mice, given repeated intravenous and intra-peritoneal injections of $(A \times C_3H)F_1$ hybrid spleen cells to a total dose of $1 \cdot 5 \times 10^9$ cells, were tolerant rather than immune to subsequent challenge with $(A \times C_3H)F_1$ skin-grafts. Furthermore [84], when the immune capacity of the adult host was depleted by prior whole-body irradiation (500 R), the dose of $(A \times CBA)F_1$ spleen cells required to induce tolerance of hybrid skin in A-strain mice could be reduced to $0 \cdot 8 \times 10^9$. Spleen cells in such tolerant A-strain mice were capable of reacting against third-party C57B1 antigens. Conversely administration of a small dose, 2×10^4 to 2×10^6, of $(A \times CBA)F_1$ spleen cells to A-strain mice on the day of birth is capable of preventing the induction of a graft-versus-host reaction in these mice, following injection of 20×10^6 adult CBA strain spleen cells 48 hours after birth [85]. It would thus seem that a very small dose of antigen administered to mice in the neonatal period is capable of inducing immunity rather than tolerance. This finding, considered in conjunction with the demonstration that it is possible to induce tolerance in an adult animal with a sufficiently high dose of antigen and the occurrence of partial tolerance with lower antigen doses, would seem to establish the hypothesis that the development of immunity or tolerance depends on the quantity of antigen administered at a given age.

A further question is whether the persistence in an animal of the tolerance-inducing antigen is necessary for the maintenance of tolerance. Chicken or turkey blood, irradiated *in vitro* with 10,000 R to destroy any leucocytes, was transfused into further chickens. Transfusions were begun before hatching and thus tolerance to the foreign, non-replicating erythrocytes was induced, as judged by the speed of elimination of a further challenge with ^{51}Cr-labelled erythrocytes of the same genotype, compared to that in non-tolerant animals. It was found that tolerance could be maintained by giving repeated injections of the appropriate erythrocytes, but that if these were omitted, so that donor antigen was gradually eliminated by natural death of the red cells, then further challenge with erythrocytes led to their immune elimination [86].

It is of interest to compare the abrogation of the homograft reaction resulting from administration of antilymphocytic serum with that seen in specific immunological tolerance.

The non-reactivity to homografts arising from antiserum treatment is non-specific, extending both to allogeneic and xenogeneic grafts, whilst immunological tolerance is specific to the inducing antigen.

Furthermore, the action of antiserum is peripheral, as is shown by its ability to prevent immunization of an animal following an orthotopic allogeneic skin-graft, but not following an intravenous injection of spleen cells of the same genotype [69]. It was also demonstrated that following the transfer of immunologically competent cells by intradermal injection (the normal lymphocyte transfer reaction) the reaction of these cells against their host, a local graft-versus-host reaction, could be prevented by a single small dose of antiserum administered to the recipient. However, relatively large and repeated doses of antiserum had to be administered to the cell donor to produce the same effect.

By contrast, specific immunological tolerance represents a central failure of the immune response, as shown by its abolition following adoptive transfer of immunologically competent cells from a non-tolerant individual.

VI. GRAFT-VERSUS-HOST REACTIONS

A. Conditions for Occurrence

A graft-versus-host (GVH) reaction can be regarded as the converse of the homograft reaction, and it occurs under conditions in which a graft of immunologically competent cells from a genetically foreign donor is able to survive and multiply in a new host. It will therefore be clear that a GVH reaction may result:—

1. When cells are grafted from an adult donor to a newborn host.

2. When cells are grafted from an adult host of a pure-line inbred strain to an F_1 hybrid host, resulting from a cross between the donor strain and a second pure-line inbred strain. In this case the hybrid host cannot reject the pure-line donor cells whose antigens are fully represented in the hybrid. On the other hand, the donor cells can react against the antigenically foreign component of the host.

3. Following transplantation of adult cells to an irradiated adult recipient. In this case the dose of irradiation must be sufficient to prevent rejection, at least for a time, of the transplanted foreign cells.

4. When animals are joined to one another in parabiosis a vascular anastomosis is formed between them with the result that considerable quantities of blood, containing immunologically competent cells, are exchanged.

B. Clinical and Pathological Features

The main clinical and pathological features in animals undergoing a GVH reaction are retardation of growth, emaciation, diarrhoea, spleno-megaly, lymphoid atrophy, hepatomegaly, and anaemia. These changes may lead to death in a few days or a few weeks or to spontaneous recovery. There is a positive correlation between both the severity of the clinical features and the mortality, on the one hand, and the number and genetic diversity of the injected cells, on the other.

The spleen goes through a phase of hyperplasia maximal 8–10 days after grafting [87] before returning to normal size or becoming atrophic. Histologically the picture is rather variable, but most workers, for example [88, 89] in mice, have noted a massive proliferation of mature and immature cells, staining with methyl-green pyronine, in the splenic red pulp and associated destruction of the Malpighian follicles. In the later stages of the reaction the splenic histology is dependent on the severity of the disease. In mild cases the spleen may return to normal, but in more severe cases, which, however, live for some time before death, atrophic changes supervene characterized by necrosis, fibrosis, and infarction.

Extreme atrophy of the lymph-nodes has been described [90] as a cardinal feature of the GVH reaction in newborn mice. More recently, however, it has been shown [91] by injection of parent line cells into irradiated adult F_1 hybrid recipients that this may be preceded by a hyper-plasic phase at 8 days after injection.

An initial proliferation of cells from the plasma-cell series in the lymphoid follicles of rabbits undergoing a GVH reaction has also been reported [92].

An increase in liver weight of chickens and mice was noted [88, 89]. The enlargement was of lesser degree than in the case of the spleen, although histologically the dominant feature was again an accumulation of plasma cells and their precursors, located in the periportal areas.

The anaemia in chickens, mice, and rats has been found to be of a haemolytic type.

It was shown [89] that in F_1 hybrid mice, undergoing a GVH reaction following injection of parental cells, there was an increased rate of clearance of intravenously injected colloidal carbon (up to ten times normal). This phagocytic activity was maximal 15 days after injection of the parental cells and returned to normal in 20–40 days. Histological examination of the livers in these mice showed a great increase in the number of carbon-containing phagocytic cells lining the sinusoids.

C. Pathogenesis

Although it has been definitely established that GVH reactions are immunological in nature, a precise explanation cannot be given for the sequence of events described under clinical and pathological features above.

Several lines of evidence prove that the GVH reactions are immunological. It is essential for a GVH reaction to be produced in newborn inbred mice that adult immunologically competent cells from a different inbred strain are injected [88]. If cells isogenic with their recipient are substituted no GVH reactions occur. Furthermore, such a reaction does not occur when the adult cell donors have been rendered specifically tolerant of the potential recipient strain [92].

Using two inbred strains of White Leghorn chickens, I and C, and their F_1 hybrid I×C, it was demonstrated [93] that a GVH reaction, as indicated by splenomegaly in the newborn recipient following injection of adult whole blood, occurs only in the combination I→(C×I)F_1, and not in either uninjected controls or in the combinations (C×I)F_1→I or I→I. From these results it may be deduced that the splenomegaly arises as a result of a reaction by the grafted cells against the antigen of the host, rather than as a result of stimulation of immature host cells by contact with adult donor cells.

As judged by the degree of splenomegaly, AKR spleen cells from adult mice produced a more marked GVH reaction in (AKR×C3H)F_1 hybrids, if the parent-line donors had been preimmunized against the F_1 hybrid antigens [87]. Furthermore, an increased mortality occurred among newborn A-strain mice injected with adult CBA-strain spleen cells when the donors had been preimmunized with A-strain tissue [90].

It may be of value to hang a discussion of the changes seen in GVH reactions mainly on events in the spleen.* Fox [94] investigated the fate

---

* This discussion will refer to events where the host has not been irradiated prior to the injection of donor cells. For a description of cell kinetics in radiation chimaeras see pp. 341–2.

of the donor cells when CBA (T6) spleen cells with two marker chromosomes were injected into adult (CBA × C57B1)F$_1$ hybrid mice. He found that at 48 hours post injection 60 per cent of the cells in the spleen were of donor origin. However, when host splenomegaly was at its height, 13 days after injection of the T6 cells, only 1 per cent of spleen cells were of donor origin. Furthermore, he demonstrated that the donor cells persisted at this diminished level until at least the sixtieth day. The idea of an initial burst of donor-cell activity is also supported by the finding that rat thoracic duct lymphocytes labelled with tritiated thymidine, on injection into allogeneic hosts, were transformed into cells indistinguishable from plasma-cell precursors [95]. These cells were located in the Malpighian follicles of the spleen.

The findings of Fox concerning the origin of the spleen cells at the height of the splenomegaly are confirmation of those previously reported [96] in connexion with experiments on the injection of adult T6 cells into newborn recipients. It is thus clear that the events in a GVH reaction including the haemolytic anaemia are determined by the initial burst of donor-cell activity, for subsequently donor cells form only a small minority of those present (at least in the spleen and probably in other organs also). It is therefore possible that the immunological activity of these donor cells may cause damage to the host, and the changes which follow, characterized by a proliferation of host cells, may be regarded as reactive hyperplasia. Depending on the degree of initial damage, this hyperplasia may restore the host to normal or may fail and be succeeded by atrophy of the lymphoid tissues and death.

The raised phagocytic activity noted [89] may be associated with the removal of damaged host cells, although the failure to find increased uptake of injected carbon in the spleen, one of the principal sites of damage, must be noted.

Much controversy has arisen concerning the nature of the pyroninophilic cells seen at the height of the host proliferative response. Howard [89] has suggested that they are members of the plasma cells series, whilst Gorer and Boyse [97] have held that they are phagocytic in nature. If one agrees with Howard, it is necessary to explain against what antigen the massive proliferation of antibody-forming plasma cells is directed—a difficult question, but it could be argued, as above, that the stimulus is the restoration of the host's damaged immunological capacity. However, it has been demonstrated [98] that the pyroninophilic lymph-node cells of mice undergoing a GVH reaction lack the endoplasmic reticulum typical of plasma cells and later develop into histiocytes.

Two reasons have been suggested [99] why host phagocytic cells might proliferate in GVH reactions. First, they might be stimulated to undergo mitosis by the action of antibody elaborated by the donor cells, and, second, having been passively sensitized by these antibodies they would proliferate under the influence of the host's own antigens.

It was further postulated that the proliferating macrophages being passive vectors of a delayed hypersensitivity response may actually play a part in the destructive effect on the host.

The above description of the cell kinetics in GVH reactions represents the situation in the case of the majority of donor–host combinations. The position is, however, made somewhat confusing by the finding [94] that following injection of CB57B1 spleen cells into (C57B1 × CBA (T6))F_1 mice, the host spleen was progressively replaced by donor cells. This replacement was 100 per cent on the thirteenth day when the splenomegaly was at its height. However, only 1 of the animals in this experiment died of a GVH reaction.

These findings raise the question of the fate of the donor cells. There are three possibilities: that they persist indefinitely with undiminished reactivity towards the antigens of the host, that they are eliminated or rendered immunologically incompetent, or that some intermediate situation exists. Using the discriminant spleen assay (*see* p. 339) it was found that in (C57B1 × CBA)F_1 mice, donor anti-host activity persisted following injection of C57B1 cells, albeit to a much decreased extent [100]. No such activity was found following injection of CBA cells.

With regard to the retardation of growth and emaciation, it is of interest to compare these clinical features with the similar picture following thymectomy in the newborn mouse. Both GVH reactions and thymectomy are associated with a destruction of host lymphocytes.

There remains the question of what causes death in some GVH reactions. The degree of anaemia encountered is scarcely sufficient to do so, whilst in contrast to what might be expected, an increased resistance to some bacteria at the height of the phagocytic response has been reported [101], although, as Simonsen [91] comments, the result may have been different at other stages of the reaction.

Another factor contributing to death may be the generalized inhibition of host mitotic activity in the later stages of the disease.

D. Prevention of Graft-versus-host Reactions

In three strain combinations injection of isogenic adult spleen cells into newborn mice, half an hour after the injection of a similar number of adult allogeneic spleen cells, caused a marked reduction in the mortality from the GVH reaction [102]. A similar observation, using weight-gain as an indication of protection against the GVH reaction, has been reported [103]. Furthermore, the degree of protection could be increased by the use of isogenic spleen cells from animals preimmunized by a graft of skin from the donor strain.

In the strain combination adult C57B1 spleen cells into DBA/2 newborn mice, significant protection against mortality from the GVH reaction was afforded by transfer of serum from DBA/2 mice preimmunized against C57B1 tissue [104]. This was true when the DBA/2 newborn mice received serum as late as 2 days after injection of allogeneic cells.

The beneficial effect of repeated small doses of methotrexate given, subcutaneously, to strain A mice which had received sublethal whole-body irradiation followed by the intravenous injection of massive doses of spleen cells from non-immunized CBA-strain mice has also been demonstrated [30].

E. The Measurement of Graft-versus-host Reactions

A crude index of the severity of GVH reactions may be had in the mortality-rate of affected animals, their time of death after injection of the donor cells, and also in terms of the degree of growth retardation in new-born animals. These parameters are of greatest value in demonstrating that GVH reactions are stronger between some strain combinations of animals than others. A more sensitive assay is based on the development of splenomegaly in mice undergoing a GVH reaction [105]. In essence it can be shown that the spleen weight in inbred chickens and mice is directly proportional to the body-weight. Furthermore, the degree of spleno-megaly at a fixed time after the injection of donor cells is an index of the magnitude of the GVH reaction.

Therefore, GVH reactions may be compared as to their intensity by means of an index obtained from the following expression:—

$$\frac{\text{Wt. of spleen/unit body-wt. in injected mouse}}{\text{Mean wt. of spleen/unit body-wt. in uninjected (control) mice}}.$$

An example of this assay is described below in the section dealing with uses of GVH reactions (see p. 340).

A practical point concerning the above assay is that it is best, when possible, to use litters of hybrid mice between 3 and 8 days old, on account of hybrid vigour, the fact that newborn animals are more sensitive to the induction of splenomegaly than older mice, and the absence of any possibility of a host-versus-graft reaction if parent-line cells are injected into an F_1 hybrid animal.

A refinement of the spleen assay is the discriminant spleen assay [87], which may be employed to estimate separately the activity of two immuno-logically competent cell populations, when these are mixed together, as in chimaeras. If the two cell populations are from inbred strains A and B, then the A component of the mixture may be assayed if the mixture is injected into an $(A \times C)F_1$ hybrid, where C is a third inbred strain whilst the B com-ponent is assayed following transplantation to a $(B \times C)F_1$ hybrid. It is obvious that this method will only afford evidence concerning the reactivity of A and B cells, separately, against antigens of the third strain C. In order to investigate the reactivity of the A and B cells in the mixture against one another, it is necessary to transfer the mixture to potentially tolerant newborn mice of both strains A and B.

The finding [89] of an increased rate of clearance from the blood of injected colloidal carbon is also the basis of an assay for GVH reactions, which has the advantage that it can be performed repeatedly on blood samples withdrawn from the same mouse without killing the animal. The blood is lysed in 0·1 per cent Na_2CO_3 and the carbon concentration determined in a photo-electric absorptiometer. The rate of carbon clearance follows an exponential function, so that the phagocytic index K is found from the expression.

$$\frac{\log \text{concentration } a - \log \text{concentration } b}{tb - ta},$$

where ta and tb are the times, in minutes, at a and b. Howard has shown that the value of K is directly proportional to the magnitude of the GVH reaction.

F. The Use of Graft-versus-host Reactions as Research Tools

The GVH reaction has been widely used to elucidate some of the fundamental problems of transplantation biology, and a number of instances have been reviewed [91]. Two illustrative examples may, however, be considered. Symes (unpublished) wished to investigate the immunological competence of mouse spleen cells after storage at 4° C. forvarying periods. He therefore injected C57Bl spleen cells from the same pool which had previously been stored for 1, 3, or 5 days into (T6 × C57B1)F$_1$ hybrid adult mice, and killed the hybrids after an interval of 14 days, to determine the several spleen indices. The results are shown in *Table XXIV*, from which it may be seen that significant immunological competence was only retained for 24 hours of storage at 4° C.

Table XXIV.—AN ASSAY OF THE IMMUNOLOGICAL COMPETENCE OF C57Bl SPLEEN CELLS FOLLOWING STORAGE FOR VARYING PERIODS OF 4° C.

C57Bl CELLS INJECTED	(C57Bl × T6)F$_1$ MICE (RECIPIENTS)		
	Spleen ratio = mg. spleen/ 10 g. mouse	Mean	Spleen index
Nil	41·3; 54·4 35·7; 40·9 37·0; 38·7 32·3; 40·6 31·6; 46·3	39·9	
Not stored	94·3; 83·9 83·1; 83·6 65·7; 70·7 89·3; 109·7 83·9		2·36; 2·10 2·08; 2·10 1·65; 1·77 2·24; 2·75 2·10
Stored for 1 day	71·5; 39·3 61·6; 84·4 55·6		1·79; 0·98 1·54; 2·12 1·39
Stored for 3 days	38·2; 33·8 48·0; 35·7		0·96; 0·85 1·20; 0·90
Stored for 5 days	37·5; 36·1 49·1; 43·3		0·94; 0·90 1·23; 1·09

Fifty million spleen cells were in each case injected intravenously into an adult (C57Bl × T6)F$_1$ adult mouse, which was killed 14 days later.

The discriminant spleen assay has been applied [92] to investigate whether adult A-strain mice, rendered tolerant of CBA-strain tissue, following neonatal injection of CBA spleen cells, can react to third-party antigens by virtue of the activity of the host A-strain cells or only by proxy through the activity of the donor CBA cells. It was found that 'activity, attributable to the host component, against third party antigens, was undiminished as compared with that of untreated A-strain mice'.

G. The Relevance of Graft-versus-host Reactions to Clinical Practice

GVH reactions present a major hazard in a variety of clinical situations. The most extensively studied of these is the question of protection against the lethal effect of whole-body irradiation by transplantation of allogeneic bone-marrow.

VII. Chimaeras

A chimaera is an animal or man in which two distinct cell populations coexist, the cells of the subject in question and those of another subject. Such a situation may arise:—

1. When cells from a donor are injected into a host during the tolerance-inducing period of the recipient's life.

2. As a variant of (1), when injection of the donor cells is made into an adult host following such a degree of immunosuppression that rejection of the graft cannot occur, or when a massive number of cells is injected so as to constitute a tolerance-inducing antigenic overload.

3. When the donor and host stand in such a genetic relationship to one another, e.g., parent line and F_1 hybrid, that rejection is impossible.

The immunological characteristics of chimaeras, arising under situations (1) and (3) above, have already been discussed, but some remarks on radiation chimaeras may be pertinent. Radiation chimaeras have been the subject of a recent monograph [106].

Jacobson et al. [107] reported that shielding of the spleen or of a whole leg during the administration of an otherwise lethal dose of whole-body irradiation to mice resulted in protection of the animals from death due to aplasia of the bone-marrow. Such protection might be the result of either the elaboration, by the shielded tissue, of a humoral factor responsible for the regeneration of the haemopoietic tissue or the seeding of viable haemopoietic cells from the protected site into the rest of the animal.

The observation [108] that removal of the shielded spleen, no more than 5 minutes after the completion of irradiation, still resulted in a significant degree of protection seemed evidence in favour of the humoral hypothesis. However, the cellular hypothesis has since been proved by several lines of evidence. It was found [109] that following the protection of lethally irradiated mice, by administration of rat bone-marrow, the majority of the recipient's haemopoietic cells were of rat origin, as shown by the distinctive arrangement of the chromosomes in metaphase plates. A similar situation was also found in allogeneic chimaeras where the donor cells were of T6 origin.

The presence of rat leucocytes in rat/mouse radiation chimaeras was demonstrated using the finding that rat granulocytes in blood-smears show positive staining for alkaline phosphatase, whilst mouse cells are negative in this respect [110].

Finally, the use of bone-marrow cells from allogeneic radiation chimaeras to restore lethally irradiated animals of either host or donor genotype revealed that a much smaller dose was necessary to save mice of the donor strain [111]. This suggested that donor-type cells formed the majority in the first chimaera. The original observations of Jacobson would therefore seem to be a reflection of the migratory potential of spleen cells.

Radiation chimaeras have been classified [106] into 'true chimaeras' which consistently show a haemopoietic cell population of exclusively donor origin, 'partial reversals' where a mixed population of donor and host-type cells coexist for a long period, and 'total reversals' in which there is complete recovery of the host's own haemopoietic tissue with total elimination of donor cells.

The establishment of 'true chimaeras' depends on the administration of a sufficiently high, usually a LD 100, dose of whole-body irradiation, and for a given radiation dose on the genetic similarity between donor and host.

The phenomenon of reversion can theoretically have two explanations: first, the rejection of the donor cells by the recovered immunological processes of the host or, secondly, competition between donor and host cells, in a milieu favourable for the proliferation of the latter.

A priori, the first explanation would seem most likely, particularly in view of the interdependence between radiation dosage and the establishment of true chimaerism. However [112], spleen cells from a second animal, isogenic with the host component in a chimaera, were no more effective in inducing a reversion if they had previously been immunized against donor-strain tissue. Furthermore, isogenic non-immunized lymph-node cells were ineffective. Finally [113], in allogeneic rat chimaeras, haemopoietic reversal could occur whilst tolerance to donor-type skin-grafts was maintained.

In the case of 'partial reversal', mutual tolerance between the donor and host cells may be established [114].

True chimaeras show immunological reactivity characteristic of the donor cells. For example [115], lethally irradiated DBA-strain mice restored with $(DBA \times BALB)F_1$ bone-marrow accepted BALB skin-grafts in the majority of cases, whilst DBA/2 mice protected with BALB/C marrow accepted BALB/C skin but rejected third-party C57Bl skin [116].

As may be expected, in the case of true chimaeras, the donor cells may launch a GVH reaction. For example [117], it was found that CBA mice repopulated, following irradiation, with BALB/C cells rejected pre-existing CBA skin-grafts.

In general GVH reactions in radiation chimaeras are similar to those described above.

There remains the question of the reactivity of true chimaeras to third-party antigens. This is delayed for varying periods of time depending on whether bone-marrow or bone-marrow plus lymphoid tissue is used in restoration. It is also dependent on the magnitude of the GVH reaction induced, which tends to diminish anti-third-party reactivity, and on the degree of 'foreignness' of the challenging antigen, which is directly related to the strength of the immune response [118].

VIII. DONOR SELECTION IN HUMAN-ORGAN TRANSPLANTATION

Assuming, as is by no means invariably true, that there is a panel of potential organ donors for a given transplant recipient, the problem is to decide which one to select.

Methods of donor selection have been divided into two broad groups, 'matching' and 'typing' [119].

Matching represents an attempt to evaluate, in terms of immunological reactivity, the sum of all the individual antigenic differences between a given donor and host. Typing is more precise in that it attempts to define the individual antigens which a given donor–host combination share and those by which they differ.

The ultimate aim of typing is to recognize and classify the individual transplantation antigens in man so that a series of antigenic profiles may be assembled and the donor selected from among those with the same profile as the intended recipient. Typing, however, suffers from the disadvantage that it only defines antigenic differences, and gives no information as to how a given transplant recipient will react thereto.

A. Matching

Matching techniques are fairly numerous, but only two will be considered here, the normal lymphocyte transfer test and mixed lymphocyte culture.

The normal lymphocyte transfer test (N.L.T.) was first described in guinea-pigs [120]. In principal, it consists in transplanting intradermally into each of the prospective donors a fixed number of lymphocytes, for example 5 million, separated from the peripheral blood of an intended recipient. At 48 hours after transfer an area of induration and erythema is observed at the site of the injection. This is thought to be due to a local GVH reaction, as it is not obtained following the injection of dead lymphocytes, and when the initial reaction has subsided it may be followed by a second reaction at between days 8 and 10. The second reaction may be host-versus-graft in character as it can be accentuated by transplanting skin from the lymphocyte donor to the recipient at the same time as the lymphocyte transfer.

The size of the reaction at 48 hours is, in principal, directly related to the degree of histo-incompatibility between the lymphocyte donor and recipients. Therefore the recipient which showed the smallest reaction would be selected to donate the organ required.

The test was applied to predict the relative times at which 16 pairs of skin-grafts to human volunteers would be rejected. It did so correctly in 9 cases and was incorrect in 2 [119]. In the other 5 cases the skin-grafts were rejected simultaneously. A positive correlation between the quality of the match and a subsequent favourable clinical course was also found in a series of 11 kidney transplants [119].

There are, however, a number of disadvantages to the N.L.T. test. The injection of lymphocytes may expose the potential donor to transmissible disease, whilst the donor may also be immunized against the recipient's tissues.

The mixed lymphocyte reaction is based on the finding that the cells in human leucocyte suspensions, when cultured in the presence of various stimuli—for example, an extract of the bean *Phaseolus vulgaris*, known as 'phytohaemagglutinin', and tuberculin (when the leucocytes come from a tuberculin-sensitive individual) [121]—undergo transformation to a more primitive state. The so-called 'transformed' lymphocytes are large cells, with a relatively small amount of strongly basophilic cytoplasm, sometimes containing a number of vacuoles of uniform size and shape, a large nucleus with a coarse chromatin pattern, and a prominent nucleolus.

Similar transformation occurred when leucocytes from two individuals were mixed together in culture [122]. It was therefore argued that the degree of transformation might be directly related to the magnitude of the histocompatibility differences between individuals.

The tedium of counting large numbers of cells was removed by adding tritiated thymidine at the beginning of culture, and subsequently digesting the washed cells, so that the incorporated radioactivity could be determined [123].

Using this modification, an accurate prediction was made of the order of skin-graft rejection in five separate experiments, where grafts were simultaneously transferred from 2 or 3 subjects to a single recipient [119].

A common failing of matching techniques is that they only discriminate between relatively large antigenic differences.

B. Typing

Dausset [124] first demonstrated that human leucocyte agglutinins were iso- rather than auto-antibodies. This finding suggested that it might be possible to group leucocyte antigens in a similar manner to that well known for erythrocyte antigens in blood grouping. In practice three immunological reactions have been used to recognize leucocyte antigens: cytotoxicity [125], agglutination [126], and complement fixation [127], arranged in ascending order of the antibody level above which the test is positive.

Antisera for use in these reactions have been obtained from women following multiple pregnancies and from patients who have received multiple blood transfusions. One major problem has been to obtain sera that are mono-specific, that is, will recognize only one antigen. As will be seen from the foregoing, this problem may be in part solved by using the complement-fixation reaction, but, on the other hand, this test is so relatively insensitive that when using it antisera will sometimes fail to detect the leucocyte antigens present. An alternative approach has been to absorb antisera with known leucocyte antigens, before using them in the cytotoxic test.

Van Rood and his colleagues have tested a considerable number of potential antisera separately against each member of a group of randomly selected individuals using the agglutination reaction. The results were fed into a computer in order to determine whether some of the sera might recognize the same antigens. This appeared to be the case. Therefore family studies were performed to determine the relative frequencies of known antigens in the leucocytes of parents and their offspring. In this way evidence for genetically controlled inheritance of the antigens was found.

On the basis of the results, the following leucocyte antigens are recognized by Van Rood et al.: 4a, 4b, 5a, 5b, 6a, 6b, 7a, 7b, 7c, 7d, 8a, and 9a. Their results have led them to suggest that groups 4, 6, 7, 8, and 9 are closely linked and may even be on the same locus, whilst group 5 is an independent system. Furthermore, antigens 4a and 4b appear to be alternatives, as do 5a and 5b, 6a and 6b, and 7b, 7c, and 7d.

In 1965 a 'workshop' was organized in Leiden to determine whether there was any relationship between the antigens described by Van Rood and colleagues and those of other workers. The plan of the study was that each participant used his own antisera and techniques to type a panel of leucocytes previously characterized by the Leiden workers, according to the leucocyte antigens listed above. The results indicated a marked correlation between the antigens of the Leiden groups and those of the other participants. The results of this workshop have been published [128].

The concept that the leucocyte antigens discussed above are related to transplantation antigens depends on whether such antigens are shared by other nucleated cells, and must be verified by comparing the fate of grafts with the degree of leucocyte compatibility between donor and recipient. Evidence in favour of leucocyte antigens being common to other nucleated cells has been reported [129].

The evidence that graft survival is related to leucocyte compatibility is suggestive but not conclusive. Skin-grafts exchanged between siblings showing compatibility for the leucocyte antigens described by the Leiden group survived for a mean of 19·4 days, whilst grafts made in the presence of leucocyte antigen incompatibility had a mean survival of 14·4 days [130]. However, it was found in the same study that the degree of leucocyte incompatibility could not be used to predict the fate of skin-grafts exchanged between unrelated individuals or between parents and offspring. In the case of the former situation, failure was ascribed to variations in the immunological reactivity of the recipient, whilst in the latter specific tolerance or immunity persisting from the intra-uterine period may be implicated. These findings serve to illustrate that factors other than leucocyte antigens may affect the fate of a graft.

In patients where leucocyte compatibility with the donor was assessed by reactivity of individual antisera against the lymphocytes of both parties, as well as by matching for six known leucocyte antigens, an improved early outcome following renal transplantation was obtained [131]. This was assessed both in terms of survival and the severity of the pathological changes in the grafted kidneys. However, the number of patients studied is still too small for the results to have reached the level of statistical significance.

Finally, it must be emphasized that erythrocyte antigens of the ABO system are also potent transplantation antigens [132].

REFERENCES

1. GORER, P. A., LOUTIT, J. F., and MICKLEM, H. S. (1961), 'Proposed Revision of Transplantese', *Nature, Lond.*, **189**, 1024.
2. MEDAWAR, P. B. (1944), 'The Behaviour and Fate of Skin Autografts and Skin Homografts in Rabbits', *J. Anat.*, **78**, 176.
3. WOODRUFF, M. F. A. (1960), *The Transplantation of Tissues and Organs*, pp. 518–19. Springfield, Ill.: Thomas.
4. BILLINGHAM, R. E., BRENT, L., and MEDAWAR, P. B. (1954), 'Quantitative Studies on Tissue Transplantation Immunity. I, The Survival Time of Skin Homografts exchanged between Different Inbred Strains of Mice', *Proc. R. Soc.*, Series B, **143**, 43.
5. WOODRUFF, M. F. A., and SIMPSON, L. O. (1955), 'Experimental Skin Grafting with Special Reference to Split Skin Grafts', *Plastic reconstr. Surg.*, **15**, 451.

6. SPARROW, E. M. (1953), 'The Behaviour of Skin Autografts and Skin Homografts in the Guinea Pig with Special Reference to the Effect of Cortisone Acetate and Ascorbic Acid on the Homograft Reaction', *J. Endocr.*, **9**, 101.
7. JAFFE, W. P., SYMES, M. O., and TERBLANCHE, J. (1967), 'Observations on the Immunological Reactions of Pigs', in *The Liver* (ed. READ, A. E.), Colston Papers, vol. 19, p. 351. London: Butterworths.
8. ANDERSON, D., BILLINGHAM, R. E., LAMPKIN, G. H., and MEDAWAR, P. B. (1951), 'The Use of Skin Grafting to distinguish between Monozygotic and Dizygotic Twins in Cattle', *Heredity*, **5**, 379.
9. WOODRUFF, M. F. A. (1960), *The Transplantation of Tissues and Organs*, p. 67. Springfield, Ill.: Thomas.
10. WOODRUFF, M. F. A., and ALLEN, T. M. (1953), 'Blood Groups and the Homograft Problem', *Br. J. plast. Surg.*, **5**, 238.
11. MEDAWAR, P. B. (1945), 'Second Study of Behaviour and Fate of Skin Homografts in Rabbits', *J. Anat.*, **79**, 157.
12. DEMPSTER, W. J. (1953), 'Kidney Homotransplantation', *Br. J. Surg.*, **40**, 447.
13. DEMPSTER, W. J. (1955), 'A Consideration of the Cause of Functional Arrest of Homotransplanted Kidneys', *Br. J. Urol.*, **27**, 66.
14. HARDIN, C. A. (1956), 'Common Antigenicity between Skin Grafts and Total Lung Transplants', *Transplantn Bull.*, **3**, 45.
15. BILLINGHAM, R. E., BRENT, L., and MEDAWAR, P. B. (1954), 'Quantitative Studies on Tissue Transplantation Immunity. II, The Origin, Strength and Duration of Actively and Adoptively Acquired Immunity', *Proc. R. Soc.*, Series B, **143**, 58.
16. BILLINGHAM, R. E., BRENT, L., and MEDAWAR, P. B. (1955), 'Acquired Tolerance of Tissue Homografts', *Ann. N.Y. Acad. Sci.*, **59**, 409.
17. MEDAWAR, P. B. (1948), 'The Cultivation of Mammalian Skin Epithelium *in vitro*', *Q. Jl Microsc. Sci.*, **89**, 187.
18. WOODRUFF, M. F. A., and WOODRUFF, H. G. (1950), 'The Transplantation of Normal Tissue with Special Reference to Auto and Homotransplants of Thyroid and Spleen in the Anterior Chamber of the Eye and Subcutaneously in Guinea Pigs', *Phil. Trans. R. Soc.*, Series B, **234**, 559.
19. ATHIAS, M., and GUIMARIAS, A. (1933), 'Graffe ovarienne intracérébrale chez des Cobayes mâles entiers et préalablement châtrés', *C. r. Séanc. Soc. Biol.*, **113**, 733.
20. PEACOCK, J. H., and TERBLANCHE, J. (1967), 'Orthotopic Homotransplantation of the Liver in the Pig', in *The Liver* (ed. READ, A. E.), Colston Papers, vol. 19, p. 333. London: Butterworths.
21. HUNT, A. C. (1967), 'Pathology of Liver Transplantation in the Pig', in *The Liver* (ed. READ, A. E.), Colston Papers, vol. 19, p. 337. London: Butterworths.
22. CALNE, R. Y., WHITE, H. J. O., YOFFA, D. E., BINNS, R. M., MAGINN, R. R., HERBERTSON, R. M., MILLARD, P. R., MOLINA, V. P., and DAVIS, D. R. (1967), 'Prolonged Survival of Liver Transplants in the Pig', *Br. med. J.*, **4**, 645.
23. KALISS, N. (1966), 'Immunological Enhancement: Conditions for its Expression and its Relevance for Grafts of Normal Tissue', *Ann. N.Y. Acad. Sci.*, **129**, 155.
24. DEMPSTER, W. J., LENNOX, B., and BOAG, J. W. (1950), 'Prolongation of Survival of Skin Homotransplants in the Rabbit by Irradiation of the Host', *Br. J. exp. Path.*, **31**, 670.
25. MEDAWAR, P. B. (1963), 'The Use of Antigenic Tissue Extracts to weaken the Immunological Reaction against Skin Homografts in Mice', *Transplantation*, **1**, 21.
26. BAKER, R., and GORDON, R. (1955), 'Effect of Total Body Irradiation on Experimental Renal Transplantation', *Surgery, St Louis*, **37**, 820.
27. WOODRUFF, M. F. A., ROBSON, J. S., McWHIRTER, R., NOLAN, B., WILSON, T. I., LAMBIE, A. T., McWILLIAM, J. M., and MacDONALD, M. K. (1962), 'Transplantation of a Kidney from a Brother to Sister', *Br. J. Urol.*, **34**, 3.
28. BERENBAUM, M. C. (1964), 'Effects of Carcinogens on Immune Processes', *Br. med. Bull.*, **20**, 159.
29. BERENBAUM, M. C. (1965), 'Immunosuppressive Agents', *Br. med. Bull.*, **21**, 140.
30. WOODRUFF, M. F. A. (1962), 'Prolonged Survival of Skin Homografts in Adult Mice following Sub-lethal Irradiation, Injection of Donor Strain Spleen Cells and Administration of Amethopterin', *Nature, Lond.*, **195**, 727.
31. RUSSELL, P. S. (1962), 'Modification of Runt Disease in Mice by Various Means', in *Ciba Foundation Symposium on Transplantation* (ed. WOLSTENHOLME, G. E. W., and CAMERON, M. P.), p. 350. London: Churchill.

32. SANTOS, G. W. (1967), 'Immunosuppressive Drugs I', *Fedn Proc. Fedn Am. Socs exp. Biol.*, **26**, 907.
33. BERENBAUM, M. C. (1964), 'Prolongation of Homograft Survival by Methotrexate with Protection against Toxicity by Folinic Acid', *Lancet*, **2**, 1363.
34. WOODRUFF, M. F. A., ROBSON, J. S., NOLAN, B., LAMBIE, A. T., WILSON, T. I., and CLARK, J. G. (1963), 'Homotransplantation of the Kidney in Patients treated by Preoperative Local Irradiation and Post Operative Administration of an Antimetabolite (Imuran)', *Lancet*, **2**, 675.
35. MILLER, J. F. A. P. (1962), 'Role of the Thymus in Transplantation Immunity', *Ann. N.Y. Acad. Sci.*, **99**, 340.
36. MILLER, J. F. A. P. (1962), 'Immunological Significance of the Thymus of the Adult Mouse', *Nature, Lond.*, **195**, 1318.
37. GLOBERSON, A., FIONE-DONATI, L., and FELDMAN, M. (1962), 'On the Role of the Thymus in Recovery of Immunological Reactivity following X-irradiation', *Expl Cell Res.*, **28**, 455.
38. GLOBERSON, A., and FELDMAN, M. (1964), 'Role of the Thymus in Restoration of Immune Reactivity and Lymphoid Regeneration in Irradiated Mice', *Transplantation*, **2**, 212.
39. LUMB, G. N., and SYMES, M. O. (1965), 'On the Value of Thymectomy in Adult Mice as a Means of potentiating the Immunosuppressive Action of Melphalan (L-Phenylalanine Mustard)', *Immunology*, **9**, 575.
40. OSOBA, D. A., and MILLER, J. F. A. P. (1963), 'Evidence for a Humoral Factor responsible for the Maturation of Immunological Faculty', *Nature, Lond.*, **199**, 653.
41. MILLER, J. F. A. P., DE BURGH, P. M., DUKOR, P., GRANT, G., ALLMAN, V., and HOUSE, W. (1966), 'Regeneration of Thymus grafts. II, Effects on Immunological Capacity', *Clin. exp. Immun.*, **1**, 61.
42. MCINTIRE, K. R., SELL, S., and MILLER, J. F. A. P. (1964), 'Pathogenesis of the Post Neonatal Thymectomy Wasting Syndrome', *Nature, Lond.*, **204**, 151.
43. MILLER, J. F. A. P., DUKOR, P., GRANT, G., SINCLAIR, N. R., and SACQUET, E. (1967), 'The Immunological Responsiveness of Germ-free Mice thymectomised at Birth. I, Antibody Production and Skin Homograft Rejection', *Clin. exp. Immun.*, **2**, 531.
44. CALNE, R. Y. (1963), 'Thymectomy in Dogs with Renal Homografts treated with Drugs', *Nature, Lond.*, **199**, 388.
45. STARZL, T. E. (1964), in *Experience in Renal Transplantation*, p. 211. Philadelphia: Saunders.
46. OLIVERAS, F. E., KELLY, W. D., MERCHANT, C., and GOOD, R. A. (1963), 'Effect of Thymectomy on Immune Reactions in Adult Dogs', *Surg. Forum*, **14**, 184.
47. MCGREGOR, D. D., and GOWANS, J. L. (1963), 'The Antibody Response of Rats depleted of Lymphocytes by Chronic Drainage from the Thoracic Duct', *J. exp. Med.*, **117**, 303.
48. WOODRUFF, M. F. A., and ANDERSON, N. F. (1964), 'The Effect of Lymphocyte Depletion by Thoracic Duct Fistula and Administration of Anti-lymphocyte Serum on the Survival of Skin Homografts in Rats', *Ann. N.Y. Acad. Sci.*, **120**, 119.
49. WOODRUFF, M. F. A., and ANDERSON, N. F. (1963), 'Effect of Lymphocyte Depletion by Thoracic Duct Fistula and Administration of Anti-lymphocytic Serum on the Survival of Skin Homografts in Rats', *Nature, Lond.*, **200**, 702.
50. MONACO, A. P., WOOD, M. L., GRAY, J. G., and RUSSELL, P. S. (1966), 'Studies on Heterologous Anti-lymphocyte Serum in Mice', *J. Immun.*, **96**, 229.
51. MONACO, A. P., WOOD, M. L., and RUSSELL, P. S. (1966), 'Studies on Heterologous Anti-lymphocyte Serum in Mice. III, Immunologic Tolerance and Chimerism produced across the H-2 Locus with Adult Thymectomy and Anti-lymphocyte Serum', *Ann. N.Y. Acad. Sci.*, **129**, 190.
52. LEVEY, R. H., and MEDAWAR, P. B. (1966), 'Some Experiments on the Action of Antilymphoid Antisera', *Ann. N.Y. Acad. Sci.*, **129**, 164.
53. NAGAYA, H., and SIEKER, H. O. (1965), 'Allograft Survival: Effect of Antiserums to Thymus Glands and Lymphocytes', *Science, N.Y.*, **150**, 1181.
54. ABAZA, H. M., NOLAN, B., WATT, J. G., and WOODRUFF, M. F. A. (1966), 'The Effect of Anti-lymphocytic Serum on the Survival of Renal Homotransplants in Dogs', *Transplantation*, **4**, 618.

55. ABBOTT, W. M., OTHERSON, H. B., MONACO, A. P., SIMMONS, R. L., WOOD, M. L., and RUSSELL, P. S. (1966), 'Prolonged Survival of Renal Allografts in Dogs treated with Anti-lymphocyte Serum', *Surg. Forum*, **17**, 228.
56. LUCKE, J. N., IMMELMAN, E. J., SYMES, M. O., and HUNT, A. C. (1968), 'Use of Horse Anti-pig Leucocyte Serum to suppress the Homograft Reaction in Pigs', *Nature, Lond.*, **217**, 560.
57. BALNER, H., and DERSJANT, H. (1967), 'Effect of Anti-lymphocytic Sera in Primates', in *Anti-lymphocytic Serum* (ed. WOLSTENHOLME, G. E. W., and O'CONNOR, M.), Ciba Foundation Study Group No. 29, p. 85. London: Churchill.
58. STARZL, T. E., PORTER, K. A., IWASAKI, Y., MARCHIORI, T. L., and KASHIWAGI, N. (1967), 'The Use of Heterologous Anti-lymphocytic Globulin in Human Renal Homotransplantation', in *Anti-lymphocytic Serum* (ed. WOLSTENHOLME, G. E. W., and O'CONNOR, M.), Ciba Foundation Study Group No. 29, p. 4. London: Churchill.
59. MONACO, A. P., WOOD, M. L., and RUSSELL, P. S. (1967), 'Some Effects of Purified Heterologous Antihuman Lymphocyte Serum in Man', *Transplantation*, **5**, 1106.
60. BALNER, H., EYSVOOGEL, V. P., and CLETON, F. J. (1968), 'Testing of Anti-human Lymphocyte Sera in Chimpanzees and Lower Primates', *Lancet*, **1**, 19.
61. SYMES, M. O., LUCKE, J. N., CLAMP, J. R., MEETEVA, G., and SELLWOOD, N. H. (1968), unpublished observations.
62. JAMES, K. (1967), 'Anti-lymphocytic Antibody—A Review', *Clin. exp. Immun.*, **2**, 615.
63. SEEGAL, B. C., HSU, K. C., ROTHENBURG, M. S., and CHAPEUA, M. L. (1962), 'Studies of the Mechanism of Experimental Nephritis with Fluorescein-labelled Antibody. II, Localisation and Persistence of Injected Rabbit or Duck Anti-rat Kidney Serum during the Course of Nephritis in Rats', *Am. J. Path.*, **41**, 183.
64. IWASAKI, Y., PORTER, K. A., AMEND, J. R., MARCHIORO, T. L., ZUHLKE, V., and STARZL, T. E. (1967), 'The Preparation and Testing of Horse Anti-dog and Anti-human Anti-lymphoid Plasma or Serum and its Protein Fractions', *Surgery Gynec. Obstet.*, **124**, 1.
65. FELDMAN, J. D. (1963), in *Immunopathology: Third International Symposium* (ed. GRABAR, P., and MIESCHER, P. A.). Basle: Schwabe & Co.
66. WOODRUFF, M. F. A., ANDERSON, N. F., and ABAZA, H. M. (1967), 'Experiments with Anti-lymphocytic Serum', in *The Lymphocyte in Immunology and Haemopoiesis* (ed. YOFFEY, J. M.), p. 286. London: Arnold.
67. GRÜSBECK, R., NORDMAN, C. T., and DE LA CHAPELLE, A. (1964), 'The Leucocyte-mitogenic Effect of Serum from Rabbits immunized with Human Leucocytes', *Acta med. scand.*, Suppl., **412**, 39.
68. LING, N. R., KNIGHT, S., HARDY, D., STANWORTH, D. R., and HOLT, P. J. L. (1967), 'Antibody Induced Lymphocyte Transformation *in vitro*', in *Anti-lymphocyte Serum* (ed. WOLSTENHOLME, G. E. W., and O'CONNOR, M.), Ciba Foundation Study Group No. 29, p. 41. London: Churchill.
69. LEVEY, R. H., and MEDAWAR, P. B. (1967), 'The Mode of Action of Antilymphocytic Serum', in *Antilymphocyte Serum* (ed. WOLSTENHOLME, G. E. W., and O'CONNOR, M.), Ciba Foundation Study Group No. 29, p. 72. London: Churchill.
70. BRENT, L., COURTNAY, T., and GOWLAND, G. (1968), 'Antilymphocytic Serum: Its Effect on the Reactivity of Lymphocytes', in *Advances in Transplantation*, Proceedings of the 1st International Congress of the Transplantation Society, Paris (ed. DAUSSET, J., HAMBURGER, J., and MATHE, G.), p. 117. Copenhagen: Munksgaard.
71. BURNET, F. M., and FENNER, F. (1948), 'Genetics and Immunology', *Heredity*, **2**, 289.
72. BURNET, F. M., and FENNER, F. (1949), in *The Production of Antibodies*, 2nd ed. Melbourne: Macmillan.
73. OWEN, R. D. (1945), 'Immunogenetic Consequences of Vascular Anastomosis between Bovine Twins', *Science, N.Y.*, **102**, 400.
74. OWEN, R. D., DAVIS, H. P., and MORGAN, R. F. (1946), 'Quintuplet Calves and Erythrocyte Mosaicism', *J. Hered.*, **37**, 209.
75. ANDERSON, D., BILLINGHAM, R. E., LAMPKIN, G. H., and MEDAWAR, P. B. (1951), 'The Use of Skin Grafting to distinguish between Monozygotic and Dizygotic Twins in Cattle', *Heredity*, **5**, 379.

76. SIMONSEN, M. (1955) 'Artificial Production of Immunological Tolerance to Heterologous Cells and Induced Susceptibility to Virus', *Nature, Lond.*, **175**, 763.
77. WOODRUFF, M. F. A., and LENNOX, B. (1959), 'Reciprocal Skin Grafting in a Pair of Twins showing Blood Group Chimaerism', *Lancet*, **2**, 476.
78. BILLINGHAM, R. E., BRENT, L., and MEDAWAR, P. B. (1953), 'Actively Acquired Tolerance of Foreign Cells', *Nature, Lond.*, **172**, 603.
79. BILLINGHAM, R. E., BRENT, L., and MEDAWAR, P. B. (1956), 'Quantitative Studies on Tissue Transplantation Immunity', *Phil. Trans. R. Soc.*, Series B, **239**, 357.
80. WOODRUFF, M. F. A., and SIMPSON, L. O. (1954), 'Induction of Acquired Tolerance to Homologous Tissue', *Proc. Univ. Otago med. Sch.*, **32**, 12.
81. BILLINGHAM, R. E., and BRENT, L. (1957), 'Acquired Tolerance of Foreign Cells in Newborn Animals', *Proc. R. Soc.*, Series B, **146**, 78.
82. WEBER, R. A., CANNON, J. A., and LONGMIRE, W. P. (1954), 'Observations on the Re-grafting of Successful Homografts in Chickens', *Ann. Surg.*, **139**, 473.
83. SHAPIRO, F., MARTINEZ, C., SMITH, J. M., and GOOD, R. A. (1961), 'Tolerance of Skin Homografts induced in Adult Mice by Multiple Injections of Homologous Spleen Cells', *Proc. Soc. exp. Biol. Med.*, **106**, 472.
84. MICHIE, D., and WOODRUFF, M. F. A. (1962), 'Induction of Specific Immunological Tolerance of Homografts in Adult Mice by Sublethal Irradiation and Injection of Donor Type Spleen Cells in High Dosage', *Proc. R. Soc.*, Series B, **156**, 280.
85. HOWARD, J. G., MICHIE, D., and WOODRUFF, M. F. A. (1962), 'Transplantation Tolerance and Immunity in Relation to Age', in *Ciba Foundation Symposium on Transplantation* (ed. WOLSTENHOLME, G. E. W., and CAMERON, M. P.), p. 138. London: Churchill.
86. MITCHISON, N. A. (1962), 'Tolerance of Erythrocytes in Poultry: Induction and Specificity', *Immunology*, **5**, 341; 'Loss and Abolition', *Immunology*, **5**, 359.
87. SIMONSEN, M., and JENSEN, E. (1959), 'The Graft-versus-host Assay in Transplantation Chimaeras', in *Biological Problems of Grafting* (ed. ALBERT, F., and LEJEUNE-LEDANT, G.), p. 214. Oxford: Blackwell.
88. SIMONSEN, M. (1957), 'The Impact on the Developing Embryo and Newborn Animal of Adult Homologous Cells', *Acta path. microbiol. scand.*, **40**, 480.
89. HOWARD, J. G. (1961), 'Changes in the Activity of the Reticulo-endothelial System following Injection of Parental Strain Spleen Cells into F_1 Hybrid Mice', *Br. J. exp. Path.*, **42**, 72.
90. BILLINGHAM, R. E., and BRENT, L. (1959), 'Quantitative Studies on Tissue Transplantation Immunity. IV, Induction of Tolerance in Newborn Mice and Studies on the Phenomenon of Runt Disease', *Phil. Trans. R. Soc.*, Series B, **242**, 439.
91. SIMONSEN, M. (1962), 'Graft-versus-host Reactions: Their Natural History and Applicability as Tools of Research', in *Progress in Allergy*, vol. 6 (ed. KALLOS, P., and WAKSMAN, B. H.), p. 349. Basle: Karger.
92. MICHIE, D., WOODRUFF, M. F. A., and ZEISS, I. M. (1961), 'An Investigation of Immunological Tolerance based on Chimaera Analysis', *Immunology*, **4**, 413.
93. COCK, A. G., and SIMONSEN, M. (1958), 'Immunological Attack on Newborn Chickens by Injected Adult Cells', *Immunology*, **1**, 103.
94. FOX, M. (1962), 'Cytological Estimation of Proliferating Donor Cells during Graft-versus-host Disease in F_1 Hybrid Mice injected with Parental Spleen Cells', *Immunology*, **5**, 489.
95. GOWANS, J. L., GESNER, B. L., and McGREGOR, D. D. (1961), 'The Immunological Activity of Lymphocytes', in *Biological Activity of the Leucocyte*, Ciba Foundation Study Group No. 10. London: Churchill.
96. DAVIES, A. J. S., and DOAK, S. M. A. (1960), 'Fate of Homologous Adult Spleen Cells injected into Newborn Mice', *Nature, Lond.*, **187**, 610.
97. GORER, P. A., and BOYSE, E. A. (1959), 'Pathological Changes in F_1 Hybrid Mice Following Transplantation of Spleen Cells from Donors of the Parental Strains', *Immunology*, **2**, 182.
98. BINET, J. L., and MATHÉ, G. (1961), 'Étude en Microscopie optique et electronique des Cellules immunologiquement competentes au Cours des Réactions de Greffe', *C. r. hebd. Séanc. Acad. Sci., Paris*, **252**, 1852.
99. MACKANESS, G. B., and BLANDEN, R. V. (1967), in *Progress in Allergy* (ed. KALLOS, P., and WAKSMAN, B. H.), vol. 11, p. 128. Basle: Karger.

100. Fox, M., and Howard, J. G. (1963), 'An Acquired Type of Refractoriness to Graft-versus-host Reaction in Adult F₁ Hybrid Mice', *Transplantation*, **1**, 2.

101. Cooper, G. N., and Howard, J. G. (1961), 'An Effect of the Graft-versus-host Reaction on Resistance to Experimental Bacteraemia', *Br. J. exp. Path.*, **42**, 558.

102. Siskind, G. W., and Thomas, L. (1959), 'Studies on the Runting Syndrome in Newborn Mice', in *Biological Problems of Grafting* (ed. Albert, F., and Lejeune-Ledant, G.), p. 176. Oxford: Blackwell.

103. Russell, P. S. (1960), 'The Weight Gain Assay for Runt Disease in Mice', *Ann. N.Y. Acad. Sci.*, **87**, 445.

104. Siskind, G. W., Leonard, L., and Thomas, L. (1960), 'The Runting Syndrome', *Ann. N.Y. Acad. Sci.*, **87**, 452.

105. Simonsen, M., Engelbreth-Holm, J., Jensen, E., and Poulsen, H. (1958), 'A Study of the Graft-versus-host Reaction in Transplantation to Embryo F₁ Hybrids and Irradiated Animals', *Ann. N.Y. Acad. Sci.*, **73**, 834.

106. Van Bekkum, D. W., and De Vries, M. J. (1967), *Radiation Chimaeras*. London: Logos.

107. Jacobson, L. O., Marks, E. K., Robson, M. J., Gaston, E. O., and Zirkle, R. E. (1949), 'Effect of Spleen Protection on Mortality following X-irradiation', *J. Lab. clin. Med.*, **34**, 1538.

108. Jacobson, L. O. (1952), 'Evidence for a Humoral Factor (or Factors) concerned in Recovery from Radiation Injury: A Review', *Cancer Res.*, **12**, 315.

109. Ford, C. E., Hamerton, J. L., Barnes, D. W. H., and Loutit, J. F. (1956), 'Cytological Identification of Radiation Chimaeras', *Nature, Lond.*, **177**, 452.

110. Vos, O., Davids, J. A. G., Weyzen, W. W. H., and Van Bekkum, D. W. (1956), 'Evidence for the Cellular Hypothesis in Radiation Protection by Bone Marrow Cells', *Acta physiol. pharmac. néerl.*, **4**, 482.

111. Van Bekkum, D. W., Vos, O., and Weyzen, W. W. H. (1956), 'Homo et hétérogreffe de Tissus hématopoiétiques chez la Souris', *Revue Hémat.*, **11**, 477.

112. Barnes, D. W. H., Ford, C. E., Gray, S. M., and Loutit, J. F. (1950), 'Spontaneous and Induced Changes in Cell Populations in Heavily Irradiated Mice', in *Progress in Nuclear Medicine*, Series VI (ed. Bugher, J. G., Coursaget, J., and Loutit, J. F.), pp. 1–10. London: Pergamon.

113. Balner, H. (1963), 'Bone Marrow Transplantation after Whole Body Irradiation: An Experimental Study in the Rat', M.D. Thesis, Municipal University, Amsterdam.

114. Davis, W. E., Tyan, M. L., and Cole, L. J. (1964), 'Mutually Tolerant Host and Donor Type Immunologically Competent Cells in Mouse Radiation Chimaeras', *Transplantation*, **2**, 21.

115. Main, J. M., and Prehn, R. T. (1955), 'Successful Skin Homografts after Administration of High Dose X-radiation and Homologous Bone Marrow', *J. natn. Cancer Inst.*, **15**, 1023.

116. Main, J. M., and Prehn, R. T. (1957), 'Fate of Skin Homografts in X-irradiated Mice treated with Homologous Marrow', *J. natn. Cancer Inst.*, **19**, 1053.

117. Koller, P. C., and Doak, S. M. A. (1960), 'The Effect of Radiation on the Immune Response in Mice and its Modification by Tissue Transplantation', in *Immediate and Low Level Effects of Ionizing Radiations* (ed. Buzatti-Traverso, A. A.), p. 326. London: Taylor & Francis.

118. Makinodan, T., and Gengozian, N. (1960), 'Effect of Radiation on Antibody Formation', in *Radiation Protection and Recovery* (ed. Hollaender, A.), p. 316. London: Pergamon.

119. Russell, P. S., Nelson, S. P., and Johnson, G. J. (1966), 'Matching Tests for Histocompatibility in Man', *Ann. N.Y. Acad. Sci.*, **129**, 368.

120. Brent, L., and Medawar, P. B. (1963), 'Tissue Transplantation: A New Approach to the "Typing" Problem', *Br. med. J.*, **2**, 269.

121. Permain, G., Lycette, R. R., and Fitzgerald, P. H. (1963), 'Tuberculin Induced Mitoses in Peripheral Blood Leucocytes', *Lancet*, **1**, 637.

122. Bain, B., Vas, M. R., and Lowenstein, L. (1964), 'The Development of Large Immature Mononuclear Cells in Mixed Leucocyte Culture', *Blood*, **23**, 108.

123. Bain, B., and Lowenstein, L. (1964), 'Genetic Studies on the Mixed Leucocyte Reaction', *Science, N.Y.*, **145**, 1315.

124. Dausset, J. (1954), 'Leucoagglutinins. IV. Leucoagglutinins and Blood Transfusion', *Vox Sang.*, **4**, 190.

125. TERASAKI, P. I., MICKEY, M. R., VREDEVOE, D. L., and GOYETTE, D. R. (1965), 'Serotyping for Homotransplantation. IV, Grouping and Evaluation of Lymphotoxic Sera', *Vox Sang.*, **11**, 350.
126. VAN ROOD, J. J., VAN LEEUWEN, A., BRUNING, J. W., and EERNISSE, J. G. (1966), 'Current Status of Human Leucocyte Groups', *Ann. N.Y. Acad. Sci.*, **129**, 446.
127. SHULMAN, N. R., MARDER, V. J., ALEDOERT, L. M., and HILLER, M. C. (1962), 'Complement-fixing Isoantibodies against Antigens Common to Platelets and Leucocytes', *Trans. Ass. Am. Phys.*, **75**, 89.
128. BRUNING, J. W., VAN LEEUWEN, A., and VAN ROOD, J. J. (1965), 'Leucocyte Antigens. A Preliminary Report of the Workshop on Histocompatibility Testing (Leiden, Aug., 1965)', *Ser. Haemat.*, **11**, 275.
129. VAN ROOD, J. J. (1962), 'Leucocyte Grouping. A Method and its Application', Thesis. Leiden.
130. VAN ROOD, J. J., VAN LEEUWEN, A., SCHIPPERS, A., CEPELLINI, R., MATTUIZ, P. L., and CURTONI, S. (1966), 'Leucocyte Groups and their Relation to Homotransplantation', *Ann. N.Y. Acad. Sci.*, **129**, 467.
131. TERASAKI, P. I., VREDEVOE, D. L., MICKEY, M. R., PORTER, K. A., MARCHIORO, T. L., FARIS, T. D., and STARZL, T. E. (1966), 'Serotyping for Homotransplantation'. VII, Selection of Kidney Donors for Thirty-two Recipients', *Ann. N.Y. Acad. Sci.*, **129**, 500.
132. CEPPELLINI, R., CURTONI, E. S., LEIGHEB, P. L., MATTUIZ, V. C., MIGGIANO, V. C., and VISETTI, M. (1965), 'An Experimental Approach to Genetic Analysis of Histocompatibility in Man. Histcompatibility Testing 1965', *Ser. Haemat.*, **11**, 13.

CHAPTER 11

TUMOUR IMMUNOLOGY*

By M. O. Symes

I. INTRODUCTION

THE idea that immunology is a discipline relevant to the study of cancer received its initial impetus from the results of work involving the transplantation of tumours. It was found that tumours arising within genetically inbred strains of laboratory animals could be transplanted successfully, so that progressive tumour growth resulted, only to animals possessing certain dominant histocompatibility antigens in common with the tumour donor.

It was subsequently found that the rejection of tumours by genetically incompatible hosts caused the latter to become actively immunized

---

* This chapter is based, in part, on a review entitled 'Some Experimental and Clinical Aspects of Neoplasia suggesting its Relationship to Reticular Tissue Function', incorporated in a Dissertation submitted by the author for the degree of Doctor of Medicine in the University of Bristol in 1963.

against the tumour in question. This immunity could be adoptively transferred by immunologically competent cell suspensions to further hosts.

It was evident that the degree of autonomy possessed by malignant cells was limited. It therefore became imperative to determine how autonomous the tumours were in the animal in which they arose, for the exploitation of any controlling influence seemed to be the best hope for the successful treatment of cancer.

Many types of experimental tumour in animals have been shown to possess 'tumour-specific antigens', that is, antigens present in the malignant cells but absent from the corresponding normal cells of the host. Such specific antigens afford the *point d'appui* for the host's immunological resistance to its tumour. But why are these host defences insufficient to destroy the tumour in every case? The precise answer to this question is unknown but it is probably a combination of three factors. These are the weak nature of specific antigens, an immunological deficiency syndrome produced in the host by progressive tumour growth, and the increasing autonomy of malignant cells with repeated division. Some of these ideas will now be considered in greater detail.

II. Transplantation of Tumours

Acceptance and Rejection by the Host

The transplantation of a tumour consists in its transfer through one or more hosts, the method dating from the latter part of the nineteenth century. The history of the subject has been reviewed [1].

If a tumour arises in a strain of genetically inbred animals, it might be postulated that within this strain its degree of autonomy towards any host would be the same as in its primary host. Progressive growth would therefore be the outcome of any transplantation within this strain. On the other hand, following transplantation to a host genetically different from that of its origin, the tumour should be rejected.

The results obtained from the transplantation of tumours arising within a given inbred strain to animals of the same strain (isogenic) and to members of different inbred strains (allogeneic) have been reviewed [2]. A study was also made on the outcome of transplanting such tumours to F_1 and F_2 hybrid hosts, raised by crossing the strain of tumour origin with another inbred strain, and to F_1 back-cross mice, where the back-cross was both to native and foreign strains relative to the tumour. As a result of these investigations, it was shown that a tumour arising in a given inbred strain, A, will grow progressively and kill all other mice of that strain, all A, F_1 hybrid mice, and all A back-cross (i.e., F_1 hybrid to A) animals. A proportion of A, F_2 hybrid mice and $F_1 \times$ foreign strain back-cross mice were also susceptible. These results were explained according to the genetic theory of tumour transplantation by assuming that a transplant will grow in a given host, only if the host carries the same dominant histocompatibility genes as the animal in which the tumour originated. It may be predicted on the basis of this theory that, in a system using two inbred lines A and B and a tumour which originated in line A, the ratio of the animals susceptible to the total number of animals will be $(\frac{3}{4})^n$ for the F_2 generation, and $(\frac{1}{2})^n$ for the F_1 $(A \times B) \times B$ back-cross generation, n being the number of dominant genes which must be present to produce susceptibility [3].

This postulate was tested [4, 5] using thirty-six different tumours: several mammary carcinomata, two leukaemias, and a melanoma. The recipient mice were bred from appropriate crosses between eight inbred strains.

Further studies along these lines were made using carcinogen-induced sarcomas [6], with a sarcoma and a leukaemia [7], and using three and eight mammary carcinomata respectively [8, 9].

Within the limits of chance, all these studies have demonstrated a good fit between the observed susceptibility of F_2 and resistant back-cross generations and that predicted above, where n is a whole number. This would be most unlikely to occur fortuitously and hence the genetic theory of tumour transplantation may be regarded as established.

It may in turn be concluded that in many cases malignant neoplasms are not totally autonomous, at least up to a certain number of transplant generations.

III. Production of Immunity to Neoplasms

Investigation in the early part of the twentieth century demonstrated that regression of a tumour transplant in a given host renders that animal resistant to a second transplant of the same tumour. The early work in this field has been reviewed [10].

Using the A, Bagg Albino, C3H, and C57B1 strains of mice, interstrain transplants were made of sarcomas induced by 1256-dibenzanthracene in the last three [11]. It was found, by removing the primary transplant at varying intervals, that strain-specific immunity to a second transplant was present by the fifth day. That damaged tumour tissue could also induce a state of active immunity was suggested by the finding that Ehrlich ascites tumour cells, irradiated *in vitro* so as to destroy their reproductive capacity, none the less retained strong auto-antigenic activity in allogeneic tumour–host systems [12].

The fundamental question of what type of antibody is concerned in the mediation of immunity to tumours must now be considered.

A direct association between the functions of the host's immunologically competent cells and the destruction of incompatible tumour grafts was suggested by experiments with diffusion chambers [13–15]. Using mice, various types of target cells—embryonic heart and lung, dissociated epidermal cells from newborn animals, and an adenocarcinoma—were placed separately in diffusion chambers composed of Millipore filters. The chambers were placed intraperitoneally in various hosts and were of two types: permeable to host leucocytes and macrophages, and impermeable save to circulating antibodies. It was found that in cell-impermeable chambers the target cells survived in both isogenic and allogeneic hosts. However, when the host cells had access to the target cells, the latter were destroyed in allogeneic and xenogeneic hosts, the process being more rapid if the foreign host had previously been immunized against the target cells. Furthermore, if the target tissue was combined, within a cell-impermeable diffusion chamber, with allogeneic non-immunized or immunized spleen cells, the whole being placed intraperitoneally in hosts isogenic with respect to the target tissue, the target was destroyed, again more rapidly, by the immune cells.

The work of Algire and his colleagues suggested the predominant position of 'cell-bound', as opposed to circulating antibody and complement, in the destruction of foreign tumour grafts [13–15]. However, it has been pointed out [16] that if tumours within diffusion chambers were susceptible to the cytotoxic effects of circulating antibody, due to the small concentration of the latter inside the chamber, this would not have been revealed by the above experiments. Of more direct relevance to the problem is the question of how and under what conditions it is possible to transfer passive immunity with antiserum to tumours.

It was possible [17] to transfer immunity to the C57B1-strain leukaemia, EL 4, by means of serum from mice of strains A, BLAB/C, and C3H, which had previously rejected subcutaneous inoculations of EL 4. In each case serum transfer was between mice of the same inbred strain, which was allogeneic with respect to the leukaemia. Protection against EL 4 was observed following serum transfer between 7 days prior to, and 2 days after, tumour challenge. That the phenomenon amounted to true passive immunity was further emphasized by a normal response to EL 4 in hosts subsequently rechallenged at a later date, when the transferred antibody had decayed.

Similar attempts to transfer passive immunity, by means of serum transfer, to tumours other than leukaemias were, however, uniformly unsuccessful.

These findings on the transfer of passive immunity may be contrasted with the results of attempts to transfer adoptive immunity to neoplasms with immunologically competent cells. Mice of strains A and C57B1 were immunized against the C3H-strain lymphoma 6C3HED by transplanting the tumour subcutaneously [18]. It was shown that a cell suspension from the draining lymph-nodes was able, on intraperitoneal injection, to transfer immunity against 63HED to further A and C57B1 hosts. The adoptive immunity was assessed by the time after which tumour 6C3HED, having been in the A or C57B1 hosts, failed to grow on further transplantation to CBA hosts.* This time was 9·9 days in non-immunized mice and 2·1 days in those to which immunity had been transferred. After a single immunizing injection, A and C57B1 lymph-nodes could transfer immunity for up to 20 days and the protection thus conferred on A or C57B1 hosts also lasted about 20 days, a most unlikely finding if the effect was due to the transfer of circulating antibody.

Subsequently it was demonstrated [19] that similar immunity to the A-strain sarcoma Sa 1 could be transferred to C57BR/a hosts. The capacity of cells from the draining nodes of C57BR/a mice to transfer immunity appeared at 3–5 days, was still present at 10 days, but disappeared 15 days after a single subcutaneous immunization. A second inoculation of Sa 1 conferred the capacity to transmit immunity within 2 days, but the response was weaker as judged by the time for which the host could transfer immunity and the degree of protection conferred.

---

* Mice of strains C3H and CBA share the same major histocompatibility antigens.

This is in direct contrast to what might be expected if the immunity conferred was due to the transfer of circulating antibody.

The power to form haemagglutinins could be adoptively transferred by immunologically competent cells from immunized hosts [20]. The antibody response in the cell recipients reached its peak titre after 4–8 days, but was still present 30 days after cell transfer. As this was far too long for any passively transferred haemagglutinins to have persisted, the results suggested antibody production by the transferred cells.

Mitchison has drawn attention to the fact that, whereas draining lymph-node cells show a relatively greater ability to confer protection against a tumour on transfer to a second animal, after 5 days' rather than 10–15 days' stimulation in the primary host, the reverse obtains in respect to haemagglutinin production. He suggested this as evidence for the dominant role of 'cell-bound' antibody in the rejection of solid-tissue grafts. However, it has been objected that in testing for transferred immunity, as shown by protection against a tumour transplant, the transferred cells are restimulated by antigen. Therefore a fairer comparison between the time of optimal protection and the production of circulating antibody would be at the total time for which the transferred cells were stimulated in both the primary and secondary hosts [16]. Allowing for this, the time relations for the production of both effects are similar.

However, further light on the importance of 'cell-bound' rather than circulating antibody, in the rejection of tumours other than leukaemias, is shed by the following experiments [21, 22]. Sera from C57B1/6Ks mice, immunized by a homogenate of A-strain spleen cells, abrogated the resistance of further C57B1/6Ks mice to the A-strain sarcoma Sa 1, such that 11 out of 30 of the challenged animals died. No deaths occurred in 15 C57B1/6Ks mice following challenge with Sa 1, after transfer of serum from non-immunized C57B1/6Ks animals.

In addition, it was shown [20] that regional lymph-node cells from C57BR/a mice, pretreated with a lyophilized preparation of sarcoma Sa 1, on adoptive transfer to further C57BR/a hosts, produced haemagglutinins but lowered resistance to subsequent challenge with Sa 1, to which these mice are normally resistant [see also 23].

These results suggested that circulating antibody, produced by allogeneic hosts in response to solid (as opposed to lymphoma) tumour transplants, may actually mitigate against the production of immunity to the latter. This leads us naturally to a discussion of the phenomenon of 'immunological enhancement'.

IV. Immunological Enhancement

Immunological enhancement has been defined [24] as 'the successful establishment or prolonged survival (conversely, the delayed rejection) of an allogeneic graft'. The phenomenon may be distinguished from other forms of prolonged graft survival by its dependence on contact between the graft and specific antigraft serum.

There are a number of possible explanations for the enhancement of tumour allografts.

1. A qualitative and/or quantitative change in the antigenicity of the tumour cells.

2. A stimulation of tumour-cell growth by contact with antiserum.

3. A 'walling off' of the iso-antigens of the tumour graft, as a result of their contact with specific antibodies. In this way effective immunization of the host against the tumour would be prevented ('afferent inhibition').

4. Antiserum acts at a 'central' level on the immune system of the host to prevent the rejection of a tumour allograft.

5. Antiserum acts by preventing the destruction of the foreign tumour cells by immune host cells ('efferent inhibition').

Theoretically, possibility 2 could be excluded if it were shown that for enhancement to occur an antiserum must be administered which was specific for the antigens possessed by the tumour and absent from the host. This requirement has been demonstrated [25], using a number of different mouse tumours and hosts of several genotypes. A direct correlation was found between the proportion of foreign-tumour antigens with which the antiserum will react and the degree of enhancement produced.

With regard to possibility 1 above, two lines of the A-strain sarcoma Sa 1 have been studied [26]. One of these, B, as a result of previous enhancement, had grown progressively through 123 passages in C57B1 mice. In the first experiment C57B1 mice received a transplant from the unenhanced line, A, of Sa 1 and 1 week later were challenged with a transplant from line B. The second transplant was rejected by the second-set response, showing that there was no change in the antigenic specificity (qualitative change) of tumour line B, due to previous enhancement.

A second experiment was similar to the first except that the enhancing antiserum was injected at the time of the second tumour transplant (of line B). The outcome was an initial regression, followed by progressive tumour growth, of the first transplant (due to enhancement), whilst in some cases the second transplant was rejected and in others enhanced. This suggested a quantitative reduction in the antigenicity of tumour line B. This conclusion was supported by a third experiment, similar to the above, in which, when both tumour transplants were from line A, no enhancement of the second transplant was seen following antiserum injection given simultaneously with the latter.

Using a variety of different tumours (lymphomata and a sarcoma), in a number of different genetic tumour–host combinations, it was shown that pretreatment of the host with antiserum directed against the foreign tumour antigens consistently resulted in tumour enhancement [27]. This was also found when the tumour cells were incubated in vitro with antiserum prior to inoculation. Enhancement was not affected by washing the preincubated tumour cells in tissue culture medium, but if trypsin was added to remove the coating antibody then the degree of enhancement was diminished. These results clearly showed the part played by afferent inhibition of the immune response in the development of enhancement.

Tumour cells coated with specific antiserum showed enhanced growth in recipients preimmunized against the foreign-tumour antigens [28]. Thus efferent inhibition was established as an effector in enhancement.

V. Tumour-specific Antigens

A tumour-specific antigen may be defined as an antigen present in malignant cells, but absent from the corresponding normal cells of the host.

It will be evident that in attempting to demonstrate the presence of tumour-specific antigens, effects due to normal tissue antigens must be excluded. In order to ensure this it is necessary to study the properties of the tumour in the animal in which it arises (the autochthonous host) or on transplantation to an isogenic host. A further problem is that inbred strains of animals over the course of many generations, and transplantable tumours on repeated passage, undergo spontaneous mutations affecting their antigenic properties. Therefore any demonstration of tumour-specific immunity based on the use of much passaged tumours should be viewed with the utmost scepticism.

Within these limitations there are a number of methods which, theoretically, might reveal the presence of tumour-specific antigens. Tumour-specific immunity would be indicated if a spontaneous tumour, or a graft thereof to an isogenic host, was caused to regress or regressed spontaneously, and subsequent to this the host was found to be refractory to further challenge with the tumour. As a modification of this approach, adoptive or passive immunity might be transferred from a host with a regressed tumour to a second isogenic host.

It will be convenient in discussing tumour-specific antigenicity to divide experimental tumours into two main groups, those of known and those of unknown aetiology. The former group may be further subdivided into carcinogen- and virus-induced tumours.

A. Carcinogen-induced Tumours

The first convincing demonstration of tumour-specific antigenicity was afforded by Foley [29, 30]. He induced fibrosarcomata in 6 C3H-strain mice by treatment with methylcholanthrene. Transplants of each tumour were then destroyed by means of a ligature tied around the base, and the host was subsequently rechallenged with a transplant of the same tumour. It was found that the animals so treated were resistant to the growth of the second tumour challenge.

A further demonstration [31] of the specific antigenicity of methylcholanthrene-induced fibrosarcomata was afforded by transplantation of a spontaneous tumour to each of a group of isogenic hosts. The tumour was subsequently excised from all but 1 of the animals, and the remaining fibrosarcoma used to rechallenge the other hosts in the group. These mice were found to be immune, as indicated by the failure of the tumours to grow in some instances and by retarded growth in others.

The technique of excision and rechallenge was also used to demonstrate the specific antigenicity of dibenzanthracene-induced fibrosarcomata in further experiments [32], in which it was shown that animals resistant to rechallenge with fibrosarcomata accepted skin-grafts from the tumour donor.

The technique of host pretreatment with lethally irradiated tumour cells has been employed to demonstrate an antigenic difference between methylcholanthrene-induced sarcomata of recent origin and their isogenic hosts [33].

The demonstration of the specific antigenicity possessed by methylcholanthrene-induced sarcomata was further extended by showing this to be true of the tumour in its autochthonous host [34]. The tumour was excised from 16 mice in which it had arisen. These animals were subsequently treated with sarcoma cells, killed by irradiation *in vitro*, prior to rechallenge with increasing doses of viable tumour cells. Twelve of the 16 mice showed increased resistance to the tumour, compared with untreated isogenic controls.

It was shown [35] that immunity against carcinogen-induced sarcomata could be adoptively transferred to prospective isogenic hosts with immunologically competent cells from the primary host, in which the tumour had been caused to regress by intradermal ligation with a thread. The secondary hosts resisted tumour growth such that progressively growing tumours were not obtained.

In further experiments [36] mice were immunized by inoculation of initially small but progressively increasing quantities of methylcholanthrene-induced tumour tissue. The lymph-node and spleen cells from such animals could transfer adoptive immunity against the tumour, on intravenous injection into further isogenic hosts. However, such immunity was only seen if the transferred cells were allowed 7 days' residence in their new hosts before the latter were challenged with the tumour.

A matter of major importance is whether there is a common tumourspecific antigen for tumours induced in similar hosts by the same carcinogen. It was shown [36] that female BALB/C-strain mice, hyperimmunized to one methylcholanthrene-induced tumour, were completely susceptible to five other tumours induced by this carcinogen in further BALB/C female mice. A similar finding has been reported for methylcholanthrene-induced breast adenoacanthomas.

B. Virus-induced Tumours

In considering the specific antigens of virus-induced tumours, the distinction between virus antigens acting in this guise and specific antigens of the neoplastic cells unrelated to those of the virus must be constantly borne in mind.

It is useful to subdivide virus-induced tumours into two groups, those arising as a result of vertical transmission of the virus from parent to offspring, and other tumours (*Table XXV*).

The significance of the distinction resides in the suggestion that in Group A, as virus infection occurs during the tolerance-inducing period of embryonic or neonatal life, any specific antigenicity demonstrable in isogenic tumour host systems must depend on tumour antigens unrelated to those of the virus.

It has been suggested[37] that tolerance to the virus antigen is maintained by residence of the virus within the lymphocytes. Recently [38–40] *in vitro* methods have been described for the demonstration of Gross, G, antigen, or antibody thereto, in the blood and tissues of mice. A positive correlation has been found between the presence of G antigen, indicating tolerance thereto, and liability to develop lymphomata. Conversely G antibody was demonstrated in those mice with a low incidence of tumours.

The Gross and Moloney virus-induced leukaemias will be taken as typical of group A.

Table XXV.—A CLASSIFICATION OF VIRUS-INDUCED MOUSE TUMOURS ACCORDING TO WHETHER OR NOT THEY ARISE AS A RESULT OF VERTICAL TRANSMISSION OF THE VIRUS FROM PARENT TO OFFSPRING

Group A	Group B
Vertical transmission	
Bittner virus-induced mouse mammary carcinomata	Tumours induced by:
Mouse leukaemia due to the following viruses:	Polyoma virus
Gross	SV 40 virus
Graffi	Adenovirus 3, 7, 12, 18,
Moloney	and 21
Friend	Shope papilloma virus
Rauscher	

It is impossible either to induce resistance in AKR mice to challenge with living isogenic Gross lymphoma cells or to demonstrate cytotoxic antibodies in the sera of AKR mice, following immunization of these animals with killed AKR tumour cells [41]. However, antisera to the lymphoma cells, raised by immunization of allogeneic hosts, and sub-sequently absorbed against normal spleen and muscle cells, caused pro-longed survival of AKR leukaemic mice, after passive transfer *in vivo*, and displayed cytotoxic effects on AKR leukaemic cells *in vitro*.

Similar demonstrations of tumour-specific antigens possessed by Gross virus-induced lymphomata have been afforded [42, 43], using allogeneic tumour–host systems.

It was found possible [44] to immunize strain C3H mice against Gross lymphomata induced in this strain, following pretreatment of the pro-spective recipient mice with either allografts of other Gross lymphomata or sub-threshold doses of cells from the same isogenic lymphoma. This work suggested that the specific antigenicity of Gross lymphomata could be expressed within the mouse strain of origin, but the question of whether this was true following vertical transmission of the virus remained.

Recently, however, it has been shown [45] that in the case of lym-phomata induced by the Moloney virus there is no correlation between the amount of tumour-specific antigen carried on different lymphoma lines (as detected by sensitivity of the tumours to rejection by immunized iso-genic hosts, or *in vitro* by susceptibility to the cytotoxic action of antibody plus complement) and the amount of infective virus released from the several tumour lines. This constitutes indirect evidence that the tumour-specific and virus antigens are distinct from one another, as does a report [46] that the degree of specific antigenicity differed among five Gross virus-induced AKR lymphomata. The degree of specific antigenicity was assessed by the time taken for the tumour to kill isogenic hosts bearing the first transplant generation from the spontaneous tumour, the positive correlation between the length of this interval and the spleen and lymph-node weight in the autochthonous host, and the occurrence of spontaneous tumour regressions in some of the animals carrying transplants of the most antigenic tumour, according to the two parameters defined above.

The polyoma virus-induced tumours will be taken as illustrative of group B (*Table XXV*).

It was shown [47] that following challenge with allogeneic transplants of non-virus-releasing polyoma-induced tumours, mice became refractory to challenge with isogenic polyoma tumour transplants. The result indicated a common tumour-specific antigen for neoplasms induced by the virus in several mouse strains. It was further suggested that, as non-virus-releasing tumours were used, the specific antigen was distinct from the virus antigen. However, infection of adult animals with the polyoma virus induced immunity to subsequent challenge with isogenic polyoma tumour transplants [48, 49]. This finding has been explained by the assumption that the virus infection leads to production of specific tumour antigen by some of the infected cells, and it is this antigen which immunizes the host. This conclusion is supported by the finding that the serum of mice pretreated with non-virus-releasing polyoma tumour cells, which was shown to contain no anti-viral antibodies, none the less impaired the plating efficiency of polyoma cells when the latter were incubated *in vitro* with the serum in the presence of complement [50]. The polyoma virus will also induce tumours in rats and hamsters. However, whilst there is a common tumour-specific antigen within a given species this uniformity does not extend across species barriers.

C. Tumours of Unknown Aetiology

In general, tumours of unknown aetiology have been found to show a much less marked specific antigenicity. The increase in the spleen and lymph-node weights of A-strain mice, in which mammary carcinomata arose spontaneously, or which had received isogenic transplants from such tumours of recent origin, was adduced as evidence for the specific antigenicity of these tumours [51]. The Bittner virus was probably not implicated in the aetiology of these tumours, as the incidence was only 10 per cent and did not rise over an observation period of 3 years. Subsequently specific antigenicity was found for 1 of 5 spontaneous mammary carcinomata, as judged by the ability of spleen cells from the autochthonous host to transfer adoptive immunity against the tumour in question to further isogenic hosts [52]. Also, in mice given an intravenous injection of a killed preparation of *Corynebacterium parvum*, a procedure which causes intense stimulation of the lymphoreticular tissue, the appearance of a palpable tumour was delayed following inoculation of viable cells from a mammary carcinoma which arose spontaneously in an isogenic host [53]. This effect was observed whether the *C. parvum* was administered 2 days before or 8–12 days after tumour transplantation and is good evidence for the specific antigenicity of the tumour.

The lesser degree of specific antigenicity shown by spontaneous tumours, as opposed to those arising from the action of carcinogens, was emphasized by attempts [54] to induce immunity to transplants of several different tumours by pretreatment of isogenic hosts with tumour cells irradiated *in vitro*.

VI. IMMUNOLOGICAL ASPECTS OF CARCINOGENESIS AND THE GROWTH OF ESTABLISHED TUMOURS

In the preceding section the evidence for the possession of specific antigens by tumours was reviewed. The important practical questions raised by the existence of such antigens are: How is it possible for an antigenic tumour to arise in spite of the host's immunological surveillance, and, further, if such a tumour does occur by what means is it able to grow until it kills the host?

Woodruff (personal communication) has suggested that many tumours may arise and be destroyed by the host before they are ever recognized clinically. Alas, however, this is by no means invariably true.

In the case of tumours caused by chemical carcinogens there is good evidence that a state of host immunosuppression exists during the latent period of tumour induction. Stjernsward [55] found that following a single exposure of mice to 3-methylcholanthrene, there was a prolonged depression of immunological responsiveness as judged by the host's reaction against weakly antigenic allografts. Subsequently [56] a similar action was demonstrated for two other carcinogens, a property not shared by non-carcinogenic hydrocarbons. The assay system in these experiments [56] was the ability of host cells presensitized to sheep red blood-cells to form lytic plaques when transferred to agar plates in which were incorporated sheep erythrocytes. Also using this assay, it was shown [57] that the carcinogen-induced immunosuppression was real, rather than being due to a mere delay in the immune response, and furthermore that an early stage in the response of mouse cells to the sheep erythrocytes was specifically sensitive. This stage was suggested as the processing of antigen by macrophages, with the result that virgin antigen came into direct contact with host lymphocytes and thereby induced partial tolerance. By analogy, the methylcholanthrene-treated host would also show tolerance to the specific antigens of its induced tumour. This was, in fact, demonstrated [58]. Sarcomata were induced in the hind-limbs of mice by injection of methylcholanthrene. The tumour was subsequently excised by amputation of the limb, and the autochthonous host was re-challenged with graded doses of its own tumour cells. It was found that a tumour grew better in its own host than in sham-amputated, non-tumour-bearing isogenic controls. Also a given tumour-bearing host, following tumour excision, supported the growth of its own tumour on rechallenge better than that of a different methylcholanthrene-induced sarcoma arising in a second isogenic host.

The phenomenon of host immunosuppression during the latent period of carcinogenesis is not limited to tumours induced by chemical carcinogens. It was shown [59] that the Gross virus depressed the immune response in mice to T2 phage or sheep erythrocytes, and similar findings have been reported by others.

In isogenic hosts a low-dose tumour transplant of a chemically induced tumour took better than a slightly higher dose of tumour cells [60]. It was suggested that the higher dose of cells evoked an effective immune response to the tumour-specific antigens carried and this led to rejection of the tumour transplant, whereas the host response was suboptimal to lower doses of tumour cells. These findings seem relevant to the induction of antigenic tumours. The small number of tumour cells initially present, coupled with the carcinogen-induced immunosuppression in the host, may allow the tumour to survive and become established [see also 61].

It has been shown [60, 62] that the shorter the latent period of tumour induction, the more antigenic are the tumour cells that arise.

There are three possible mechanisms whereby an established tumour may progress until it kills its host, in spite of any immune response by the latter:—

1. The tumour may induce 'self-enhancement'.

2. The tumour may induce a state of non-reactivity in the host, which can be either specific for the tumour antigens or a general reduction in immunological responsiveness.

3. The tumour may delete its specific antigens on progressive growth, thus removing the *point d'appui* of the host's immune response.

The work [58] cited above affords strong evidence for a tumour antigen-specific component in the host immunosuppression associated with a progressively growing tumour. This concept is supported by the finding [63] that in an isogenic tumour–host system there was a positive correlation between the dose of methylcholanthrene-induced tumour cells administered and decrease in resistance to the tumour. Also, when a benzpyrene-induced rat sarcoma was partially removed, the animal was more susceptible to a second transplant of its own tumour cells than a non-tumour bearing control [64].

A number of studies have demonstrated a depression of the host's immune response to third-party antigens, associated with progressive tumour growth. For example, a prolonged survival of skin-allografts was found in mice with spontaneous mammary carcinomata [65].

The complementary mechanism of tumour-specific antigen deletion as a means of progressive tumour growth has been proposed [66]. When spontaneously occurring mouse mammary carcinomata were transplanted serially in isogenic hosts, the tumour progressively lost its capacity to evoke an immunological response as judged by host spleen and lymph-node weight. It was suggested that during serial passage the tumour-specific antigens had been deleted, so that an immunological response of the host thereto was no longer evoked. Subsequently it was shown [67] that this phenomenon was associated with a decrease in the time taken by the tumour to kill its host in successive transplant generations. Furthermore, in animals dying from tumour growth there was gross atrophy of the lymphoid tissues. This is additional evidence for the theory of host immunosuppression, discussed above.

Two mechanisms seem possible to account for antigen deletion. They are illustrated in *Fig. 62*.

Evidence in favour of hypothesis B (*Fig. 62*) has been provided by the following experiment [68]. Two spontaneous A-strain mouse mammary carcinomata were each maintained in two groups of isogenic hosts by serial transplantation. The first group of mice was untreated; the second received 15 mg. per kg. body-weight of L-phenylalanine mustard, as an immunosuppressant, 1 day before tumour transplantation. At each passage a portion of tumour from each group of hosts was transplanted to further normal mice, the tumour growth-rates and ability to produce evidence of immunological stimulation being compared after 14 days.

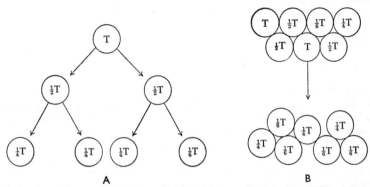

Fig. 62.—Possible mechanisms for the deletion of tumour-specific antigens. A, The antigens may be progressively diluted out by division of the tumour cells. B, The tumour may initially consist of a mosaic of cells with varying degrees of specific antigenicity. The most antigenic cells are eliminated by the immune response of the host, leaving the others free to proliferate.

Successive passages of the tumour, obtained from the immunosuppressed hosts, grew more slowly on transplantation into normal hosts, and this finding was correlated with a more persistent immunological response by the latter. Thus it would seem that a tumour protected from the immunological attack of the host may retain its specific antigens longer.

The findings cited on p. 359 [34] tell against the idea of 'self-enhancement' as a means of tumour progression, otherwise it would be difficult to account for the increased resistance to an autochthonous tumour, conferred by treatment of the host with irradiated tumour cells.

The second mechanism of specific antigen deletion postulated above [*see* 68] would account for the greater malignancy of tumours in young patients compared with old, for immunological competence declines with age.

VII. Immunotherapy for Experimental Neoplasms

In general, attempts to treat neoplasms by immunological means may be divided into two groups: those which aim at increasing the host's resistance to the tumour, and those wherein an extrinsic immunological attack is mounted against the tumour.

Theoretically increasing the host's immunological response might be most effective for relatively early neoplasms with specific antigens, whilst extrinsic attack is especially applicable in the treatment of more advanced tumours.

It was found [69] that stimulation of the reticulo-endothelial system (R.E.S.) by administration of BCG vaccine caused regression of some allogeneic tumours, and retarded the growth-rate of certain isogenic tumours in inbred mice. Similar observations were subsequently reported [53] using *C. parvum* as a R.E.S. stimulant (*see* p. 361). As a variant of this approach it was shown that the radiosensitivity of 3,4-benzpyrene-induced sarcomata in rats could be increased by implantation of an irradiated biopsy of the tumour to be treated, 2–4 hours before administration of local irradiation to the main tumour [70]. Only a proportion of the tumours so treated were, however, favourably affected, and the efficacy of the method was not increased by treatment of the tumour-bearing rats with BCG 1 week beforehand. It is possible that host immunosuppression associated with the presence of a tumour (*see preceding section*) may mitigate the effectiveness of this type of therapy.

It will be clear that all the above methods depend on the presence of tumour-specific antigens against which an immunological reaction of the autochthonous or isogenic host can be stimulated. Such a situation is unlikely to exist in animals with more advanced tumours, for the twin reasons of tumour antigen deletion and host immunosuppression. Therefore the suggestion was made [71] that it might be possible to transfer adoptive immunity, directed against established tumours, using transplants of allogeneic immunologically competent cells. For this purpose spleen and lymph-node cells from either normal hosts or animals which had been immunized against the tumours to be treated were used. It was found that the growth of subcutaneous mouse mammary carcinoma transplants in isogenic hosts could be retarded by the administration of sublethal whole-body irradiation followed by intravenous injection of immunologically competent cells. The whole-body irradiation, which was given to suppress, for a time, the host's reaction against the allogenic cells, exerted no restraining influence on the tumour when given in isolation.

A major limitation to this form of therapy is the concomitant induction of graft-versus-host disease in the tumour-bearing animals treated. Various methods have been explored to overcome this difficulty.

Woodruff, Symes, and Boak (unpublished) repeated the experiments cited above [71] with the difference that allogeneic immunologically competent cells, from donors preimmunized against the tumour, were injected intraperitoneally in the treatment of intraperitoneal tumour transplants. The result of this immediate intimate contact between the donor cells and the tumour was a significant prolongation of host survival with minimal graft-versus-host disease.

Further experiments [72] investigated the effect of treating subcutaneous mouse mammary carcinoma transplants in isogenic hosts by subcutaneous injection of L-phenylalanine mustard (given as an immunosuppressant in place of whole-body irradiation), and intravenous injection of allogeneic immunologically competent cells from donors previously immunized against the tumour. It was found that splenectomy immediately before the start of treatment focused the action of the donor cells on the tumour, and that under these conditions the larger the tumour treated the greater the therapeutic effect in terms of host survival.

That an immunological reaction by the lymphoid cells was responsible for the anti-tumour effect is shown by the following evidence:—

15

1. The effect of immunologically competent cells from donors previously immunized against the tumour was greater than that of non-immunized cells.

2. In experiments where tumour transplants of a parent line strain, growing in F_1 hybrid hosts, were treated by injection of immunized spleen cells from donors of the opposite parent line, thus eliminating the necessity for giving whole-body irradiation, a significant anti-tumour effect was obtained [73].

Evidence that the small lymphocyte was the cell responsible for the anti-tumour effect was afforded in further experiments [74, 75]. An attempt was made to treat intraperitoneal transplants of the Landschutz ascites tumour (of mouse origin) by intraperitoneal injection of equivalent numbers of either spleen cells or thoracic duct lymphocytes from rats preimmunized against the tumour. The therapeutic superiority of the duct lymphocytes was clearly shown; indeed, some of the animals treated thereby remained free from tumour. Undue optimism should not, however, arise from this result, as the Landschutz tumour, although growing progressively in 100 per cent of the mice used, is, in fact, an allograft therein. It follows that there is a greater antigenic difference between tumour and host than occurs in isogenic tumour–host systems, and therefore a greater potential for specific immunization of the rat lymphoid cells against the tumour.

Recently a powerful anti-tumour effect has been obtained by treating primary carcinogen-induced rat sarcomata with RNA obtained from the cells in the efferent lymph from sheep lymph-nodes preimmunized by transplantation of a biopsy from the sarcoma [76]. Confirmation of this result will be awaited with interest. A similar claim has been made in the field of delayed hypersensitivity.

At a clinical level 9 patients were treated by administration of a small dose of a radiomimetic drug and subsequent intravenous infusion of non-immunized allogeneic spleen cells [77]. Some regression of the tumours occurred with this form of treatment. A similar finding was reported in a further study [78]. However, the results were not felt sufficiently encouraging to continue the trial of this therapy. Mesenteric lymph-node cells from a pig, preimmunized against the tumour to be treated, were therefore substituted for allogeneic spleen cells [78]. In 3 patients treated thus, massive tumour necrosis occurred, and the method may hold promise for the future.

REFERENCES

1. LITTLE, C. C. (1947), 'The Genetics of Cancer in Mice', *Biol. Rev.*, **22**, 315.
2. LITTLE, C. C. (1941), 'The Genetics of Tumour Transplantation', in *Biology of the Laboratory Mouse* (ed. SNELL, G. D.), p. 279. Philadelphia: Blakiston.
3. SNELL, G. D. (1958), in *Physiopathology of Cancer* (ed. HOMBURGER, F.), pp. 302–308. London: Cassell.
4. MACDOWELL, E. C., and RICHTER, N. M. (1930), 'Studies on Mouse Leukaemia. II, Hereditary Susceptibility to Inoculated Leukaemia', *J. Cancer Res.*, **14**, 434.
5. MACDOWELL, E. C., and RICHTER, N. M. (1932), 'Studies on Mouse Leukaemia. V, A Genetic Analysis of Susceptibility in Inoculated Leukaemia of Line I', *Biol. Zbl.*, **52**, 266.
6. FURTH, J., BOON, M. C., and KALISS, N. (1944), 'On Genetic Character of Neoplastic Cells as determined in Transplantation Experiments, with Notes on the Somatic Mutation Theory', *Cancer Res.*, **4**, 1.

7. GORER, P. A. (1937), 'The Genetic and Antigenic Basis of Tumour Transplantation', *J. Path. Bact.*, **44**, 691.

8. BITTNER, J. J. (1933), 'Genetic Studies on Transplantation of Tumours. VII, Comparative Study of Tumours 19308 A, B, and C', *Am. J. Cancer*, **17**, 724.

9. CLOUDMAN, A. M. (1932), 'A Comparative Study of Transplantability of Eight Mammary Gland Tumours arising in Inbred Mice', *Am. J. Cancer*, **16**, 568.

10. WOGLOM, W. H. (1929), 'Immunity to Transplantable Tumours', *Cancer Rev.*, **4**, 129.

11. LEWIS, M. R. (1940), 'Immunity in Relation to 1256, Dibenzanthracene Induced Sarcomata', *Johns Hopkins Hosp. Bull.* **67**, 325.

12. REVEZ, L. (1955), 'Effect of X Irradiation on the Growth of the Ehrlich Ascites Tumour', *J. natn. Cancer Inst.*, **15**, 1691.

13. ALGIRE, G. H., WEAVER, J. M., and PREHN, R. T. (1954), 'Growth of Cells *in vivo* in Diffusion Chambers. I, Survival of Homografts in Immunized Mice', *J. natn. Cancer Inst.*, **15**, 493.

14. PREHN, R. T., WEAVER, J. M., and ALGIRE, G. H. (1954), 'The Diffusion Chamber Technique applied to a Study of the Nature of Homograft Resistance', *J. natn. Cancer Inst.*, **15**, 509.

15. WEAVER, J. M., ALGIRE, G. H., and PREHN, R. T. (1955), 'The Growth of Cells *in vivo* in Diffusion Chambers. II, The Role of Cells in the Destruction of Homografts in Mice', *J. natn. Cancer Inst.*, **15**, 1737.

16. GORER, P. A. (1956), 'Some Recent Work on Tumour Immunity', in *Advances in Cancer Research* (ed. GREENSTEIN, J. P., and HADDOW, A.), vol. 4, p. 169. New York: Academic.

17. GORER, P. A., and AMOS, D. B. (1956), 'Passive Immunity in Mice against C57B1 Leukosis EL 4 by Means of Iso-immune Serum', *Cancer Res.*, **16**, 338.

18. MITCHISON, N. A. (1954), 'Passive Transfer of Transplantation Immunity', *Proc. R. Soc.*, Series B, **142**, 72.

19. MITCHISON, N. A. (1955), 'Studies on the Immunological Response to Foreign Tumour Transplants in the Mouse. I, The Role of Lymph Node Cells in conferring Immunity by Adoptive Transfer', *J. exp. Med.*, **102**, 157.

20. MITCHISON, N. A., and DUBE, O. L. (1955), 'Studies on the Immunological Response to Foreign Tumour Transplants in the Mouse. II, The Relation between Haemagglutinating Antibody and Graft Resistance in the Normal Mouse and Mice Pretreated with Tissue Preparation', *J. exp. Med.*, **102**, 179.

21. KALISS, N., and MOLOMUT, N. (1952), 'The Effect of Prior Injections of Tissue Antiserums on the Survival of Cancer Homografts in Mice', *Cancer Res.*, **12**, 110.

22. KALISS, N., MOLOMUT, N., HARRIS, J. L., and GAULT, S. D. (1953), 'Effect of Previously Injected Immune Serum and Tissue on the Survival of Tumour Grafts in Mice', *J. natn. Cancer Inst.*, **13**, 847.

23. SNELL, G. D. (1954), 'The Enhancing Effect (or Actively Acquired Tolerance) and the Histocompatibility-2 Locus in the Mouse', *J. natn. Cancer Inst.*, **15**, 665.

24. KALISS, N. (1958), 'Immunological Enhancement of Tumour Homografts in Mice. A Review', *Cancer Res.*, **18**, 992.

25. MOLLER, G. (1963), 'Studies on the Mechanism of Immunological Enhancement of Tumour Homografts. I, Specificity of Immunological Enhancement', *J. natn. Cancer Inst.*, **30**, 1153.

26. KALISS, N. (1962), 'The Elements of Immunological Enhancement: A Consideration of Mechanisms', *Ann. N.Y. Acad. Sci.*, **101**, 64.

27. MOLLER, G. (1963), 'Studies on the Mechanisms of Immunological Enhancement of Tumour Homografts. II, Effect of Isoantibodies on Various Tumour Cells', *J. natn. Cancer Inst.*, **30**, 1177.

28. MOLLER, G. (1963), 'Studies on the Mechanism of Immunological Enhancement of Tumour Homografts. III, Interaction between Humoral Isoantibodies and Immune Lymphoid Cells', *J. natn. Cancer Inst.*, **30**, 1205.

29. FOLEY, E. J. (1953), 'Attempts to induce Immunity against Mammary Adenocarcinoma in Inbred Mice', *Cancer Res.*, **13**, 578.

30. FOLEY, E. J. (1953), 'Antigenic Properties of Methylcholanthrene Induced Tumours in Mice of the Strain of Origin', *Cancer Res.*, **13**, 835.

31. PREHN, R. T., and MAIN, J. M. (1957), 'Immunity to Methylcholanthrene Induced Sarcomas', *J. natn. Cancer Inst.*, **18**, 769.

32. PREHN, R. T. (1960), 'Tumour-specific Immunity to Transplanted Dibenzanthracene induced Sarcomas', *Cancer Res.*, **20**, 1614.

33. REVEZ, L. (1960), 'Detection of Antigenic Differences in Isologous Host-tumour Systems by Pretreatment with Heavily Irradiated Tumour Cells', *Cancer Res.*, 20, 443.
34. KLEIN, G., SJOGREN, H. O., KLEIN, E., and HELLSTROM, K. E. (1960), 'Demonstration of Resistance against Methylcholanthrene Induced Sarcomas in the Primary Autochthonous Host', *Cancer Res.*, 20, 1561.
35. KOLDOVSKÝ, P. (1961), 'Passive Transfer of Anti-tumour Isoimmunity', *Folia biol., Praha*, 7, 157.
36. OLD, L. J., BOYSE, E. A., CLARKE, D. A., and CARSWELL, E. A. (1962), 'Antigenic Properties of Chemically Induced Tumours', *Ann. N.Y. Acad. Sci.*, 101, 80.
37. ALLISON, A. C. (1967), 'Cell Mediated Immune Responses to Virus Infections and Virus Induced Tumours', *Br. med. Bull.*, 23, 60.
38. AOKI, T., BOYSE, E. A., and OLD, L. J. (1968), 'Wild Type Gross Leukaemia Virus. I, Soluble Antigen (GSA) in the Plasma and Tissues of Infected Mice', *J. natn. Cancer Inst.*, 41, 89.
39. AOKI, T., BOYSE, E. A., and OLD, L. J. (1968), 'Wild Type Gross Leukaemia Virus. II, Influence of Immunological Factors on Natural Transmission and on the Consequences of Infection', *J. natn. Cancer Inst.*, 41, 97.
40. AOKI, T., BOYSE, E. A., and OLD, L. J. (1968), 'Wild Type Gross Leukaemia Virus. III, Serological Tests as Indications of Leukaemia Risk', *J. natn. Cancer Inst.*, 41, 103.
41. BUBENÍK, J., ADAMCOVA, B., and KOLDOVSKÝ, P. (1964), 'A Contribution to the Question of the Antigenicity of Spontaneous Lymphoid AKR Leukaemia', *Folia biol., Praha*, 10, 293.
42. OLD, L. J., BOYSE, E. A., and STOCKERT, E. (1965), 'The G (Gross) Leukaemia Antigen', *Cancer Res.*, 25, 813.
43. WAHREN, B. (1966), 'Demonstration of Tumour Specific Antigen in Spontaneously Developing AKR Lymphomas', *Int. J. Cancer*, 1, 41.
44. KLEIN, G., SJOGREN, H. O., and KLEIN, E. (1962), 'Demonstration of Host Resistance against Isotransplantation of Lymphomas induced by the Gross Agent', *Cancer Res.*, 22, 955.
45. KLEIN, G., KLEIN, E., and HAUGHTON, G. (1966), 'Variation of Antigenic Characteristics between Different Mouse Lymphomas induced by the Moloney Virus', *J. natn. Cancer Inst.*, 36, 607.
46. DENTON, P. M., and SYMES, M. O. (1968), 'Observations on the Changing Behaviour of AKR Mouse Lymphomas serially transplanted in the Strain of Origin', *Immunology*, 15, 371.
47. SJOGREN, H. O. (1961), 'Further Studies on the Induced Resistance against Isotransplantation of Polyoma Tumours', *Virology*, 15, 214.
48. HABEL, K. (1961), 'Resistance of Polyoma Virus Immune Animals to Transplanted Polyoma Tumours', *Proc. Soc. exp. Biol. Med.*, 106, 722.
49. SJOGREN, H. O., HELLSTROM, I., and KLEIN, G. (1961), 'Resistance of Polyoma Virus Immunized Mice to Transplantation of Established Polyoma Tumours', *Expl Cell Res.*, 23, 204.
50. HELLSTROM, I. (1965), 'Distinction between the Effects of Antiviral and Anticellular Polyoma Antibodies on Polyoma Tumour Cells', *Nature, Lond.*, 208, 652.
51. WOODRUFF, M. F. A., and SYMES, M. O. (1962), 'The Significance of Splenomegaly in Tumour Bearing Mice', *Br. J. Cancer*, 16, 120.
52. SYMES, M. O. (1966), 'Further Observations on the Growth of Mouse Mammary Carcinomata in the Strain of Origin. Attempts to transfer Adoptive Immunity against the Tumour, to Isogenic Hosts, with Spleen Cells from Tumour Bearing Mice', *Br. J. Cancer*, 20, 356.
53. WOODRUFF, M. F. A., and BOAK, J. L. (1966), 'Inhibitory Effect of Injection of Corynebacterium parvum on the Growth of Tumour Transplants in Isogenic Hosts', *Br. J. Cancer*, 20, 345.
54. REVEZ, L. (1960), 'Detection of Antigenic Differences in Isologous Host–tumour Systems by Pretreatment with Heavily Irradiated Tumour Cells', *Cancer Res.*, 20, 443.
55. STJERNSWARD, J. (1965), 'Immunodepressive Effect of 3-Methylcholanthrene. Antibody Formation at the Cellular Level and Reaction against Weak Antigenic Homografts', *J. natn. Cancer Inst.*, 35, 885.
56. STJERNSWARD, J. (1966), 'Effect of Non-carcinogenic and Carcinogenic Hydrocarbons on Antibody Forming Cells measured at the Cellular Level *in vivo*', *J. natn. Cancer Inst.*, 36, 1189.

57. STJERNSWARD, J. (1967), 'Further Immunological Studies on Chemical Carcinogenesis', *J. natn. Cancer Inst.*, **38**, 515.
58. STJERNSWARD, J. (1968), 'Immune Status of the Primary Host toward its own Methylcholanthrene Induced Sarcomas, *J. natn. Cancer Inst.*, **40**, 13.
59. PETERSON, R. D., HENDRICKSON, R., and GOOD, R. A. (1963), 'Reduced Antibody Forming Capacity during the Incubation Period of Passage A Leukaemia in C_3H Mice', *Proc. Soc. exp. Biol. Med.*, **114**, 517.
60. OLD, L. J., BOYSE, E. A., CLARKE, D. A., and CARSWELL, E. A. (1962), 'Antigenic Properties of Chemically Induced Tumours', *Ann. N.Y. Acad. Sci.*, **101**, 80.
61. OLD, L. J., and BOYSE, E. A. (1964), 'Immunology of Experimental Tumours', *Ann. Rev. Med.*, **15**, 167.
62. PREHN, R. T. (1963), 'The Role of Immune Mechanisms in the Biology of Chemically and Physically Induced Tumours', in *Conceptual Advances in Immunology and Oncology*, Sixteenth Annual Symposium on Fundamental Cancer Research, p. 475. New York: Hoeber.
63. BUBENÍK, J., KRYSTOFOVÁ, H., and KOLDOVSKÝ, P. (1965), 'Quantitative Aspects of Resistance and Tolerance to Methylcholanthrene Induced Tumours', *Folia biol.*, *Praha*, **11**, 415.
64. MIKULSKA, Z. B., SMITH, C., and ALEXANDER, P. (1966), 'Evidence for an Immunological Reaction of the Host directed against its own Actively Growing Primary Tumour', *J. natn. Cancer Inst.*, **36**, 29.
65. LINDER, O. E. A. (1962), 'Survival of Skin Homografts in Methylcholanthrene-treated Mice and in Mice with Spontaneous Mammary Cancers', *Cancer Res.*, **22**, 380.
66. WOODRUFF, M. F. A., and SYMES, M. O. (1962), 'Evidence of Loss of Tumour-specific Antigen on repeatedly transplanting a Tumour in the Strain of Origin', *Br. J. Cancer*, **16**, 484.
67. SYMES, M. O. (1965), 'Further Observations on the Growth of Mouse Mammary Carcinomata in the Strain of Origin. The Relation between the Degree of Tumour Specific Antigenicity and Malignancy', *Br. J. Cancer*, **19**, 189.
68. SYMES, M. O. (1965), 'Further Observations on the Growth of Mouse Mammary Carcinomata in the Strain of Origin. The Influence of the Host's Immunological Resistance on the Deletion of Tumour Specific Antigens', *Br. J. Cancer*, **19**, 181.
69. OLD, L. J., BENACERAFF, B., CLARKE, D. A., CARSWELL, E. A., and STOCKERT, E. (1961), 'The Role of the Reticuloendothelial System in the Host Reaction to Neoplasia', *Cancer Res.*, **21**, 1281.
70. HADDOW, A., and ALEXANDER, P. (1964), 'An Immunological Method of Increasing the Sensitivity of Primary Sarcomas to Local Irradiation with X-rays', *Lancet*, **1**, 452.
71. WOODRUFF, M. F. A., and SYMES, M. O. (1962), 'The Use of Immunologically Competent Cells in the Treatment of Cancer. Experiments with a Transplantable Mouse Tumour', *Br. J. Cancer*, **16**, 707.
72. SYMES, M. O. (1967), 'The Use of Immunologically Competent Cells in Treatment of Cancer: Further Experiments with a Transplantable Mouse Tumour', *Br. J. Cancer*, **21**, 178.
73. WOODRUFF, M. F. A., and BOAK, J. L. (1965), 'Inhibitory Effect of Pre-immunized CBA Spleen Cells on Transplants of A-strain Mouse Mammary Carcinoma in $(CBA \times A)F_1$ Hybrid Recipients', *Br. J. Cancer*, **19**, 411.
74. WOODRUFF, M. F. A., SYMES, M. O., and STUART, A. E. (1963), 'The Effect of Rat Spleen Cells on Two Transplanted Mouse Tumours', *Br. J. Cancer*, **17**, 320.
75. WOODRUFF, M. F. A., SYMES, M. O., and ANDERSON, N. F. (1963), 'The Effect of Intraperitoneal Injection of Thoracic Duct Lymphocytes from Normal and Immunized Rats in Mice inoculated with the Landschutz Ascites Tumour', *Br. J. Cancer*, **17**, 482.
76. HALL, J. G., ALEXANDER, P., DELORME, E. J., and HAMILTON, L. D. G. (1968), 'The Effect of Nucleic Acids extracted from Lymph Nodes of Specifically Immunized Sheep on the Growth of Rat Sarcomata', in *Advances in Transplantation* (ed. DAUSSET, J., HAMBURGER, J., and MATHE, G.), p. 545. Copenhagen: Munksgaard.
77. WOODRUFF, M. F. A., and NOLAN, B. (1963), 'Preliminary Observations on Treatment of Advanced Cancer by Injection of Allogeneic Spleen Cells', *Lancet*, **2**, 426.
78. SYMES, M. O., RIDDELL, A. G., IMMELMAN, E. J., and TERBLANCHE, J. (1968), 'Immunologically Competent Cells in the Treatment of Malignant Disease', *Lancet*, **1**, 1054.

CHAPTER 12

AUTO-IMMUNITY

By W. J. Harrison

I. INTRODUCTION

DURING its early years immunology was devoted largely to studying the response to bacterial infection and it therefore appeared that the immune response had evolved because of its protective value against bacteria and their toxins. It was Ehrlich who, at the turn of the century, introduced the concept of auto-immunity. He showed that goats would produce antibodies against the red cells of other goats, but not against their own, and regarded this as illustrating a fundamental law of nature embodied in the term 'horror autotoxicus' [1]. He did not, however, regard this law as inviolable and clearly realized the possibility that some diseases might be due to breakdown of the mechanisms which, in health, prevent auto-immune reactions: 'In the explanation of many disease phenomena it will in the future be necessary to consider the possible failure of the internal regulations.'

The possibility that auto-immunity might be a pathogenetic mechanism in disease has stimulated much of the interest in the subject. During the decade which followed Ehrlich's observations autohaemolysins and autohaemagglutinins were described in haemolytic anaemia, but the subject was then largely forgotten until 1938 when auto-immune haemolytic anaemia was rediscovered [2]. Globulin was demonstrated on the red-cell surface in this condition by the Coombs test in 1946 [3] and during the ensuing 10 years major advances were made in other fields: Freund's complete adjuvant was used to facilitate the production of various experimental auto-immune diseases, and antibodies against gamma-globulin were described in rheumatoid arthritis, against cell nuclei in systemic lupus erythematosus, and against thyroglobulin in Hashimoto's thyroiditis.

The main purpose of this chapter is twofold. First, to consider how these and other auto-immune phenomena arise and, secondly, to consider their significance in the pathogenesis of disease.

II. CAUSES OF AUTO-IMMUNIZATION

Theoretically there are two main ways in which auto-immunization might arise. It might be due to antigenic stimuli able to overcome tolerance to body components. Alternatively, there might be an abnormality of the immunological apparatus resulting in loss of tolerance.

A. Auto-immunization following Antigenic Stimulation

1. TOLERANCE TO BODY CONSTITUENTS

Whether or not an antigenic stimulus elicits auto-immunization will depend on the degree of tolerance which already exists towards the corresponding determinant groups no less than on the nature of the stimulus itself. Since much of our knowledge of tolerance and its termination is derived from the study of acquired tolerance to foreign antigens, it is pertinent to ask whether this serves as a valid model of natural tolerance to autologous antigens. Boyden and Sorkin [4] found that, in rabbits made tolerant to human serum albumin (HSA) at birth, the subsequent injection of sulphanilazo-HSA did not lead to the production of antibodies against the hapten (or the protein), whereas following the injection of the sulphanil conjugate of rabbit serum albumin (RSA) the expected antibodies to sulphanilic acid were produced. This suggested that, contrary to what had been generally assumed, there was a basic difference between natural tolerance to RSA and acquired tolerance to HSA. However, this far-reaching conclusion was not substantiated by later work in which rabbits were made tolerant to HSA in adult life by repeated injections after whole-body irradiation. Both the foreign and the homologous proteins acted as effective carriers of the hapten in inducing anti-hapten antibodies [5].

The principal factors affecting the induction and maintenance of tolerance have been discussed in Chapter 4 and will now be considered in relation to autologous antigens.

a. Antigen Dosage

It has been clearly established that for foreign antigens the dosage is crucial in determining whether there is immunization or tolerance. It is interesting to speculate as to whether tolerance to plasma albumin, which is present in high concentration, represents Mitchison's 'high-dose paralysis' and whether tolerance to insulin or thyroglobulin, which are present in much lower concentrations, represents 'low-dose paralysis'. However, in attempting such comparisons, there are considerable problems, such as the fluctuating levels of the foreign proteins due to intermittent injection in these model experiments and the fact that the endogenous substances are present at much higher concentrations near their sites of synthesis than in the circulation [6].

b. Seclusion of Antigen

As with the soluble, circulating antigens considered above, so with cellular components; tolerance is presumably determined partly by the amount reaching the lymphoid tissues. In the latter case, however, actual measurements are not feasible. Some of these antigens, such as surface components of circulating cells, would be expected to have ready access to the lymphoid tissues and to establish full tolerance. At the other end of the scale antigens with no such access ('secluded' or 'hidden' antigens) would fail to establish tolerance. Possible examples are found in the eye and in a few other sites. In between these two extremes there are many body constituents to which there is some degree of tolerance. Intracellular antigens are secluded to some extent, but they presumably reach the immunological apparatus after cell death provided they are not degraded too rapidly by lysosomal or other enzymes.

c. Persistence of Antigen

This is really an aspect of dosage and is necessary for the maintenance of acquired tolerance. Loss of tolerance to the pituitary has been reported in frogs hypophysectomized in foetal life [7]. It would be interesting to study the response to thyroid antigens following total thyroidectomy.

d. Physical State of Antigen

Soluble extrinsic antigens will readily induce tolerance, especially when freed of aggregated molecules by centrifugation, but it is very difficult to induce tolerance to particulate antigens. This, rather than seclusion within cells, may explain why tolerance does not seem to develop to some particulate tissue antigens. Thus antibodies directed mainly against mitochondria occur naturally in rats and tolerance to mitochondria with respect to IgM antibody has not been induced despite intensive courses of injections in newborn animals [8].

e. Chemical Structure of Antigen

The influence of chemical structure, molecular rigidity, and related factors in determining antigenicity and tolerance induction have been discussed in Chapter 2.

f. Age

The relationship between antigen dosage, on the one hand, and immunization and tolerance, on the other, is very different in foetal life from that in the adult. In general, tolerance is most easily induced in the foetus and it is at this stage that most auto-antigens first make contact with the immunological apparatus.

2. THE NATURE OF THE ANTIGENIC STIMULUS

The stimulus necessary to cause auto-immunization will depend on the degree of tolerance (if any) to be overcome. If, because of complete seclusion, tolerance is totally lacking, the release of an adequate quantity of native (unaltered) antigen will be sufficient. Where partial tolerance exists this might be lost if an alteration in the rate of release of antigen produced a change from a tolerance-inducing to an immunizing level. Experimentally, however, immunization with the native antigen is often ineffective, but success may then be achieved with a cross-reacting antigen. Breakdown of tolerance may also be facilitated by the use of adjuvants, but whether the adjuvant effect of bacterial products plays any part in the production of spontaneous auto-immune disease is unknown.

a. The Release of Secluded Antigens

The eye has been mentioned as a possible site of secluded antigens. Penetrating injuries to one eye are sometimes followed several weeks later by uveitis in the other eye. It has been postulated that this is due to an immunological reaction stimulated by uveal antigen liberated by the injury since delayed hypersensitivity to uveal tissue has been demonstrated [9]. Another form of sterile inflammation in the eye, believed to be due to an immunological reaction to escaped lens protein, occasionally follows surgery for cataract. The auto-antigenicity of the lens has been demonstrated experimentally and supports the concept that it is a secluded structure. However, leakage of lens antigens must occur frequently since antibodies to lens have been found in 50 per cent of human sera [10].

The first example of auto-immunization was described in 1900 by Metalnikoff, who showed that guinea-pigs immunized with their own sperm produced sperm-immobilizing antibodies [11]. In man antibodies to spermatozoa may occur as a result of damage to the genital tract with the release of sperm into the tissues [12]. These observations suggest that spermatozoa may not induce tolerance because they are secluded behind the basement membrane of the genital tract, but, as in the case of the lens, seclusion is apparently not complete because antibodies occur normally in various animal species. A more important factor than seclusion may be the late development of antigen. Spermatozoa contain an antigen which is not found in immature germinal cells and is therefore absent in foetal and neonatal life when tolerance to most body constituents is being acquired [13].

When Roitt and his colleagues [14] first detected antibodies to thyroglobulin in Hashimoto's thyroiditis they were believed to result from their release from seclusion within the thyroid follicles. However, it has since been found that thyroglobulin is normally present in lymph draining from the gland and, in small amounts, in the blood of many healthy human adults without eliciting antibodies [15]. There is further evidence that tolerance is at least partially developed and that antibody formation does not result simply from the release of native thyroglobulin from the thyroid: first, unless Freund's complete adjuvant is added, animals usually cannot be immunized with homologous* thyroglobulin prepared in such a way as to avoid denaturation [16]; secondly, there is no antibody response to experimental thyroid injury; and, lastly, thyroid damage in man by irradiation [17] or surgery or in the course of viral thyroiditis does not provoke thyroglobulin antibodies in patients with previously negative tests.

It is probable that very few antigens are completely secluded in the sense in which the word is used in the preceding paragraphs, but there is evidence that some antigenic determinants are concealed within macromolecules or by some adjacent molecular arrangement and do not establish tolerance. Examples of such seclusion at the molecular level will be found in a later section.

b. Cross-reacting Antigens

Acquired tolerance to bovine serum albumin (BSA) in rabbits may be overcome by the injection of cross-reacting albumins from other species [18]. A certain degree of cross-reactivity with BSA is necessary but beyond this point the more marked the cross-reactivity the less effective is a given albumin in terminating tolerance. Tolerance to a foreign protein

---

* The terminology used in this chapter is that generally used in the literature on auto-immunity. It is given below, followed by the equivalent terms used in Chapter 10 on transplantation (p. 320): isologous (isogenic); homologous (allogeneic); heterologous (xenogeneic).

may also be terminated by the same protein coupled to a synthetic hapten provided it is still cross-reactive with the native protein [6]. Under these conditions most of the antibody formed initially is directed exclusively against the 'new' determinant. Breakdown of tolerance may depend on antibody subsequently becoming adapted to a wider area which includes adjacent determinants common to the native and conjugated proteins (*see Fig.* 63). Conjugation can, however, alter the structure of the carrier protein other than merely by the addition of a haptenic group. Thus rabbits immunized with sulphanilazo rabbit serum albumin (RSA)

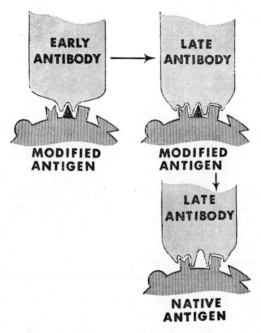

Fig. 63.—A scheme proposed by Cinader [6] to account for breakdown of tolerance to a native antigen following immunization with that protein modified by conjugation to a synthetic hapten. (*Reproduced from B. Cinader (ed.) in 'Regulation of the Antibody Response', Springfield, Illinois, Thomas, 1968.*)

produce antibodies which cross-react with native human serum albumin (HSA), a phenomenon most easily explained by the unmasking of determinants normally concealed in native RSA but accessible in native HSA [5].

These observations suggest that natural tolerance might be broken by antigens similar, but not too similar, to native autologous components. There are two likely sources of suitable antigens: first, body components altered in the course of inflammation, trauma, or even normal wear and tear; secondly, micro-organisms with antigens which cross-react with tissue antigens.

i. Altered Body Components

Weigle [16] has shown that, whereas native homologous thyroglobulin without an adjuvant is not antigenic in rabbits, when coupled to certain haptens or modified by heating it elicits antibodies to normal thyroglobulin. Sometimes thyroiditis is also produced. Moreover, if immunization is continued with *normal* thyroglobulin, the antibody titre and the severity of the thyroiditis are increased [19]. There is no evidence, however, that in man thyroglobulin becomes auto-antigenic through structural modification. Nevertheless, there are instances of autologous macromolecules which do indeed become suitably altered *in vivo*. Alteration of immunoglobulins and complement, eliciting rheumatoid factors and immunoconglutinin respectively, is discussed earlier in this book (pp. 109, 224). In both cases auto-antigenicity appears to depend on the exposure of hidden determinants as a result of unfolding of the molecules concerned during immunological reactions.

There are many examples of tissue damage causing auto-immunization, but it is often not clear whether this is due to alteration of antigenic structure or to the release of native antigen. Antibodies to heart muscle have been found after cardiac surgery and myocardial infarction [20] and antibodies to cytoplasmic components of various organs after toxic liver injury in rats [21]. The latter observation appears to represent the enhancement of a low level of naturally occurring antibody rather than the termination of tolerance [22]. Tissue damage by *in vivo* freezing has also been found to induce auto-antibodies [23]. Another way in which body components may be made auto-antigenic is by the action of enzymes. Thus neuraminidase produced by certain myxoviruses and bacteria acts on the erythrocyte surface, unmasking the 'T' antigen, and the almost universal occurrence of T agglutinin in adult human sera appears to represent a harmless auto-immune response following natural infection [24]. It has been suggested that in the human connective-tissue diseases such as systemic lupus erythematosus (p. 387) lysosomes are abnormally fragile and that the resulting release of enzymes modifies tissue antigens and so stimulates auto-antibody production [25].

The induction of auto-immunity has been studied by immunizing animals with tissues of other species. Auto-antibodies against lens, uvea, cornea, brain, liver, kidney, heart, adrenal, colonic mucosa, and thyroglobulin [16] can all be produced more readily by immunizing with the appropriate heterologous tissue than with homologous tissue [see 26]. The reason may be that the heterologous tissues contain haptens linked to proteins to which there is no tolerance whereas the homologous tissues contain the same haptens linked to proteins to which there is at least partial tolerance. Thus the efficacy of a foreign protein in potentiating the immune response to a simple chemical hapten is reduced if tolerance to the protein is first established [27]. Similarly, acquired tolerance to a synthetic hapten conjugated to a foreign protein can be terminated by injections of the same hapten conjugated to another foreign protein (to which there is no tolerance) but not to a host protein [28]. These observations suggest that auto-immunity could arise if host haptens became coupled to foreign carriers such as micro-organisms or their products. For instance, the Wassermann antibody might be elicited by autologous lipids carried on *Treponema pallidum*.

ii. Antigens of Micro-organisms

Micro-organisms provide the second main source of antigens which might be able to terminate self-tolerance because of their similarity to tissue antigens. This subject has recently been reviewed [29]. It is fortunate that apparently suitable situations do not always lead to auto-immunization; the exact extent of cross-reactivity between the pairs of antigens concerned and the degree of tolerance to be overcome must both be relevant. There is strong evidence that antibodies against cardiac muscle in patients with rheumatic fever arise as a result of stimulation by related streptococcal antigens [30] and anti-colon antibodies in ulcerative colitis may be provoked by bowel organisms (p. 389).

The existence of bacterial antigens similar to body constituents raises two interesting problems. The first is that if the immune mechanism did not respond to these extrinsic antigens there would be no specific immunological defence against organisms whose main surface antigens resemble those of the host [31]. On the other hand, a vigorous response might carry the risk of producing auto-immunization. This dilemma may be resolved partly by the phenomenon of immune deviation (p. 380). The second problem is that of how small a divergence from the structure of a normal auto-antigen can be recognized by the immunological apparatus. Variation in the sensitivity of such discrimination would result in auto-immunity developing in one individual in response to an antigenic stimulus which another would ignore.

B. Auto-immunization due to Abnormality of the Immunological Apparatus

Auto-immunity could arise not only through abnormal antigenic stimuli in the various ways discussed above but also through the loss of tolerance resulting from a primary abnormality of the antibody-forming apparatus. In the clonal selection theory of antibody production Burnet postulated that lymphoid cells reacting with auto-antigens arise in normal subjects as a result of somatic mutations, but are suppressed by a control mechanism dependent on the presence of antigen [32]. A failure of this suppressive mechanism would lead to the proliferation of clones of auto-reactive cells. This was suggested as the underlying defect in diseases such as systemic lupus erythematosus and auto-immune haemolytic anaemia where auto-antibodies are directed against readily accessible antigens to which tolerance appears to be well developed. Auto-immune haemolytic anaemia sometimes occurs in malignant diseases of lymphoid tissue such as lymphosarcoma and chronic lymphatic leukaemia. Dameshek and Schwartz [33] ascribed this to somatic mutation in the rapidly proliferating neoplastic lymphoid cells. Auto-reactive cells arising in this way could be regarded as the equivalent of a tolerated graft of genetically dissimilar lymphoid cells capable of mounting an attack upon the host. In other words, the auto-immune disease is the equivalent of graft-versus-host disease (*see* Chapter 10). The latter is associated with Coombs-positive haemolytic anaemia [34] and skin, heart, and joint lesions histologically nbling those seen in various human diseases which are thought to an auto-immune basis.

Although somatic mutation, whether in normal or neoplastic lymphoid tissue, provides an attractively simple explanation for auto-immunity, this hypothesis does not lend itself to experimental verification. There is, however, some preliminary evidence to suggest that certain auto-immune processes may result from viral transformation of lymphoid cells. For instance, mice surviving the acute stage of infection with reovirus 3 develop a chronic disease in which infectious virus can no longer be detected [35]. This chronic stage may be auto-immune because it resembles graft-versus-host disease and a similar syndrome can be transmitted to isologous new-born mice by spleen cells from affected adults. Lymphoma may develop in mice which survive the transmitted disease and it has been suggested that viruses might cause both auto-immune disease and lymphoma [35]. This is of particular interest in view of the possibility that an auto-immune disease of New Zealand Black mice, some of which develop lymphomas, is caused by a virus (p. 381).

III. EXPERIMENTAL AUTO-IMMUNE DISEASE

A. Production of Auto-immune Disease

A wide range of organ-specific auto-antibodies may be produced by immunization with extracts of the corresponding organs, either alone or with incomplete adjuvant. However, except when the antigen is chemically altered [16, 36], tissue damage rarely occurs unless many immunizing injections are given over a long period of time or unless a bacterial adjuvant is incorporated into the injection mixture. Thus in order to produce encephalomyelitis in monkeys Rivers and Schwentker [37] gave 46–85 intramuscular injections of cerebral tissue during periods of 5–9 months. The introduction of Freund's complete adjuvant greatly facilitated the production of encephalomyelitis [38, 39], and led to the production of further experimental diseases such as uveitis [40], orchitis [41], thyroiditis [42], and adrenalitis [43] in a similar manner.

The exact course of events following immunization depends on the species and strain, the antigen, the adjuvant, and the route of administration. Following the intradermal injection of antigen with Freund's complete adjuvant, delayed hypersensitivity to the homologous antigen usually appears after 5–10 days, although in the case of adrenalitis delayed skin reactions have not been obtained [44]. Shortly after this the organ concerned becomes infiltrated by lymphocytes, histiocytes, and sometimes plasma cells, except in orchitis where cellular infiltration is absent or minimal. This is soon followed by parenchymal tissue damage and humoral antibodies may appear at about this time.

Although Freund's complete adjuvant has been the most widely used, several organisms have been substituted for mycobacteria in mineral oil emulsions and there is considerable variation in the effectiveness of various adjuvants in different animal species [45]. Thus for the production of auto-immune disease in the guinea-pig incomplete adjuvant is ineffective and mycobacteria or other bacteria such as *Bordetella pertussis* or *Corynebacterium rubrum* are mandatory. On the other hand, in the case of encephalitis in the rat, a bacterial component is not required and mineral oil alone is an adequate adjuvant as is aqueous pertussis vaccine without mineral oil [45].

Adjuvants appear to promote the production of auto-immune diseases in two ways. First, they facilitate the breakdown of tolerance; this has been clearly shown in the case of acquired tolerance to bovine serum albumin in rabbits [46] and applies equally to natural tolerance. Secondly, they enhance the development of delayed hypersensitivity which is probably the main pathogenetic mechanism in most of the experimental diseases.

The intradermal route is the most effective route of immunization, as was first demonstrated for encephalomyelitis [47]. This is probably a function of the rate of release of antigen from the injection site and the nature of the lymphatic drainage. Excision of the injection site within an hour does not prevent the appearance of encephalitis, some of the injected material having already reached the regional lymph-nodes [48]. Encephalitis is prevented by excision of these nodes [49] and its production is greatly enhanced if injections are given directly into lymph-nodes [50].

Most experimental auto-immune diseases can be produced by immunization with autologous tissue. For instance, in rabbits immunized with thyroid tissue obtained by surgical excision of one lobe, thyroiditis occurs in the other lobe [51]. However, isologous, homologous, or heterologous tissue is usually used. The relative efficacy of tissue from different species in producing disease varies according to the organ being studied and the species of the recipient, and may be unrelated to its efficacy in stimulating auto-antibody formation. Thus, in the rabbit, immunization with heterologous thyroglobulin in Freund's incomplete adjuvant results in the production of antibodies to rabbit thyroglobulin but not thyroiditis [16]. The fact that an antigen capable of eliciting antibody may be incapable of producing tissue damage has important implications for the possible auto-immune pathogenesis of some human diseases.

Some progress has been made towards the identification of antigens responsible for experimentally induced tissue damage. Thyroglobulin was soon identified as the component of thyroid extracts active in producing thyroiditis, but the nature of the encephalitogenic factor in brain tissue has proved more elusive. Lipid–protein complexes, collagen-like protein, and water-soluble basic protein have all been championed [52]. It has recently been suggested that a polypeptide component of myelin, which may have a molecular weight as low as 3000, accounts for the activity of these fractions [53, 54]. The antigenicity of such a small molecule is of great interest, especially in the light of the observation that synthetic polypeptides can elicit delayed hypersensitivity [55].

B. Prevention of Experimental Auto-immune Disease

Auto-immune disease following immunization with the appropriate organ extract in Freund's complete adjuvant may be prevented in various ways. Some of these, such as excision of the draining lymph-nodes, the use of antimitotic drugs, and neonatal thymectomy, are mentioned elsewhere in this chapter. Corticosteroids and antilymphocyte serum have also been used.

Other methods include previous experience of the specific antigen, previous production of the same disease, and immunization with unrelated antigens. These will now be considered according to the probable mechanisms involved.

1. TOLERANCE

The injection of brain [56], thyroid [57], or testis [13] in saline or incomplete adjuvant can inhibit the development of auto-immune disease after a later challenge by antigen in Freund's complete adjuvant. Similarly, thyroiditis produced by chemically altered thyroglobulin without adjuvant is suppressed by the prior injection of unaltered thyroglobulin [58]. Two different mechanisms, induction of tolerance and production of protective antibody, may account for the prevention of auto-immune disease in this way.

In this type of experiment it is common for the inhibition of the disease to be accompanied by the appearance of the corresponding circulating antibody, so it is evident that tolerance as it is usually understood, affecting all forms of immune response, both humoral and cellular, is not induced. In the guinea-pig inhibition of orchitis is accompanied by the production of antibody to testis (presumably gamma-1) demonstrable by passive cutaneous anaphylaxis, but the delayed hypersensitivity and cytotoxic (presumably gamma-2) antibody responses are suppressed [59, 60]. This is probably an example of 'split tolerance' or 'immune deviation', a phenomenon which has been elicited in the guinea-pig using extrinsic antigens (p. 150). Thus prior or concurrent treatment with antigen, either soluble, alum-precipitated, or in Freund's *incomplete* adjuvant, modifies the responses to the same antigen given in Freund's *complete* adjuvant [61, 62]. Delayed hypersensitivity is greatly depressed and gamma-2 antibody moderately depressed, while the gamma-1 response is depressed only slightly or not at all. The responses most easily depressed, delayed hypersensitivity and gamma-2 antibody, are those considered able to cause tissue damage. This may be of importance for the limitation of spontaneous auto-immune disease since it would allow harmless gamma-1 responses to tissue antigens but prevent damaging responses [63].

2. PROTECTIVE ANTIBODY

Rats which have recovered from encephalomyelitis are resistant to further challenge. Their serum contains a complement-fixing antibody against alcoholic brain extracts and will protect other rats from developing the disease [64], probably by blocking the induction of delayed hypersensitivity or the peripheral action of sensitized cells. This mechanism is analogous to that of the immune enhancement of tumour growth (p. 356).

3. ANTIGENIC COMPETITION

Animals which have been treated with either Freund's complete adjuvant or pertussis vaccine and then challenged with brain extract in complete adjuvant are protected against the development of encephalomyelitis. This is probably the result of antigenic competition [65].

C. The Spontaneous Auto-immune Disease of New Zealand Black Mice

In mice of the inbred New Zealand Black (NZB) strain and in crosses between this and other strains there arises spontaneously a disease which is a remarkably close model of systemic lupus erythematosus (p. 387). These mice develop an auto-immune haemolytic anaemia, circulating antinuclear antibodies which include the lupus erythematosus (LE) factor [66], and glomerulonephritis (p. 383).

There is also striking proliferation of plasma cells and reticulum cells in many organs, especially the spleen and lymph-nodes, and malignant lymphoma may develop. This observation led to the identification by electron microscopy of particles resembling murine leukaemia virus not only in tumour cells but also in other tissues [67]. Similar particles are even present in foetuses and in germ-free older mice [68]. The possibility that these particles are indeed viral and that they are the cause of the auto-immune disease as well as the lymphoma is supported by a claim to have transmitted both conditions from NZB mice to mice of another strain by inoculation in infancy with cell-free filtrates [69]. The virus may be acquired by NZB mice in utero and persist into adult life as a tolerated infection as in the case of lymphocytic choriomeningitis.

D. Mechanisms of Tissue Damage

1. CELLULAR IMMUNITY IN ENCEPHALOMYELITIS AND THYROIDITIS

It is generally considered that cellular rather than humoral mechanisms play a major role in causing the tissue lesions of encephalomyelitis and thyroiditis. The evidence may be summarized as follows:—

a. The histological picture of the early lesions is one of perivascular cuffing and parenchymal infiltration by lymphoid cells as seen in a delayed hypersensitivity reaction to the intradermal injection of antigen.

b. There is a parallel between the ability of Freund's complete adjuvant to enhance the production of auto-immune tissue damage and its promotion of delayed hypersensitivity. However, antibody production is also enhanced.

c. The severity of the disease correlates better with delayed skin reactions to the immunizing antigen than with antibody titres both in thyroiditis [70] and encephalomyelitis [71]. In the latter disease exceptions may be due to the use of crude preparations containing multiple antigens some of which, although not encephalitogenic, may be capable of eliciting delayed hypersensitivity [72]. Conversely, a role for humoral immunity cannot be excluded by a lack of correlation between a given antibody and disease activity because of the possibility that other, tissue-damaging antibodies are present but not detected by the methods used.

d. The effects of both serum and lymphoid cells from animals with experimental auto-immune diseases on cell cultures of the target organs have been studied. In thyroiditis cytotoxic antibodies have not been detected in any species except the monkey [73], but negative results have also been obtained with lymphocytes [74] in spite of earlier claims of success. On the other hand, in encephalomyelitis both serum [75] and lymphoid cells [76] appear to be toxic to cultures of nervous tissue, raising the possibility of synergism between humoral and cellular factors.

e. Blast-cell transformation and inhibition of macrophage migration in the presence of antigen are discussed fully in Chapter 8.

f. Passive transfer: neither encephalomyelitis nor thyroiditis has been transferred from affected animals to recipients with serum even in large quantities. A claim to have transferred encephalomyelitis by injecting serum directly into the lateral ventricles of the brain [77] has not been substantiated. However, encephalomyelitis can be transferred with lymphoid cells provided the recipient is tolerant to them. Patterson [78] originally achieved this in outbred rats by first inducing tolerance to normal cells from the prospective donor and then injecting sensitized cells. Transfer with lymphoid cells has subsequently been demonstrated in inbred, histocompatible strains. The transfer of thyroiditis with lymphoid cells was claimed in a preliminary report in 1961 [79], but this has not been confirmed.

g. Dissociation of cellular and humoral responses: in guinea-pigs immunized with small doses of homologous thyroglobulin heavily conjugated with picryl groups humoral antibody production is greatly decreased, but the incidence of thyroiditis and delayed skin reactions is not affected [80]. Conversely delayed hypersensitivity to thyroglobulin and the severity of thyroiditis are reduced by 6-mercaptopurine while the antibody response is undiminished [81]. In the chicken neonatal thymectomy, which impairs cellular but not humoral immunity, prevents the appearance of thyroiditis [82] and encephalomyelitis [83], and diminishes delayed skin reactions but not antibody production to the corresponding antigens. On the other hand, neonatal bursectomy, which impairs humoral but not cellular immunity, does not inhibit these diseases or the skin reactions, although antibody production is reduced.

In summary, there is evidence that tissue damage in experimental allergic encephalomyelitis is due to auto-aggressive lymphoid cells rather than antibody. In thyroiditis the case for cellular immunity is less compelling, the main gaps in the evidence being the lack of any convincing demonstration that sensitized lymphocytes will specifically attack thyroid cells *in vitro* or that they will transfer the disease.

2. SYNERGISM BETWEEN HUMORAL AND CELLULAR IMMUNITY IN ORCHITIS

Cellular infiltration is absent in the early stages of experimental autoimmune orchitis and this must raise some doubt as to whether cellular mechanisms are solely or principally involved in the production of the lesion. Under certain conditions it is possible to elicit anti-testis antibodies without delayed hypersensitivity, while under different conditions delayed hypersensitivity can be elicited without circulating antibodies [84]. In neither of these two sets of circumstances is there any evidence of testicular damage. However, lesions develop when animals with delayed hypersensitivity alone are given serum containing antibody or when animals with antibody alone are given sensitized lymphoid cells. The presence of humoral antibody has been shown to potentiate the passive transfer of delayed hypersensitivity to various extrinsic antigens [85] and synergism of this type may well prove to be concerned in the pathogenesis of other diseases, both experimental and human.

3. ANTIBODIES

Auto-antibodies against red blood-cells cause haemolytic anaemia in NZB mice and are more fully discussed in connexion with human disease (p. 384).

Recent work has shown that humoral antibodies are also responsible for the glomerulonephritis which follows immunization with glomerular basement membrane (GBM) material, either heterologous, homologous, or autologous [86]. Anti-GBM antibodies, together with complement, localize as a linear deposit along the GBM from which they can be recovered by acid elution. In animals whose kidneys have been removed following the development of nephritis, the antibodies accumulate in the serum in sufficient amounts to permit the passive transfer of the disease to normal homologous recipients. Anti-GBM antibodies are also involved in some types of glomerulonephritis in man (p. 388).

4. IMMUNE COMPLEXES

The tissue lesions of serum sickness have been shown to result from the deposition of complexes of foreign antigen, antibody, and complement (p. 247). In the kidney these complexes form discrete masses on the outer (epithelial) side of the glomerular basement membrane and the lesions are therefore readily distinguished from those due to anti-GBM antibodies. The fact that the kidney bears the brunt of the attack, although the antigens concerned are unrelated to kidney, is probably due to its filtering function, the pores in the glomerular capillary endothelium providing direct contact between blood and basement membrane.

When renal damage occurs by this mechanism and the antigen is either autologous or cross-reacts with autologous components it is justifiable to describe the lesions as auto-immune. The glomerulonephritis produced by immunizing rats with homologous whole-kidney homogenates in Freund's complete adjuvant is of this type and anti-GBM antibodies are not involved [86]. The antigen is not a constituent of the glomerulus but of the brush border of the cells lining the proximal convoluted tubule. Not only homologous antigen used for immunization but also circulating autologous tubular antigen, together with antibody and complement, are deposited on the outer side of the glomerular basement membrane [87] in the lumpy manner characteristic of serum sickness nephritis. A similar glomerular lesion develops spontaneously in NZB mice (p. 381) as a result of the deposition of immune complexes involving nuclear antigens and antinuclear antibodies [88].

IV. AUTO-IMMUNITY AND DISEASE IN MAN

Much of the interest in auto-immunity stems from its possible clinical importance as a mechanism causing human disease. However, auto-antibodies may occur in the serum of healthy individuals. Thus antibodies against various tissue components occur in normal animals [22] and antibodies against immunoglobulin fragments are found in both animals and human beings. Sometimes auto-antibodies are merely the *consequence* of tissue damage (p. 376). It has even been suggested that auto-immunity plays a normal, physiological role in the removal of tissue debris [89]. On the other hand, auto-antibodies arising in response to tissue damage could cause further damage leading to a vicious circle. Finally, an auto-immune process might be solely responsible both for initiating and perpetuating disease.

Many diseases of man have been labelled 'auto-immune' on insufficient evidence, and it may therefore be helpful to have certain criteria to be fulfilled before a given disease can be said to be the result of auto-immunity. The main criteria are as follows:—

a. There is auto-antibody and/or delayed hypersensitivity against the diseased tissue.

b. Auto-antibody or lymphoid cells specifically attack cells of the target organ in tissue culture. Even more convincing is the passive transfer of the disease to an experimental animal, a human volunteer, or a grafted human organ (p. 388).

c. As an alternative to (*a*) and (*b*), immune complexes are found at the sites of tissue lesions. The complexes may be composed of auto-antigen and auto-antibody unrelated to the tissue in which they are deposited.

d. An experimental model can be produced by active immunization with the appropriate organ extract, usually in Freund's complete adjuvant, or else a similar disease occurs spontaneously in animals.

Other features, common to many supposedly auto-immune diseases, are sometimes cited as additional criteria for an auto-immune pathogenesis. These provide at best very indirect evidence, but may be useful as indicating that immunological investigation is warranted. They include: (i) raised serum immunoglobulin levels; (ii) tissue infiltration by lymphocytes, plasma cells, and histiocytes; (iii) familial incidence of the disease; (iv) an association with other possibly auto-immune diseases in patients and their relatives; (v) abnormality of the thymus; and (vi) beneficial effect of corticosteroids and cytotoxic agents.

Some examples of human disease, selected mainly on the strength of the evidence for auto-immunity as the cause of the tissue damage, will now be considered. Understanding of aetiology, the underlying cause of auto-immunization, has not advanced in step with that of pathogenesis and is still largely at the stage of speculation.

A. The Auto-immune Haemolytic Anaemias

Auto-immune haemolytic anaemia is due to auto-antibodies against red blood-cells. It may be either primary, occurring in the absence of any other disease process, or secondary to an underlying disease such as chronic lymphatic leukaemia, lymphosarcoma, systemic lupus erythematosus, mycoplasmal pneumonia, or glandular fever.

Serologically there are two major groups, characterized by 'warm' and 'cold' antibodies respectively [90]. Warm antibodies are most active at 37° C., are usually incomplete, do not fix complement, and belong to the IgG class. However, incomplete IgM and IgA warm antibodies and IgM warm haemolysins also occur [91]. Cold antibodies are most active at 4° C., become progressively less active at higher temperatures, and, in most cases, are inactive above 32° C. They are complete IgM antibodies which cause haemolysis in the presence of complement at temperatures somewhat higher than the optimum for agglutination.

Although the antiglobulin reaction shows that immunoglobulin is present on the red-cell surface, it is necessary to have proof that this represents antibody specifically combined with antigen since adsorption of globulins can occur non-immunologically [92]. Proof has been provided by eluting the antibody and showing that it will then react with other cells of the same specificity. In some cases it has even been possible to show that, following recovery, the patient's 'healthy' cells can be sensitized by his own serum taken during the active phase of the disease [93].

Rhesus specificity has been demonstrated for at least 70 per cent of warm antibodies. Some are directed against well-known antigens such as 'e', others against antigens of the Rh system which are not recognized by the usual Rh iso-antibodies and appear to be universally distributed [94]. The cold antibodies are of completely different specificity and this usually involves the Ii blood-group system, most being anti-I but a few being anti-i [95].

Paroxysmal cold haemoglobinuria is a syndrome which is rare nowadays. In the past it was often secondary to congenital syphilis, but primary cases also occur. In 1904, in the first published report of an auto-immune disease in man, Donath and Landsteiner [96] described an autohaemolysin which explained the pathogenesis of this condition. It is an IgG antibody which combines with red cells at low temperatures (around 2° C.) but does not cause lysis until the temperature is raised to above 30° C. It is specific for the blood-group antigen P [97].

An interesting example of warm-antibody haemolytic anaemia has recently been described in patients taking the anti-hypertensive agent α-methyldopa [98]. Up to one-third of those treated develop positive direct antiglobulin tests, but only a very small proportion of these have evidence of increased red-cell destruction. In haemolytic anaemia due to certain other drugs, such as Fuadin (stibophen) and in thrombocytopenia due to Sedormid (apronal), the antibodies are directed against the drug or the drug–cell complex [99]. However, in α-methyldopa-induced anaemia the antibodies are directed against intrinsic red-cell antigens (usually of Rh specificity) and are true auto-antibodies.

Although haemolytic antibodies, especially when present in high titre, may cause lysis in the blood-stream, they usually cause red-cell destruction in a more indirect way. When coated with warm antibody, red cells are mainly removed from the circulation by the spleen and, when coated with cold antibody, by the reticulo-endothelial system in general, especially in the liver.

There is no evidence that alterations to the red-cell surface are the cause of auto-immunization except perhaps in the case of anti-I antibodies following mycoplasmal infection which may be due to alteration of the I antigen by the organism [100]. There is also nothing to implicate cross-reacting antigens of micro-organisms. It is therefore possible that there is a loss of tolerance due to a primary abnormality of lymphoid cells.

B. Hashimoto's Thyroiditis and Related Conditions

Hashimoto's thyroiditis, idiopathic adrenal atrophy, hypoparathyroidism, and the atrophic gastritis of pernicious anaemia form a group of conditions characterized by lymphoid-cell infiltration of a particular organ and the presence in the serum of antibodies specific for that organ. These conditions are found together in one patient or in members of a family more often than could occur by chance, either as overt clinical disease or as subclinical disease detectable only by the presence of antibodies or of histological changes at biopsy.

In Hashimoto's disease the thyroid is invaded by large numbers of lymphocytes, plasma cells, and histiocytes. The acini are destroyed and if the damage is severe enough hypothyroidism develops. Antibodies against three different thyroid antigens have been fully documented; thyroglobulin [14], a second antigen of the acinar colloid distinct from thyroglobulin [101], and the microsomes of thyroid epithelial cells [102]. Virtually all patients have at least one of these antibodies in their serum, but the titres do not correlate well with the severity of the disease process.

Experimental thyroiditis is a good model of Hashimoto's disease and strengthens the evidence that the latter has an auto-immune pathogenesis. There are, however, differences between the two conditions, such as the absence of a microsomal antigen–antibody system in most animal species and the usually self-limiting course of the experimental disease.

In the presence of complement the microsomal antibody rapidly kills thyroid cells in tissue culture [103]. For three reasons it appears unlikely that this antibody is solely responsible for the tissue damage in Hashimoto's disease. First, the cytotoxic effect can only be demonstrated in cultures prepared from cells dispersed by proteolytic enzymes, suggesting that prior alteration of the cell surface is necessary. Secondly, although it is often an IgG antibody and able to cross the placenta, it does not appear to damage the thyroids of infants whose mothers have the disease. Lastly, it reacts with monkey thyroid microsomes *in vitro*, but no effect has been detected following infusion of serum into a monkey.

The heavy infiltration of the thyroid by lymphoid cells and the analogy with experimental thyroiditis both suggest a role for delayed hypersensitivity in Hashimoto's disease, but there is little direct evidence for this [104]. Skin reactions to the injection of thyroid extracts have been studied in a few cases and, when positive, have been of Arthus type, probably due to the presence of high titres of antithyroglobulin antibody. Experiments on blast-cell transformation of patients' lymphocytes in response to thyroid antigens have given conflicting results and lymphocytes do not appear to damage thyroid cells in culture. Perhaps the thyroid lesions are the result of synergism between cellular and humoral mechanisms as in experimental orchitis, sensitized lymphocytes rendering thyroid cells susceptible to the cytotoxic antibody.

Thyrotoxicosis (Graves' disease) is clinically and serologically associated with other members of the Hashimoto group of diseases. The thyroid is hyperplastic and secretes an excess of thyroxine. Lymphocytic thyroiditis is usually present but, unlike that of Hashimoto's disease, it is confined to small, scattered foci and is usually not progressive. The antibodies characteristic of thyroiditis are frequently present, but recent interest has centred on a further serum factor which, when injected intravenously, stimulates the thyroids of assay animals [105] and human volunteers [106]. It is known as the long-acting thyroid stimulator (LATS) because its effect is more prolonged than that of thyroid-stimulating hormone. LATS appears to be an antibody since activity is confined to IgG, is absorbed by thyroid tissue, and can then be recovered by acid elution [107]. The precise antigenic site in the thyroid is unknown but it may be in the cell membrane. LATS probably accounts entirely for the thyroid overactivity in thyrotoxicosis and is of particular interest as an auto-antibody which stimulates rather than damages its target.

There is no evidence that thyroid auto-immunization is the result of excessive leakage of antigens from the gland (p. 374) or of the formation of abnormal, cross-reacting thyroglobulin (p. 376). The frequent coexistence of multiple organ-specific antibodies in a single individual is more readily explained as a disturbance of tolerance than as the result of abnormal antigenic stimuli arising in multiple organs. The familial incidence of organ-specific auto-immunity indicates that, whatever the nature of the underlying disturbance, it is genetically determined. In the case of the thyroid there appears to be a dominant mode of inheritance [108].

C. Systemic Lupus Erythematosus

Systemic lupus erythematosus (SLE) resembles the disease of NZB mice (p. 381) in many respects. Lesions are found in the skin, joints, serous membranes, blood-vessels, and renal glomeruli, those in the glomeruli being a major cause of death. There is a remarkable range of circulating antibodies against various nuclear and cytoplasmic components which are neither organ nor species-specific [109, 110]. Nuclear antigens include deoxyribonucleoprotein (DNP), both double and single-stranded deoxyribonucleic acid (DNA), histone, a soluble nuclear protein distinct from histone, and ribonucleic acid of the nucleolus. Antibodies may also be directed against antigens of mitochondria, ribosomes, lysosomes, and a soluble cytoplasmic fraction. The incidence of these antibodies varies; thus antibody to DNP is present in virtually all cases of SLE whereas antibody to nucleoli is only found in a small minority. Rheumatoid factor is found in about one-third of cases.

The LE-cell phenomenon, first described in 1948 [111], was largely responsible for the subsequent interest in immunological aspects of SLE and has been shown to depend on the antibody to DNP. This antibody cannot, of course, enter healthy cells, but it can reach the nuclei of damaged leucocytes and causes them to swell and become homogeneous. In the presence of complement these altered nuclei (LE bodies) are then phago-cytosed by healthy polymorphonuclear leucocytes or monocytes which, with their contained LE bodies, are known as LE cells.

Although antibodies against erythrocytes, leucocytes, platelets, and blood-clotting factors occur in some cases and are responsible for haemo-lytic anaemia, leucopenia, thrombocytopenia, and clotting defects respectively, there is no evidence that any of the antibodies to nuclear or cytoplasmic components mentioned earlier are directly cytotoxic. Indeed, their targets, being intracellular, are presumably inaccessible to antibody. However, deposits of immunoglobulin and complement have been found at the sites of tissue lesions, especially in renal glomeruli, and are believed to represent immune complexes formed elsewhere. The glomerular deposits have the distribution characteristic of immune-complex nephritis (p. 383) and appear to be composed of nuclear and cytoplasmic antigens and the corresponding auto-antibodies [112].

A number of observations, some still unconfirmed, suggest that cellular immunity may also be concerned in the pathogenesis of SLE [104]. Patients' lymphocytes are transformed to blast cells by DNA [113] and it has been claimed that they will destroy homologous fibroblasts in tissue culture. Delayed skin reactions to the injection of autologous leucocytes and of purified nuclear antigens have also been described [104].

In view of the wide distribution of the non-organ specific antigens, their presence in the antibody-forming cells themselves, and, compared with organ-specific antigens, their poor antigenicity when injected into experimental animals it appeared until recently that tolerance towards them was well established. This suggested that there was loss of tolerance in SLE because of a primary abnormality of lymphoid cells.

However, there is increasing evidence that both nuclear and cytoplasmic constituents are in fact antigenic in individuals with a normal immune mechanism. Antinuclear antibodies have been produced experimentally by immunization with nucleoproteins and with nucleic acids and purine and pyrimidine bases coupled to carrier proteins [114]. They also occur after pulmonary infarction in man. Moreover, antibodies to non-organ-specific cytoplasmic components are stimulated by toxic liver injury in rats and viral hepatitis in man. The underlying abnormality in SLE could therefore be a state of hyperreactivity to cell-breakdown products. The suggestion that the disease of NZB mice is due to a virus raises a similar possibility in SLE but there is no evidence for this at present.

D. Glomerulonephritis

There are several types of glomerulonephritis in addition to that seen in SLE. Perhaps the commonest is acute glomerulonephritis following infection with certain serotypes of group A, beta-haemolytic streptococci. The presence in the serum of low complement levels and of an altered complement component C'_{3A} [115] and the deposition of immunoglobulin and complement in the glomeruli suggest an immunological mechanism for this disease, but the exact role of the streptococcus is uncertain. An antigenic relationship has been reported between a strain of nephritogenic streptococci and human glomeruli and on this basis acute glomerulonephritis has been attributed to auto-immunization by cross-reactive antigen [116]. However, this cross-reactivity is not clearly established [117], and there is evidence that the glomerular lesions are due to the deposition of immune complexes which may contain streptococcal antigen [88].

On the other hand, some forms of human glomerulonephritis appear to be genuinely auto-immune [88] and to be due to antibodies against the glomerular basement membrane (GBM), as in the experimental disease produced by immunization with GBM material (p. 383). Antibodies eluted from affected kidneys will transfer the disease to monkeys. Moreover, in one patient antibodies appeared in the serum following bilateral nephrectomy but then rapidly disappeared after renal allotransplantation due to fixation to the GBM of the graft in which glomerulonephritis then developed. The cause of auto-immunization against GBM antigens is unknown, but it could well be due to previous renal damage.

E. Ulcerative Colitis

In this disease the mucosa of the large intestine becomes inflamed and ulcerated. There are auto-antibodies against mucus-secreting cells of both large and small intestine but they are not related to the severity of the disease [118, 119]. The fact that their incidence and titre are not raised in amoebic colitis indicates that they are not merely the result of damage to the colon [120]. Perlmann and Broberger [121] found that patients' blood lymphoid cells, but not serum, were toxic to fresh suspensions of homologous colon cells in the presence of complement. The necessity for complement in this reaction is rather surprising and has been both confirmed [122] and denied [123] by other workers.

There is evidence that auto-immunity in ulcerative colitis may arise through stimulation by a bacterial antigen in the bowel flora. Experiments with patients' sera have shown cross-reactions between an antigen in lipopolysaccharide extracts of colon from germ-free rats and one in *Escherichia coli* 014 which is common to most Enterobacteriaceae [120]. Moreover, auto-antibodies against colon have been produced by immunization of rabbits with another strain of *E. coli* in Freund's complete adjuvant [124].

F. Myasthenia Gravis and the Role of the Thymus in Auto-immune Disease

Myasthenia gravis is a disease in which there is excessive fatigue of voluntary muscles due to impaired neuromuscular transmission. Auto-antibodies against an antigen common to skeletal muscle A bands and the epithelial cells of the thymus are found in 30 per cent of patients [125]. The antibodies do not appear to be responsible for the neuromuscular block since they show no correlation with its severity and are not directed against the motor end-plate. However, some other humoral factor is probably involved since a transient neonatal myasthenia unrelated to the transfer of antimuscular antibody is seen in infants born of myasthenic mothers [126] and globulin fractions of patients' serum inhibit neuromuscular transmission in the rat [127]. In the majority of patients lymphoid follicles with germinal centres are seen in the thymus in large numbers. Some of the remaining cases are associated with a thymic tumour and follicles are then found in the adjacent thymic tissue.

It was recently claimed that an experimental model of myasthenia gravis had been produced by immunizing guinea-pigs with skeletal muscle or thymus extracts in Freund's complete adjuvant [128]. Changes were described in the thymus which were considered to represent an auto-immune thymitis and a neuromuscular block developed. In addition, following immunization with muscle, antibodies against muscle and thymic epithelial cells appeared in the serum. The neuromuscular block was prevented by thymectomy on the day before immunization and it was suggested that a blocking agent was released from the damaged thymus.

Lymphoid follicles are a feature of the thymus not only in myasthenia gravis but also in Hashimoto's thyroiditis, thyrotoxicosis, systemic lupus erythematosus, and the disease of NZB mice and related strains. It has been generally believed that thymic follicles are not present in normal individuals and their presence in these diseases has given rise to speculation as to whether thymic abnormalities are in any way responsible for the development of auto-immunity. One hypothesis is that these follicles are the sites of formation of auto-reactive lymphoid cells [129]. However, neonatal thymectomy fails to prevent the appearance of auto-immune disease in NZB mice [130]. This is not surprising since the thymus is concerned mainly in the development of the ability to manifest cellular immunity (p. 311), while the disease of NZB mice is mediated by anti-bodies. Neonatal thymectomy does, however, prevent the subsequent production of experimental auto-immune encephalomyelitis and thyroiditis, diseases in which cellular immunity appears to play a dominant role (p. 381). An alternative hypothesis is that the thymic changes indicate damage to the organ because of which it is unable to perform a postulated normal function of eliminating autoreactive cells [131].

The significance which has hitherto been attached to the finding of lymphoid follicles in the thymus in various diseases will have to be reassessed in the light of a recent autopsy study of the 'normal' thymus [132]. Thymic follicles were found in 70 per cent of patients under 40 years of age who died after accidents. However, following terminal illness of more than a few days' duration and with advancing age, follicles were rarely found.

V. CONCLUSIONS

It is evident from this brief account that, in spite of much experimental work in animals and much speculation, the origin of auto-immunity in human disease is still largely obscure, except in certain conditions in which it may be provoked by bacterial antigens which cross-react with body constituents. On the other hand, although auto-immunization may occur in health or simply as a *result* of tissue damage, its importance as a pathogenetic mechanism in certain diseases is becoming increasingly clear. This is of practical importance as well as of academic interest since it provides a rational basis for treatment with the immunosuppressive agents which are used to inhibit the allograft reaction (p. 323). Corticosteroids are of value in a number of auto-immune diseases and have been widely used for some years. Cytotoxic drugs such as azathioprine have been introduced more recently and are still being assessed. Antilymphocyte serum has been found to be effective in treating experimental auto-immune encephalomyelitis [133], but its use in human disease is a matter for future investigation.

REFERENCES

1. EHRLICH, P. (1906), *Collected Studies on Immunity* (translated by BOLDUAN, C.). New York: Wiley.
2. DAMESHEK, W., and SCHWARTZ, S. O. (1938), 'The Presence of Hemolysins in Acute Hemolytic Anaemia', *New Engl. J. Med.*, **218**, 75.
3. BOORMAN, K. E., DODD, B. E., and LOUTIT, J. F. (1946), 'Haemolytic Icterus (Acholuric Jaundice); Congenital and Acquired', *Lancet*, **1**, 812.
4. BOYDEN, S. V., and SORKIN, E. (1962), 'Effect of Neonatal Injections of Protein on the Immune Response to Protein–hapten Complexes', *Immunology*, **5**, 370.
5. NACHTIGAL, D., and FELDMAN, M. (1964), 'The Immune Response to Azo-protein Conjugates in Rabbits unresponsive to the Protein Carriers', *Immunology*, **7**, 616.
6. CINADER, B. (1968), 'Immunogenicity and Tolerance to Autologous Macro-molecules', in *Regulation of the Antibody Response* (ed. CINADER, B.), p. 3. Springfield, Ill.: Thomas.

7. TRIPLETT, E. L. (1962), 'On the Mechanism of Immunologic Self-recognition', *J. Immun.*, **89**, 505.
8. WEIR, D. M., and PINCKARD, R. N. (1967), 'Failure to induce Tolerance to Rat Tissue Antigens', *Immunology*, **13**, 373.
9. WOODS, A. C., and LITTLE, M. F. (1933), 'Uveal Pigment. Hypersensitivity and Therapeusis', *Archs Ophthal.*, *N.Y.*, **9**, 200.
10. HACKETT, E., and THOMPSON, A. (1964), 'Anti-lens Antibody in Human Sera', *Lancet*, **2**, 663.
11. METALNIKOFF, S. (1900), 'Etudes sur la Spermotoxine', *Annls Inst. Pasteur, Paris*, **14**, 577.
12. RUMKE, P. (1965), 'Autospermagglutinins: A Cause of Infertility in Men', *Ann. N.Y. Acad. Sci.*, **124**, 696.
13. BROWN, P. C., GLYNN, L. E., and HOLBOROW, E. J. (1963), 'The Pathogenesis of Experimental Allergic Orchitis in Guinea-pigs', *J. Path. Bact.*, **86**, 505.
14. ROITT, I. M., DONIACH, D., CAMPBELL, P. N., and HUDSON, R. V. (1956), 'Auto-antibodies in Hashimoto's Disease (Lymphadenoid Goitre)', *Lancet*, **2**, 820.
15. ROITT, I. M., and TORRIGIANI, G. (1967), 'Identification and Estimation of Undegraded Thyroglobulin in Human Serum', *Endocrinology*, **81**, 421.
16. WEIGLE, W. O. (1965), 'The Induction of Autoimmunity in Rabbits following Injection of Heterologous or Altered Homologous Thyroglobulin', *J. exp. Med.*, **121**, 289.
17. IRVINE, W. J. (1964), 'Thyroid Auto-immunity as a Disorder of Immunological Tolerance', *Q. Jl exp. Physiol.*, **49**, 324.
18. WEIGLE, W. O. (1961), 'The Immune Response of Rabbits Tolerant to Bovine Serum Albumin to the Injection of Other Heterologous Serum Albumins', *J. exp. Med.*, **114**, 111.
19. WEIGLE, W. O. (1965), 'The Production of Thyroiditis and Antibody following Injection of Unaltered Thyroglobulin without Adjuvant into Rabbits previously stimulated with Altered Thyroglobulin', *J. exp. Med.*, **122**, 1049.
20. VAN DER GELD, H. (1964), 'Anti-heart Antibodies in the Postpericardiotomy and the Postmyocardial-infarction Syndromes', *Lancet*, **2**, 617.
21. WEIR, D. M. (1963), 'Liver Autoantibodies in the Rat', *Immunology*, **6**, 581.
22. WEIR, D. M., PINCKARD, R. N., ELSON, C. J., and SUCKLING, D. E. (1966), 'Naturally Occurring Anti-tissue Antibodies in Rat Sera', *Clin. exp. Immun.*, **1**, 433.
23. YANTORNO, C., SOANES, W. A., GONDER, M. J., and SHULMAN, S. (1967), 'Studies in Cryo-immunology. I, The Production of Antibodies to Urogenital Tissue in Consequence of Freezing Treatment', *Immunology*, **12**, 395.
24. ISACSON, P. (1967), 'Myxoviruses and Autoimmunity', *Prog. Allergy*, **10**, 256.
25. WEISSMANN, G. (1964), 'Lysosomes, Autoimmune Phenomena and Diseases of Connective Tissue', *Lancet*, **2**, 1373.
26. ASHERSON, G. L., and DUMONDE, D. C. (1964), 'Autoantibody Production in Rabbits. V, Comparison of the Autoantibody Response after the Injection of Rat and Rabbit Liver and Brain', *Immunology*, **7**, 1.
27. CINADER, B., and DUBERT, J. M. (1955), 'Acquired Immune Tolerance to Human Albumin and the Response to Subsequent Injections of Diazo Human Albumin', *Br. J. exp. Path.*, **36**, 515.
28. WEIGLE, W. O. (1965), 'The Immune Response of Rabbits tolerant to One Protein Conjugate following the Injection of Related Protein Conjugates', *J. Immun.*, **94**, 177.
29. ASHERSON, G. L. (1968), 'The Role of Micro-organisms in Autoimmune Responses', *Prog. Allergy*, **12**, 192.
30. KAPLAN, M. H. (1965), 'Autoantibodies to Heart and Rheumatic Fever: The Induction of Autoimmunity to Heart by Streptococcal Antigen Cross-reactive with Heart', *Ann. N.Y. Acad. Sci.*, **124**, 904.
31. ROWLEY, D., and JENKIN, C. R. (1962), 'Antigenic Cross-reaction between Host and Parasite as a Possible Cause of Pathogenicity', *Nature, Lond.*, **193**, 151.
32. BURNET, F. M. (1959), 'Autoimmune Disease. I, Modern Immunological Concepts. II, Pathology of the Immune Response', *Br. med. J.*, **2**, 645, 720.
33. DAMESHEK, W., and SCHWARTZ, R. S. (1959), 'Leukaemia and Auto-immunisation—Some Possible Relationships', *Blood*, **14**, 1151.
34. STASTNY, P., STEMBRIDGE, V. A., VISCHER, T. L., and ZIFF, M. (1965), 'Homologous Disease, a Model for Autoimmune Disease', *Ann. N.Y. Acad. Sci.*, **124**, 158.

35. JOSKE, R. A., LEAK, P. J., PAPADIMITRIOU, J. M., STANLEY, N. F., and WALTERS, M. N.-I. (1966), 'Murine Infection with Reovirus. IV, Late Chronic Disease and the Induction of Lymphoma after Reovirus Type 3 Infection', *Br. J. exp. Path.*, **47**, 337.
36. POKORNÁ, Z., and VOJTÍŠKOVA, M. (1964), 'Autoimmune Damage of the Testes induced with Chemically Modified Organ Specific Antigen', *Folia biol., Praha*, **10**, 261.
37. RIVERS, T. M., and SCHWENTKER, F. F. (1935), 'Encephalomyelitis accompanied by Myelin Destruction experimentally produced in Monkeys', *J. exp. Med.*, **61**, 689.
38. KABAT, E. A., WOLF, A., and BEZER, A. E. (1947), 'The Rapid Production of Acute Disseminated Encephalomyelitis in Rhesus Monkeys by Injection of Heterologous and Homologous Brain Tissue with Adjuvants', *J. exp. Med.*, **85**, 117.
39. MORGAN, I. M. (1947), 'Allergic Encephalomyelitis in Monkeys in Response to Injection of Normal Monkey Nervous Tissue', *J. exp. Med.*, **85**, 131.
40. COLLINS, R. C. (1949), 'Experimental Studies on Sympathetic Ophthalmia', *Am. J. Ophthal.*, **32**, 1687.
41. FREUND, J., LIPTON, M. M., and THOMPSON, G. E. (1953), 'Aspermatogenesis in the Guinea Pig induced by Testicular Tissue and Adjuvants', *J. exp. Med.*, **97**, 711.
42. ROSE, N. R., and WITEBSKY, E. (1956), 'Studies on Organ Specificity. V, Changes in the Thyroid Glands of Rabbits following Active Immunisation with Rabbit Thyroid Extracts', *J. Immun.*, **76**, 417.
43. COLOVER, J., and GLYNN, L. E. (1958), 'Experimental Iso-immune Adrenalitis', *Immunology*, **1**, 172.
44. BARNETT, E. V., DUMONDE, D. C., and GLYNN, L. E. (1963), 'Induction of Autoimmunity to Adrenal Gland', *Immunology*, **6**, 382.
45. WHITE, R. G. (1967), 'Role of Adjuvants in the Production of Delayed Hypersensitivity', *Br. med. Bull.*, **23**, 39.
46. SMITH, R. T., and BRIDGES, R. A. (1958), 'Immunological Unresponsiveness in Rabbits produced by Neonatal Injection of Defined Antigens', *J. exp. Med.*, **108**, 227.
47. LIPTON, M. M., and FREUND, J. (1953), 'The Efficacy of the Intracutaneous Route of Injection and the Susceptibility of the Hartley Strain of Guinea Pigs in Experimental Allergic Encephalitis', *J. Immun.*, **70**, 326.
48. FREUND, J., and LIPTON, M. M. (1955), 'Experimental Allergic Encephalomyelitis after the Excision of the Injection Site of Antigen–adjuvant Emulsion', *J. Immun.*, **75**, 454.
49. CONDIE, R. M., KELLY, J. T., THOMAS, L., and GOOD, R. A. (1957), 'Prevention of Experimental Allergic Encephalomyelitis by Removal of the Regional Lymph Node' (Abstract), *Anat. Rec.*, **127**, 405.
50. NEWBOULD, B. B. (1965), 'Production of Allergic Encephalomyelitis in Rats by Injections of Spinal Cord in Adjuvant into the Inguinal Lymph Nodes', *Immunology*, **9**, 613.
51. WITEBSKY, E., ROSE, N. R., TERPLAN, K., PAINE, J. R., and EGAN, R. W. (1957), 'Chronic Thyroiditis and Autoimmunisation', *J. Am. med. Ass.*, **164**, 1439.
52. PATERSON, P. Y. (1966), 'Experimental Allergic Encephalomyelitis and Autoimmune Disease', *Adv. Immun.*, **5**, 131.
53. LUMSDEN, C. E., ROBERTSON, D. M., and BLIGHT, R. (1966), 'Chemical Studies on Experimental Allergic Encephalomyelitis. Peptide as the Common Denominator in all Encephalitogenic "Antigens"', *J. Neurochem.*, **13**, 127.
54. CARNEGIE, P. R., and LUMSDEN, C. E. (1967), 'Fractionation of Encephalitogenic Polypeptides from Bovine Spinal Cord by Gel Filtration in Phenol–acetic acid–water', *Immunology*, **12**, 133.
55. BEN-EFRAIM, S., FUCHS, S., and SELA, M. (1963), 'Hypersensitivity to a Synthetic Polypeptide: Induction of a Delayed Reaction', *Science, N.Y.*, **139**, 1222.
56. SHAW, C.-M., ALVORD, E. C., jun., FAHLBERG, W. J., and KIES, M. W. (1962), 'Specificity of Encephalitogen-induced Inhibition of Experimental "Allergic" Encephalomyelitis in the Guinea Pig', *J. Immun.*, **89**, 54.
57. JANKOVIĆ, B. D., and FLAX, M. H. (1963), 'Alterations in the Development of Experimental Allergic Thyroiditis induced by Injection of Homologous Thyroid', *J. Immun.*, **90**, 178.
58. WEIGLE, W. O. (1967), 'Inhibition of the Production of Autoimmune Thyroiditis in the Rabbit', *Immunology*, **13**, 241.

59. CHUTNÁ, J., and RYCHLÍKOVÁ, M. (1964), 'Prevention and Suppression of Experimental Autoimmune Aspermatogenesis in Adult Guinea Pigs', *Folia biol., Praha*, **10**, 177.

60. CHUTNÁ, J., and RYCHLÍKOVÁ, M. (1964), 'A Study of the Biological Effectiveness of Antibodies in the Development and Prevention of Experimental Autoimmune Aspermatogenesis', *Folia biol., Praha*, **10**, 188.

61. ASHERSON, G. L., and STONE, S. H. (1965), 'Selective and Specific Inhibition of 24-hour Skin Reactions in the Guinea Pig. I, Immune Deviation: Description of the Phenomenon and the Effect of Splenectomy', *Immunology*, **9**, 205.

62. DVORAK, H. F., BILLOTE, J. B., McCARTHY, J. S., and FLAX, M. H. (1966), 'Immunologic Unresponsiveness in the Adult Guinea Pig. III, Variation of the Antigen and Vehicle of Suppression. Induction of Unresponsiveness in the Adult Rat', *J. Immun.*, **97**, 106.

63. ASHERSON, G. L. (1967), 'Antigen-mediated Depression of Delayed Hypersensitivity', *Br. med. Bull.*, **23**, 24.

64. PATERSON, P. Y., and HARWIN, S. M. (1963), 'Suppression of Allergic Encephalomyelitis in Rats by Means of Antibrain Serum', *J. exp. Med.*, **117**, 755.

65. LUMSDEN, C. E. (1964), 'The Problem of Prevention and Control of Auto-allergic Inflammation in the Nervous System', *Z. Immun. Allergie-Forsch.*, **126**, 209.

66. HELYER, B. J., and HOWIE, J. B. (1963), 'Spontaneous Autoimmune Disease in NZB/BL Mice', *Br. J. Haemat.*, **9**, 119.

67. MELLORS, R. C., and HUANG, C. Y. (1966), 'Immunopathology of NZB/BL Mice. V, Virus-like (Filtrable) Agent separable from Lymphoma Cells and identifiable by Electron Microscopy', *J. exp. Med.*, **124**, 1031.

68. PROSSER, P. R. (1968), 'Particles resembling Murine Leukaemia Virus in New Zealand Black Mice', *Clin. exp. Immun.*, **3**, 213.

69. MELLORS, R. C., and HUANG, C. Y. (1967), 'Immunopathology of NZB/BL Mice. VI, Virus Separable from Spleen and Pathogenic for Swiss Mice', *J. exp. Med.*, **126**, 53.

70. LERNER, E. M., McMASTER, P. R. B., and EXUM, E. D. (1964), 'The Course of Experimental Autoallergic Thyroiditis in Inbred Guinea Pigs. The Pathologic Changes and their Relationship to the Immune Response over a 2-year Period', *J. exp. Med.*, **119**, 327.

71. SHAW, C. M., ALVORD, E. C., jun., KAKU, J., and KIES, M. W. (1965), 'Correlation of Experimental Allergic Encephalomyelitis with Delayed-type Skin Sensitivity to Specific Homologous Encephalitogen', *Ann. N.Y. Acad. Sci.*, **122**, 318.

72. CASPARY, E. A., and FIELD, E. J. (1963), 'Encephalitogenic Factor in Experimental "Allergic" Encephalomyelitis', *Nature, Lond.*, **197**, 1218.

73. ROSE, N. R., SKELTON, F. R., KITE, J. H., jun., and WITEBSKY, E. (1966), 'Experimental Thyroiditis in the Rhesus Monkey. III, Course of the Disease', *Clin. exp. Immun.*, **1**, 171.

74. LING, N. R., ACTON, A. B., ROITT, I. M., and DONIACH, D. (1965), 'Interaction of Lymphocytes from Immunised Hosts with Thyroid and other Cells in Culture', *Br. J. exp. Path.*, **46**, 348.

75. APPEL, S. H., and BORNSTEIN, M. B. (1964), 'The Application of Tissue Culture to the Study of Experimental Allergic Encephalomyelitis. II, Serum Factors Responsible for Demyelination', *J. exp. Med.*, **119**, 303.

76. BERG, O., and KÄLLÉN, B. (1963), 'White Blood Cells from Animals with Experimental Allergic Encephalomyelitis tested on Glia Cells in Tissue Culture', *Acta path. microbiol. scand.*, **58**, 33.

77. JANKOVIĆ, B. D., DRASKOCI, M., and JANJIC, M. (1965), 'Passive Transfer of "Allergic" Encephalomyelitis with Antibrain Serum injected into the Lateral Ventricle of the Brain', *Nature, Lond.*, **207**, 428.

78. PATTERSON, P. Y. (1960), 'Transfer of Allergic Encephalomyelitis in Rats by Means of Lymph Node Cells', *J. exp. Med.*, **111**, 119.

79. FELIX-DAVIES, D., and WAKSMAN, B. H. (1961), 'Passive Transfer of Experimental Immune Thyroiditis in the Guinea Pig', *Arthritis Rheum.*, **4**, 416.

80. MIESCHER, P., GORSTEIN, F., BENACERRAF, B., and GELL, P. G. H. (1961), 'Studies on the Pathogenesis of Experimental Immune Thyroiditis', *Proc. Soc. exp. Biol. Med.*, **107**, 12.

81. SPIEGELBERG, H. L., and MIESCHER, P. A. (1963), 'The Effect of 6-Mercaptopurine and Aminopterin on Experimental Immune Thyroiditis in Guinea Pigs', *J. exp. Med.*, **118**, 869.
82. JANKOVIĆ, B. D., IŠVANESKI, M., POPESKOVIĆ, L., and MITROVIĆ, K. (1965), 'Experimental Allergic Thyroiditis (and Parathyroiditis) in Neonatally Thymectomized and Bursectomized Chickens', *Int. Archs Allergy appl. Immun.*, **26**, 18.
83. JANKOVIĆ, B. D., and IŠVANESKI, M. (1963), 'Experimental Allergic Encephalomyelitis in Thymectomised, Bursectomised and Normal Chickens', *Int. Archs Allergy appl. Immun.*, **23**, 188.
84. BROWN, P. C., GLYNN, L. E., and HOLBOROW, E. J. (1967), 'The Dual Necessity for Delayed Hypersensitivity and Circulating Antibody in the Pathogenesis of Experimental Allergic Orchitis in Guinea Pigs', *Immunology*, **13**, 307.
85. ASHERSON, G. L., and LOEWI, G. (1966), 'The Passive Transfer of Delayed Hypersensitivity in the Guinea-pig. I, The Synergic Effect of Immune Cells and Immune Serum on the 24-hour Skin Reaction and a Study of the Histology', *Immunology*, **11**, 277.
86. UNANUE, E. R., and DIXON, F. J. (1967), 'Experimental Glomerulonephritis: Immunological Events and Pathogenetic Mechanisms', *Adv. Immun.*, **6**, 1.
87. EDGINGTON, T. S., GLASSOCK, R. J., and DIXON, F. J. (1967), 'Autologous Immune-complex Pathogenesis of Experimental Allergic Glomerulonephritis', *Science, N.Y.*, **155**, 1432.
88. DIXON, F. J. (1968), 'The Pathogenesis of Glomerulonephritis', *Am. J. Med.*, **44**, 493.
89. BOYDEN, S. (1964), 'Autoimmunity and Inflammation', *Nature, Lond.*, **201**, 200.
90. DACIE, J. V. (1962), *The Haemolytic Anaemias: Congenital and Acquired*, 2nd ed., Part 2—'The Auto-immune Haemolytic Anaemias'. London: Churchill.
91. ENGELFRIET, C. P., VAN DER BORNE, A. E. G. Kr., VAN DER GIESSEN, M., BECKERS, Do., and VAN LOGHEM, J. J. (1968), 'Autoimmune Haemolytic Anaemias. I, Serological Studies with Pure Anti-immunoglobulin Reagents', *Clin. exp. Immun.*, **3**, 605.
92. PIROFSKY, B. (1965), 'The Structure and Specificity of Erythrocyte Autoantibodies', *Ann. N.Y. Acad. Sci.*, **124**, 448.
93. WITEBSKY, E. (1965), 'Acquired Hemolytic Anaemia', *Ann. N.Y. Acad. Sci.*, **124**, 462.
94. WEINER, W., and VOS, G. H. (1963), 'Serology of Acquired Hemolytic Anaemias', *Blood*, **22**, 606.
95. JENKINS, W. J., KOSTER, H. G., MARSH, W. L., and CARTER, R. L. (1965), 'Infectious Mononucleosis: An Unsuspected Source of Anti-i', *Br. J. Haemat.*, **11**, 480.
96. DONATH, J., and LANDSTEINER, K. (1904), 'Ueber paroxysmale Hämoglobinurie', *Münch. med. Wschr.*, **51**, 1590.
97. WORLLEDGE, S. M., and ROUSSO, C. (1965), 'Studies of the Serology of Paroxysmal Cold Haemoglobinuria (P.C.H.) with Special Reference to its Relationship with the P Blood Group System', *Vox Sang.*, **10**, 293.
98. WORLLEDGE, S. M., CARSTAIRS, K. C., and DACIE, J. V. (1966), 'Autoimmune Haemolytic Anaemia associated with α-Methyldopa Therapy', *Lancet*, **2**, 135.
99. ACKROYD, J. F., and ROOK, A. J. (1968), 'Allergic Drug Reactions' in *Clinical Aspects of Immunology* (ed. GELL, P. G. H., and COOMBS, R. R. A.), 2nd ed., p. 693. Oxford: Blackwell.
100. SCHMIDT, P. J., BARILE, M. F., and McGINNISS, M. H. (1965), 'Mycoplasma (Pleuropneumonia-like Organisms) and Blood Group I; Associations with Neoplastic Disease', *Nature, Lond.*, **205**, 371.
101. BALFOUR, B. M., DONIACH, D., ROITT, I. M., and COUCHMAN, K. G. (1961), 'Fluorescent Antibody Studies in Human Thyroiditis: Autoantibodies to an Antigen of the Thyroid Colloid distinct from Thyroglobulin', *Br. J. exp. Path.*, **42**, 307.
102. HOLBOROW, E. J., BROWN, P. C., ROITT, I. M., and DONIACH, D. (1959), 'Cytoplasmic Localisation of "Complement-fixing" Auto-antigen in Human Thyroid Epithelium', *Br. J. exp. Path.*, **40**, 583.
103. FORBES, I. J., ROITT, I. M., DONIACH, D., and SOLOMON, I. L. (1962), 'The Thyroid Cytotoxic Auto-antibody', *J. clin. Invest.*, **41**, 996.
104. ROITT, I. M., and DONIACH, D. (1967), 'Delayed Hypersensitivity in Auto-immune Disease', *Br. med. Bull.*, **23**, 66.

105. ADAMS, D. D. (1965), 'Pathogenesis of the Hyperthyroidism of Graves's Disease', *Br. med. J.*, **1**, 1015.
106. ARNAUD, C. D., KNEUBUHLER, H. A., SEILING, V. L., WIGHTMAN, B. K., and ENGBRING, N. H. (1965), 'Responses of the Normal Human to Infusions of Plasma from Patients with Thyrotoxicosis', *J. clin. Invest.*, **44**, 1287.
107. BENHAMOU-GLYNN, N., EL KABIR, D. J., DONIACH, D., and ROITT, I. M. (1968), 'Inhibition of the Thyroid-stimulating Globulin (LATS) by Particulate and Soluble Cell Fractions', *Proc. R. Soc. Med.*, **61**, 1303.
108. HALL, R., and STANBURY, J. B. (1967), 'Familial Studies of Autoimmune Thyroiditis', *Clin. exp. Immun.*, **2**, 719.
109. HOLMAN, H. R., DEICHER, H. R. G., and KUNKEL, H. G. (1959), 'The L.E. Cell and the L.E. Serum Factors', *Bull. N.Y. Acad. Med.*, **35**, 409.
110. WIEDERMANN, G., and MIESCHER, P. A. (1965), 'Cytoplasmic Antibodies in Patients with Systemic Lupus Erythematosus', *Ann. N.Y. Acad. Sci.*, **124**, 807.
111. HARGRAVES, M. M. (1949), 'Production in vitro of the L.E. Cell Phenomenon: Use of Normal Bone Marrow Elements and Blood Plasma from Patients with Acute Disseminated Lupus Erythematosus', *Proc. Staff Meet. Mayo Clin.*, **24**, 234.
112. KOFFLER, D., SCHUR, P. H., and KUNKEL, H. G. (1967), 'Immunological Studies concerning the Nephritis of Systemic Lupus Erythematosus', *J. exp. Med.*, **126**, 607.
113. PATRUCCO, A., ROTHFIELD, N. F., and HIRSCHHORN, K. (1967), 'The Response of Cultured Lymphocytes from Patients with Systemic Lupus Erythematosus to DNA', *Arthritis Rheum.*, **10**, 32.
114. PLESCIA, O. J., and BRAUN, W. (1967), 'Nucleic Acids as Antigens', *Adv. Immun.*, **6**, 231.
115. SOOTHILL, J. F. (1967), 'Altered Complement Component C'_{3A} (β_{1C}–β_{1A}) in Patients with Glomerulonephritis', *Clin. exp. Immun.*, **2**, 83.
116. MARKOWITZ, A. S., and LANGE, C. F. (1964), 'Streptococcal related Glomerulonephritis. I, Isolation, Immunochemistry and Comparative Chemistry of Soluble Fractions from Type 12 Nephritogenic Streptococci and Human Glomeruli', *J. Immun.*, **92**, 565.
117. ZABRISKIE, J. B. (1967), 'Mimetic Relationships between Group A Streptococci and Mammalian Tissues', *Adv. Immun.*, **7**, 147.
118. BROBERGER, O., and PERLMANN, P. (1959), 'Autoantibodies in Human Ulcerative Colitis', *J. exp. Med.*, **110**, 657.
119. HARRISON, W. J. (1965), 'Autoantibodies against Intestinal and Gastric Mucous Cells in Ulcerative Colitis', *Lancet*, **1**, 1346.
120. LAGERCRANTZ, R., HAMMARSTROM, S., PERLMANN, P., and GUSTAFSSON, B. E. (1968), 'Immunological Studies in Ulcerative Colitis. IV, Origin of Autoantibodies', *J. exp. Med.*, **128**, 1339.
121. PERLMANN, P., and BROBERGER, O. (1963), '*In vitro* Studies of Ulcerative Colitis. II, Cytotoxic Action of White Blood Cells from Patients on Human Fetal Colon Cells', *J. exp. Med.*, **117**, 717.
122. SHORTER, R. G., SPENCER, R. J., HUIZENGA, K. A., and HALLENBECK, G. A. (1968), 'Inhibition of in vitro Cytotoxicity of Lymphocytes from Patients with Ulcerative Colitis and Granulomatous Colitis for Allogenic Colonic Epithelial Cells using Horse Anti-human Thymus Serum', *Gastroenterology*, **54**, 227.
123. WATSON, D. W., QUIGLEY, A., and BOLT, R. J. (1966), 'Effect of Lymphocytes from Patients with Ulcerative Colitis on Human Adult Colon Epithelial Cells', *Gastroenterology*, **51**, 985.
124. ASHERSON, G. L., and HOLBOROW, E. J. (1966), 'Autoantibody Production in Rabbits. VII, Autoantibodies to Gut produced by the Injection of Bacteria', *Immunology*, **10**, 161.
125. VAN DER GELD, H. W. R., and STRAUSS, A. J. L. (1966), 'Myasthenia Gravis—Immunological Relationship between Striated Muscle and Thymus', *Lancet*, **1**, 57.
126. OOSTERHUIS, H. J. G. H., FELTKAMP, T. E. W., and VAN DER GELD, H. W. R. (1966), 'Muscle Antibodies in Myasthenic Mothers and their Babies', *Lancet*, **2**, 1226.
127. PARKES, J. D., and McKINNA, J. A. (1966), 'Neuromuscular Blocking Activity in the Blood of Patients with Myasthenia Gravis', *Lancet*, **1**, 388.
128. GOLDSTEIN, G., and WHITTINGHAM, S. (1967), 'Histological and Serological Features of Experimental Autoimmune Thymitis in Guinea Pigs', *Clin. exp. Immun.*, **2**, 257.

129. BURNET, F. M., and HOLMES, M. C. (1964), 'Thymic Changes in the Mouse Strain NZB in Relation to the Auto-immune State', *J. Path. Bact.*, **88**, 229.

130. HOWIE, J. B., and HELYER, B. J. (1966), 'The Influence of Neonatal Thymectomy and Thymus Grafting on Spontaneous Auto-immune Disease in Mice', in *The Thymus: Experimental and Clinical Studies* (ed. WOLSTENHOLME, G. E. W., and PORTER, R.), p. 360. London: Churchill.

131. DE VRIES, M. J., and HIJMANS, W. (1967), 'Pathological Changes of Thymic Epithelial Cells and Autoimmune Disease in NZB, NZW and (NZB × NZW) F$_1$ Mice', *Immunology*, **12**, 179.

132. MIDDLETON, G. (1967), 'The Incidence of Follicular Structures in the Human Thymus at Autopsy', *Aust. J. exp. Biol. med. Sci.*, **45**, 189.

133. LEIBOWITZ, S., KENNEDY, L. A., and LESSOF, M. H. (1968), 'Antilymphocyte Serum in the Later Stages of Experimental Allergic Encephalomyelitis', *Lancet*, **1**, 569.

INDEX